What families who are dealing with a brain tumor have to say about
Brain Tumors-Leaving the Garden of Eden

...explains the complex issues of brain tumors in a manner that the general public can understand - without 'talking down' to us... the tone is crisp and reads well... Ray G, Albany NY

Written well from the beginning... you can ... see this book is not like a Physician's Desk Reference. Patty A, a survivor in NJ

I was struck by how much I did not know even though I have been researching brain mets on behalf of several friends with melanoma and breast cancer brain mets. Helen S, NY

... a roadmap through what is complicated and scary to the lay reader. The Checklist To Assess My Team & Care is empowering, challenging and clear ....and will piss off lots of doctors! ... in a good way. Shira G, TV writer, CA

Inspiringly hopeful...so admirable - coming from a physician instead of an on-line bulletin board or support group. Katie C, UCLA, Los Angeles

I have wished for this book. The chapter on the Team is probably the best thing I have read on this... ever! "... successful patients not only learn how to 'work the system' but they also learn how to live in this foreign land." This book shows you how. Loice, Philadelphia, PA

You can take comfort in having Dr. Zeltzer with you during your brain tumor journey. Naomi Berkowitz, Executive Director, American Brain Tumor Association, Chicago, IL

More comments from readers who are dealing with a brain tumor and what they have to say about
Brain Tumors-Leaving the Garden of Eden

The personal e-mail comments express familiar situations I'm sure will strike a vote with all those who read the book...it connects on a personal level. Christine D, Austin, TX

A "how to" book when your world is falling apart... you're a person... not a patient or a statistic. A lot of great information how to get to the right place. Alan A, Newberry Park , CA

We really like the conversational tone. The subject is so serious...it is so nice to read something that is not too technical, not condescending. '...this was written for me.' Lindsay F, Los Angeles, CA

What physicians are saying about
Brain Tumors-Leaving the Garden of Eden

Informative...written with ...a nice blend of compassion... providing sensitive information and respecting the patients' intelligence.
Dr Maria Bishop, Arizona Cancer Center, Tucson

Packed with practical information and inspiring stories from patients and families who have "been there,..."

Like a compass in the wilderness, ... a user-friendly tool for plotting an early course through the uncertainties of diagnosis and treatment of a brain tumor. Dr. Henry Friedman & Bebe Guill, Tug Mcgraw Neuro-Oncology Quality Of Life Center, Duke University, Durham, NC (See page 396 for additional comments from professionals).

BRAIN TUMORS
LEAVING THE GARDEN OF EDEN

BRAIN TUMORS
LEAVING THE GARDEN OF EDEN

A Survival Guide to Diagnosis, Learning the Basics, Getting Organized and Finding Your Medical Team

BY PAUL M. ZELTZER MD

S P
Shilysca Press
Encino, California

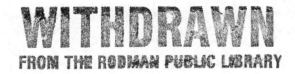

Zeltzer, Paul M. 1942-

Brain Tumors – Leaving the Garden of Eden: *A Survival Guide to Diagnosis, Learning the Basics, Getting Organized & Finding Your Medical Team*

1. Health   2. Illness   3. Brain Tumors   4. Faith

Library of Congress Control Number: 2004097100
ISBN 0-9760171-0-5

Layout and design: Apron Strings Design & Katja Loesch

Cover picture: <u>Expulsion from the Garden of Eden</u>, John Storrs (Am. 1885-1956) 4 1/4" x 3 1/2" woodcut, 1934. Courtesy of Estate of John Storrs. Thanks to Valerie Carberry Gallery, Chicago, IL.

Questions about the book contents?
Go to Q & A section of <u>www.survivingbraincancer.com</u> and e-mail your specific question to the author: <u>info@survivingbraincancer.com</u>

Printed in Canada on acid-free paper

Published by:

S P

Shilysca Press
Encino, California

Shilysca Press
5041 Valjean Avenue
Encino, California 91436

www.braincancersurvivors.com
www.survivingbraincancer.com
e-mail address: <u>info@survivingbraincancer.com</u>

DEDICATION

To Lonnie for your love, affection, and support in my calling to write the book.

To my daughters: Shira for helping me find the voice to tell the story; Alysa for her comments and critique; Carin for helpful comments and organization of the major Centers' tables.

Finally, to my high school English teacher Phyllis Bartine Clemens who opened my mind to think about the power and meanings of words.

ACKNOWLEDGMENTS

This book would not have been possible without three people who saw the vision of the project in its initial stages: George Diaz, Mary Naughton, and Lucy Gonda. Al Musella and Neal Levitan understood the need and also provided constructive criticism and welcome support. Neopharm Inc. (Ken Johnson) and Guilford Pharmaceuticals also supported this work. Rick Sontag, Kay Verble, and The Sontag Foundation responded to the need and have enabled distribution of the book in a major way.

My writing plan included editorial input from people affected by and committed to the subject – the group to whom this book is directed. Many of my lay colleagues are spouses or people I've met on the Internet or talked with on the phone but never actually met. Others have been my patients or we have talked at National meetings. I am indebted for both kind words and harsh critiques to the following: Patty Adorno, MaryJane Brant, Sandi Cantor, Rose Cohen, Katie Couturier, Melinda Crosby, Christine and John Dallio, Kathleen Davis, Stephen Duffy, David Edge, Pepper Edmiston, Michele Gabay, Dennis Kilroy, Neal Levitan, Ed Martin, Pamela Mathers, Leigh Meissner, Linda Needham, Murray and Lenore Neidorf, Craig Norton, Stina O'leary, Larry Phemeister, Chris Quatrocci, Jeremy Shatan, Sheryl Shetsky, Nan Silver, Helen Sloniker, Maria Sansalone, and Phill Weissman.

Many of my professional colleagues gave unselfishly of their time to make insightful commentary and point out inaccuracies: Loice Swisher (Chapters 1, 3, 5, 22); Elana Faraci and Linda O Connor (Chapter 2); Patricia McGrath (Chapter 6); Maria Bishop, Deborah Blumenthal, Jon Finlay (Chapters 5,10); Brian Pikul, Moise Danielpour, Susan Panullo, and Larry Seigler (Chapters 6 and 17); Michele Burnison, Melvin Deutsch, Minesh Mehta (Chapters 10 and 17); Victor Levin (Chapter 17); Marsha Drozdoff, Deana Luchs, Julie McKay, Cynthia Meyers, Evan Ross, Jean Wallace (Chapter 18); Dan von Hoff (Chapter 21); Leland Albright, Archie Bleyer, Finn Bretnach, Leah Ellenberg, Mark Greenberg, Tania Maher-Shiminski (Chapter 22); Dennis Kilroy, Ruth Hoffman of CandleLighters (Chapter 23); Scott Pomeroy, Ian Pollack, Margot Scheuner (Chapter 24); Bill Duke, (Chapter 25). I thank Toni Bernay, Jon Finlay, Lloyd Fischel, Valerie and Victor Ostrower, Rochelle Simmons, and Jacob Zighelboim for helpful conversations and insights.

I have been blessed with wonderful editors. Ping Ho, my content editor, provided critique on language and organization. I discovered (painfully) that writing for the public was much more challenging and difficult compared with my previous science writing. Caryn Freeman, my line editor and proofreader, undertook the daunting task of correcting my non-parallel constructions and misuse of bulleting in producing a clearer manuscript. Kristin Loberg completed the editing and provided insightful commentary. Julie-Beenhower-Macht of Apron Strings provided layout counsel and creativity in developing a meaningful theme and cover design. Katja Loesch completed the layout and added line art and drawings.

The book was developed in part from answering questions about brain tumors posted on websites over a seven-year period. I have borrowed quotations from those sites and e-mails sent to me about a variety of brain tumor-associated issues. Most quotations have been made anonymous, though I have tried to remain true to their content. I am deeply indebted to all whose words expressed, in such pristine ways, the complex medical and emotional issues confronting them. You are my heroes.

CONTENTS

CHAPTER 11
TUMORS ORIGINATING IN THE BRAIN – MEDULLOBLASTOMAS, PNETS AND EPENDYMOMAS   *273*

PREFACE

You experienced some alarming symptoms and now have been through a series of tests for brain cancer. You may be thinking with dread, "what if I really have a brain tumor!" You are not sure what lies ahead.

I have been a physician for children and adults with brain tumors since 1978. I know firsthand how the suspicion of a tumor, or the fear of hearing "You have a brain tumor" can cause an emotional train wreck. Many people freeze and cannot listen after that news. Both shock and panic set in. A sense of urgency descends upon you immediately. You wonder if it's too late to "fix" the problem, or if you're doomed for a slow and painful death. No one, myself included, can guarantee you survival, or that you will live for another 20 years. We all face Fate's uncertainties every day whether we have a brain tumor or not.

What I can say to you is that this book can be a pathway to help you cope, function, gather intelligent information, and work more effectively with your physicians. I have listened to thousands of people, like yourself, both in person and over the Internet. I understand the confusion and what it is like to have to master the language of doctors and fight the healthcare system. With this book, you will understand the technical information and its implications, learn to view your physicians as team players, and then put together a game plan for dealing with this new and unexpected challenge in your life.

I always find it interesting how one family can "work the system", seek and find useful information, not be intimidated by the doctors and nurses, and be successful. These patients and their families maximize their chances for survival. Others seem more dependent on the doctors and don't know which questions to ask. It's not necessarily their lack of education or being rich versus poor. They simply don't know how or feel equipped to take charge of their situation. I want all my patients to be successful and get the best care available. This book will show you how.

The perspective I used in writing this book came about after reading *Genesis: A Living Conversation*,[1] a work that started as a Public Television series in 1996. Acclaimed television journalist Bill Moyers gathered prestigious writers, film critics, clergy, scientists, physicians, and philosophers from many cultures and moderated a round table dialogue. This diverse group studied the stories of Genesis and discussed how our reactions to ordinary and familiar situations echoed many themes of those stories. Rarely mentioned was our response to illness as part of those themes, however.

Making sense out of our experiences often relies on storytelling. And when you look at the large themes in Genesis—creation, authority, temptation, exile, and family strife-you can see those same themes repeated throughout history. Evolution of man and his culture parallels the themes found in the stories of Genesis that most of us have known since childhood. For example, Genesis describes Eve questioning the highest authority figure. This parallels an individual's instinctual need to question a doctor's authority about diagnosis or treatment… and risk the consequences. Other examples include the story of Noah's Ark: ordinary people today caught up in a torrential flood (in our case, following a diagnosis of a brain tumor) and reaching for the Ark of safety during the long journey toward health. Or a son, Isaac, "going under the knife" by his father's own hand: he is giving up his autonomy (the special reverential and dependent relationship that a cancer patient has when in the hands of the neurosurgeon). The emotional, gut reactions to power and authority figures have been so integrated into our secular culture that we do not recognize their linkage to the Genesis stories heard in our youth.

Many of my patients tell me about seeing their lives as divided into "before the brain tumor" (Eden) and "after the diagnosis of the brain tumor" (The Fall) as their punishment and pain. People with cancer often ask, "What did I do so wrong to deserve this?" They think cancer is their punishment. But punishment for what?

Two common reactions occur upon the diagnosis of a brain tumor that are similar to events in the Garden of Eden: a sense of mortality and fear of challenging authority. My patients also tell me of their discomfort in questioning the physician's diagnosis or his treatment recommendations because they do not want to be abandoned or cause their doctor to be angry with them. Rational? No. Real? Yes. Adam and Eve were expelled from the Garden of Innocence precisely because Eve wanted knowledge (of good and evil) equal to that of the supreme authority figure. The higher source was questioned… and look what happened! Eve and Adam were expelled with three fates: pain for Eve, toil and hard work for Adam, and mortality for them both.

In spite of the diagnosis, many people plunge into a search for knowledge, questioning and sometimes challenging their physicians. Others choose to follow their doctors' recommendations without question and believe that Fate will determine the outcome. Which pathway is preferable for you?

Resolving that conflict is the subtext of this book. How can you work with and understand those feelings, so that you receive the best care, are aware of the choices and alternatives, and do not feel punished? How do you learn to manage the chaos you feel and minimize the confusion so that you can make good decisions? I plan to teach you how. I hope to accomplish this with advice from people who have traveled the same path as you, with specific questions to ask of your physicians, and with information about your own type of tumor. I also use artwork that connects those feelings to actions.

This work is not meant to be an encyclopedia. When I set out to write this book, I didn't expect so many pages of useful information to come out. Over eight hundred pages are too daunting when you have just been diagnosed with a serious illness. So, I divided the original manuscript into two user-friendly and comprehensive books. There is considerable restatement throughout the books. I did not eliminate this repetition because the material can be difficult to digest, and reiteration clarifies nuances and details that require more background and supplementary information.

I have included more than 250 web links, helpful foundation contacts, books, and other information so that more details can be accessed easily. Soon a CD-ROM edition will be available so you can access these resources in real time, as you read the chapters of interest to you.

When it comes to people with cancer, time is of the essence - no matter what your prognosis. It's okay to feel overwhelmed, panicky, or even devastated or defeated. Many of these emotions are natural and inevitable. But beyond the great unknowns, there are many things you can control that ultimately ease your journey. You can channel those negative feelings into positive energy. The greater your sense of control over this situation, the greater your ability to fight.

This first book is called *Brain Tumors - Leaving the Garden of Eden: A Survival Guide to Learning the Basics, Getting Organized & Finding Your Medical Team*. It contains the basics, including information about surfing the Internet, facts about your specific brain tumor, ensuring your correct diagnosis, medications you may be taking, obtaining second opinions, and the referral medical center. The sequel and second book, *Brain Tumors - Finding the Ark: Meeting the Challenges of Treatment Choices, Side Effects, Healthcare Costs & Long Term Survival* contains information you need once you have been diagnosed. It has action-oriented, problem-solving tools about your therapies, medications and their side effects, insurance, clinical trials, inherited aspects of brain tumors, information specific to children, and a discussion about your legacy.

Each chapter is organized around a similar model and starts with a quotation that brings up an image related to the theme of the chapter. Contents and key search words for surfing the Internet are next. The last table following the text in each chapter contains a summary of all the websites and contact information in that chapter.

The audience for these two books is mostly people more than 40 years old. My graphics consultant, Julie Macht of Apron Strings Design, has chosen text and fonts of a size and quality most helpful for those with visual difficulties. The dimensions of the book also were chosen with this in mind. The special binding will allow you to open the book, flatten it out, and keep it open, as though it were a manual.

I want to clarify my chapter titled "Your Legacy." According to author Arthur Frank, when you are confronted with a serious health threat, a necessary part of the recovery is telling the story - not of who you were, but who you have become because of this illness.[2] Your personal story is called a narrative. Your story or thoughts about the changes that have occurred may be logical, full of chaos and panic, or even heroic at any given moment. I see this every day in my patients or with people communicating on the Internet, as they share experience, confusion, pain, and triumph. These stories are also expressed in drawings and paintings by people touched with cancer.

One of the problems of modern medicine is that we physicians try to get patients to tell their stories in terms of MRI scans, blood counts, and symptoms - all things familiar to us. But each individual is changed in unique ways that do not fit this medical model. You, the patient and family, need to be treated and appreciated for your uniqueness. I think your personal story is something that is important to share with family and loved ones. It can be part of your recovery and healing process. In these books, I hope to provide you with some tools to understand and tell your story.

Paul Zeltzer, M.D.
June 1, 2004

CHAPTER 1

I Have a Brain Tumor

Newly diagnosed brain tumor patients are like people who don't know how to swim being thrown into deep water with no flotation device.

Kathleen, aunt to Kyra, a child with a brain tumor

WHY PREPARE AND BE ORGANIZED?

Here you are. You, your spouse, your child, or loved one has a serious illness. It is a disease with a medical name that you may not recognize, something you thought only other people got. It is a BRAIN TUMOR.

The diagnosis makes it sound like "it's all over." You may feel numb, helpless, and unsure of where or to whom to turn. Your family and friends stare in disbelief. Your primary doctor, on whom you trust and depend, is not familiar with its treatment; so you are sent off to a specialist at a well-known medical center or institute. Now what?

Brain Tumors – Leaving the Garden of Eden will help you – as patient, caregiver, or friend – to
- Feel more in control of the situation and less like a victim.
- Organize your strategy for traveling the difficult road ahead.
- Identify the right "experts."
- Navigate through the maze of specialists who you will encounter.
- Ask the right questions about your diagnosis and tests to ensure that you receive the proper care.
- Find important facts and answers, so that you can make informed decisions about your treatment options. (Yes, there ARE options.)

My secretary, Kimba, tells me that brain tumors are "funky, unpredictable things." It is precisely because of this that you will need to develop a strategy and organize. You will find out exactly how to get started in Chapters 2 and 3, but first let me give three reasons to explain why you need to prepare and get organized.

REASON 1
BRAIN TUMORS CAN BE DIFFICULT TO DIAGNOSE CORRECTLY

One of my colleagues, Dr. Jonathan Finlay of the University of Southern California, conducted a clinical study of almost 200 patients with *malignant* gliomas (also called astrocytomas) from the U.S.A and Canada who were diagnosed at their local hospital. We submitted all their pathology slides to an "expert" panel of neuropathologists (physicians who specialize in diagnosing diseases of the nervous system through analysis of brain and spinal cord tissues.) Guess what? The experts disagreed 25 percent of the time on the exact diagnosis; and some patients placed on the study had low grade, not more malignant tumors[1]. This points out that a second opinion may

> Brain Tumors can be difficult to diagnose correctly.

be essential to your treatment. Often, the treating doctor does not think about questioning the diagnosis, especially if it is a low-grade tumor. This is why you must ask questions to ensure that you receive the care that you need and deserve.

REASON 2
THESE DARN THINGS ARE NOT ALWAYS PREDICTABLE

I usually refrain from statistics because they apply to populations, not individuals. However, there is one fact that I want you to remember: no matter how smart any doctor or healer may be, no one can predict for how long any one person will live! We are capable of predicting what will happen to hundreds of people with brain tumors, but we cannot predict what will happen to you.

Prognosis is what a doctor says might happen. It is the odds. This can be based on true statistics or a physician's personal experience. However, when looking at one person, it's like flipping a coin. In 100 tries, the theoretical odds are 50-50 heads/tails each time. In actuality, we may get six straight heads; hence, the attraction to gambling. There are many accounts of people beating the "statistics" with successful fights against brain tumors.

> These darn things are not always predictable.

Even with the same pathology, what happens can be markedly different among patients. For example, two of my patients, Evan and Jeanne, have the most malignant type of astrocytoma called a glioblastoma multiforme. Both tumors look identical under a microscope. After surgery and other treatments, Evan's tumor responds to treatments for over 10 years. He becomes an acupuncturist and helps a lot of people with cancer. Jeanne's tumor initially responds but then grows in spite of treatment. This is only one of many examples of how brain tumors can behave differently.

How can the course of the same type of brain tumor be so variable? Until a few years ago, we did not understand why similar-looking tumors behaved differently. New research suggests that within each brain tumor cell there are "messenger" molecules that activate growth signals inside it. The amount and type of these may differ among tumors that look alike. Understanding the "messengers" may be the key to new therapies. What your tumor cells look like under the microscope may not be the whole story.

Reason 3
Brain Tumor Treatment Can Be Complex

In the "normal world," a doctor will have a thousand patients. In the brain tumor world, you may have a thousand doctors – and it might seem like that many healthcare professionals! After surgery you may see neurosurgeons, radiation oncologists, neuro-oncologists, neuro-ophthalmologists, rehabilitation doctors, nutritionists, therapists, audiologists, radiologists, as well as other health-care providers. Excellent organization ensures that the correct medical information is shared and it establishes you as the CEO (chief executive officer) of your body (Chapter 3).

> Brain tumor treatment can be complex.

You may be thinking, "This author is so calm, but I am the one with the brain tumor... and I am panicking!" Remember, this book did not spring from an ivory-tower view. I based it on real and successful experiences of many families. My examples include successful appeals to reverse HMO or insurance claims and other successes in coping from the actual patients.

Did every patient live to a ripe old age? No. Did tumors come back? Yes, sometimes. But these families learned to do everything they could; they did not let this "thing" tear away at their fabric. They had weeks, months, and years living fully, with the tumor taking a back seat. And yes, many lived much longer than any expert of statistics would have predicted.

Don't just take my word for it. Go to the Internet, click on www.tbts.org or http://www.virtualtrials.com/survive.cfm and read stories[2] written by people like Ben Williams,[3] or M.L. Dubay,[4] both of whom have had brain tumors and traveled the path you are on right now.

In the previous section I gave examples of how being prepared will help you regain control. But you may still be feeling like this tumor is some form of punishment and the whole experience has left you powerless and out of control. On the first page of this book, Kathleen's words likened a brain tumor diagnosis to being tossed in water without a floatation device. This made me think of a famous painting of Noah and the FLOOD (Figure 1-1). In it there is a churning river awash with people struggling to take a breath; others are drowning. Floating in the middle is a plain wooden ark-no rudder, no windows, with a large lock on the door, being carried along by the torrent. One man is trying to climb up on it for safety. Many of my patients have told me that is exactly what their struggle felt like – in a torrent being tossed around and hoping to find a place to get out from under the storm. They also secretly felt like this brain tumor was a kind of punishment. We are so used to things being under our control. Akin to a cataclysmic flood, a brain tumor changes that and puts us in the middle of a torrent, out of reach from the Ark.

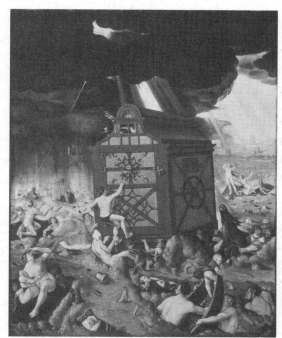

Figure 1-1 Hans Baldung Grien: The Flood, 16th Century

So, where is your Ark? How can one regain control? When we are ill, we want to find the key, unlock the ark so we can climb to safety and wait out the storm. In the past, the medical system – the hospitals, doctor, nurses – could let us in. Today's health care system has put us more on our own; but we have ever increasing opportunities to help ourselves with knowledge.

In this book, *Brain Tumors – Leaving the Garden of Eden*, I detail basic information about brain tumors – from getting organized, to diagnosis, second opinions, and health professionals you will meet along the way. In the companion book, *Brain Tumors – Finding the Ark*, I include more problem – solving approaches to understand and deal with specifics of treatment, insurance companies and HMOs, special considerations for children, long-term effects, and understanding effects and side effects of your medications.

Remember that you were a person – not a patient – before your symptoms alerted you to a problem. Apart from doctors and the medical system, you are still a person with a life that may include family, loved ones, a pet dog or fish. There is still someone who inside

> You were a person-not a patient-before your symptoms.

is whole and well – capable of pursuing life, love and things that feel good. As that person, you have choices. They may not be the choices that you want, but you do have choices. You can choose whether to go on a clinical trial. You can choose how to spend each day in hope... or with fear. The power to make choices is still yours.

One of the choices patients and caretakers may make is to connect with others. This can be one-on-one, in a local support group, or even through a computer-based Internet group. For many, the discovery of not being alone on this journey is freeing. One can share the doubts, angst and fears as well as celebrations of small successes that only people in the same situation would understand. The feeling of being connected and genuinely heard cannot be underestimated.

Before we end this chapter, let me say something about attitude. One of my patients, Al, a retired Los Angeles area career fireman who had saved more lives than I, taught me something about his brain tumor. He regarded it as just a "thing" with no more status than that. "It could make me sick, cause seizures, and weaken my limbs," he reflected; but "it alone did not have the power to cripple my Love, corrode my Faith, or kill a Friendship. It might kill me but not my spirit." He regarded his situation like, "OK, what can I do now?" Al lived a lot longer than anyone thought he would. Food for thought.

Yes, brain tumors are serious, but take a deep breath and pause. There are many long-term survivors of brain tumors, even of the type that you have. A number of survivors have gone on to become directors of brain tumor foundations and societies. You have time to learn and plan so as not to let this tumor rule your life. You will learn to preserve wholeness and gain control over your situation through knowledge and awareness. My hope is that this book, and the resources that can be accessed through it, will bring you to quieter, safer waters until the storm calms down.

> You may not have the choices you want, but you do have choices.

It is time to begin the climb and learn more about brain tumors in general and your tumor specifically. Then you can ask the right questions and understand the choices ahead.

CHAPTER 2

Beginning Your New Journey – The Basics About Brain Tumors

Do not get bogged down with the "why me" question - even if you knew, it wouldn't change anything. The better question is "what now?" Ask that question every morning and look for answers all day.

David Bailey. Musician, GBM survivor

THE BASICS ABOUT BRAIN TUMORS

Key search words

- cancer
- secondary brain tumors
- eloquent areas
- prognosis
- cancer center
- primary brain tumors
- metastases
- knowledge
- cancer susceptibility
- gliomas
- brain functions
- empowerment
- statistics

This chapter answers the questions most frequently asked by people diagnosed with brain tumors. Before you begin your quest for knowledge, remember: not all brain tumors behave in the same way. How fast a tumor grows can depend on its location in the brain, your age, general health, and other conditions as yet unknown. You'll find a very brief description of 25 common types of brain tumors in the Glossary of the book.

HOW DO I BEGIN THIS JOURNEY?

First, take a break and look where you have been. You were told that you have a brain tumor. It's normal to feel overwhelmed, sad, angry, depressed and even ashamed. You are worried about the future and what will happen next. The design of each chapter in this book is to take you, step-by-step, through the challenges you might face.

Your first step in regaining control is to acquire knowledge about your tumor and then to organize yourself for the journey ahead. (See Chapter 3.) Being as informed and aggressive as you can be about your specific brain tumor is

> Your first step in regaining control is to acquire knowledge and organize yourself.

critical to your journey. Even if you never had any interest in the biology of the brain and various symptoms, now is the time to become acquainted with all that relates to your tumor.

It's important to first understand where your tumor is located in your brain. Using the pictures of the brain in Table 2-1, find the

> A website for basic information about the nervous system: **http://www.cancerindex.org/medterm/medtm13.htm**

location of your tumor in Figure 2-3 and, in pen or pencil, place a mark on that area of the brain. This exercise might seem strange, even uncomfortable, and a little like being back in grade school… but it will help you focus, become aware of choices, and be proactive. It will also help you to monitor your progress and be aware of your symptoms, something that most people do anyway.

HOW COMMON ARE BRAIN TUMORS?

Primary brain tumors, which originate inside the brain itself, are the fifth most common type of cancer in adults. They are more likely to occur as people age.

> Annually 150,000 people have a metastasis that spreads to the brain from another place in the body.

Table 2-1 Brain Areas of the Cortex

Hemispheres	Frontal Lobes	Parietal Lobe & Occipital Lobe	Temporal Lobe

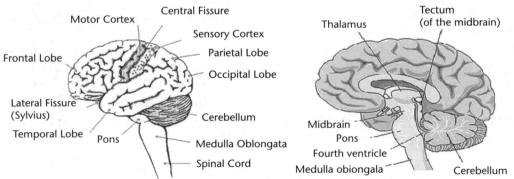

(Bottom up view)

Prefrontal areas

Parietal

(bottom view)

cerebellum w/ lines
Brainstem

The cortex does not
include cerebellum or
brain stem.

motor strip

(side view)

Occipital Lobe

Outer Side View of Brain

Motor Cortex
Central Fissure
Sensory Cortex
Parietal Lobe
Occipital Lobe
Frontal Lobe
Lateral Fissure
(Sylvius)
Cerebellum
Temporal Lobe   Pons
Medulla Oblongata
Spinal Cord

Cut Away Side View

Thalamus
Tectum
(of the midbrain)
Midbrain
Pons
Fourth ventricle
Medulla obiongala
Cerebellum

The Brain Stem

32

Roughly speaking, each year about 17,000 people are diagnosed with *malignant* (rapidly growing) types and about the same number are diagnosed with *low-grade* (slower growing) forms. Each year about 150,000 people have a metastasis that has spread to the brain from another place in the body. For example, a cancer of the lung spreads to the brain. The most frequent tumor types in adults and children are shown (Figures 2-1, 2-2).

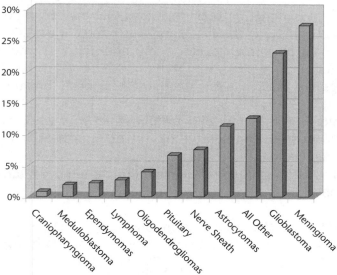

Figure 2-1 Relative frequency of brain tumors in adults (CBTRUS - 1995 - 1999)

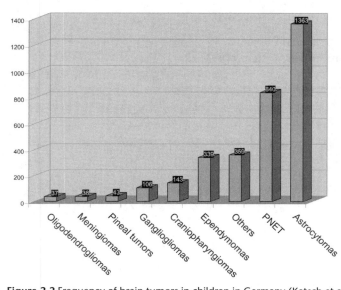

Figure 2-2 Frequency of brain tumors in children in Germany (Katsch et al 2001)

HOW DOES TUMOR LOCATION AFFECT MY SYMPTOMS & TREATMENT CHOICES?

Your different functions are controlled by separate portions of the brain. Not unlike the real estate adage "Location, Location, Location," your symptoms and treatment options also depend on the tumor's location. The brain locations that control important functions are listed (Table 2-2) and Illustrated (Figure 2-3). For example:

> Your symptoms and treatment options depend on the tumor's location.

- One area controls some speech and understanding and finding words (temporal lobe).
- Other areas are packed with functions: heartbeat, breathing, movement (brain stem).
- If your tumor is in the outer parietal lobe, then your vision field may be cut and you will need to compensate by turning your head and not relying on your peripheral vision.
- The brain has silent areas with "wiggle room" to remove a tumor (frontal and temporal lobes).

I have omitted details of the limbic system and corpus callosum, which connects the two halves of the brain. Symptoms occur when brain pathways are disrupted. Examples of symptoms that might occur depend on which lobe or hemisphere is involved (Table 2-3).

This website has more detail on anatomy and functions of the brain:
http://www.neurosurgery.org/health/ patient/answers.asp?DisorderID=51

For anatomy & brain tumors, see this link:
http:// www.oncolink.com/types/article.cfm?c=2 &s=4&ss=25&id=102

Table 2-2 Brain Areas And Normal Functions of Cerebral Cortex

Hemispheres	Frontal Lobes	Parietal & Occipital	Temporal
Memory; learning, making thoughts and decisions. **Motor/ sensory strips** **Right Side** "Big" picture of environment. Visual spatial skills. Memory storage of hearing, sight, smell sense; spatial forms. **Left Side** **Language Memory** Logical interpretation of information of symbols like: language, math, abstract reasoning.	**Prefrontal area:** Concentration & original thoughts. The "Gatekeeper" (judgment, inhibition). Personality and emotional traits. **Pre-motor strip:** Storage of motor patterns and voluntary activities. Language: act of speaking **Motor Strip** Movement	**Parietal** = Process sensory input and discrimination. Feeling of Body orientation. **Occipital** = Primary visual reception and association areas: Allows for visual interpretation.	**Receptive hearing** and association areas. **Expressed behavior** **Language:** Receptive speech. **Memory:** Right side: pictures / and faces. Left side: words and names.

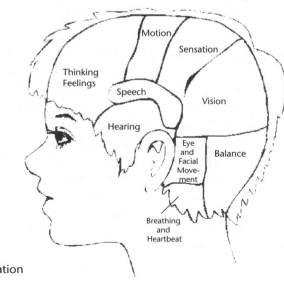

Figure 2-3 Brain Function and Location

Table 2-3 Symptoms or Loss of Function in Areas of the Cerebra Cortex

Frontal Lobes	Parietal & Occipital	Temporal
Thought areas - Impaired recent memory - Inability to concentrate confused thinking - Inattentiveness, Forgetfulness - Difficulty in learning new information **Languages** - Expressive or motor aphasia **Behavior areas** - Lack of inhibition (inappropriate social and/ or sexual behavior) - Emotional highs/ lows - Looking and feeling "Flat" **Motor Strip** - Opposite side weakness/ paralysis - Seizures, headache	**Parietal** Inability to: - Discriminate among sensory stimuli - Locate/ recognize parts of body (Neglect) - Recognize self - Orient self to environmental space - Write **Occipital** Loss of - Vision in opposite field - Ability to recognize object seen in opposite field of vision.	- Hearing deficits - Agitation, irritability, or childish behavior - Memory or expression of objects or words

WHY DO THE WORDS *CANCER & BRAIN TUMOR* MAKE ME UNEASY?

You have made a big first step in confronting your tumor by knowing its location. But just the word "tumor" or "cancer" frightens many people. Although words by themselves are not harmful, our mind and experiences give them meaning or "emotional value." Cancer typically connotes something bad, painful, and lethal. This, in turn, can trigger stomachaches, sweating, tears, and heart palpitations. Over 200 years ago, physicians knew of the brain's influence on what our gut feels (Figure 2-4). The accompanying picture appears in a Turkish medical textbook from around 1800. It shows a mountain and a valley. Look at the brain on the mountaintop and how it connects to the valley by a river (stomach) leading to trees, which become part of the intestines. This is the mind-body or mind-gut connection.

> The mind-body or mind-gut connection can affect how we respond to the tumor.

The *cancer* word is the subject of a recent e-mail on a brain tumor chat group:

> *I've been wondering if most people are using the cancer word with their sick child and their other children. Once in a while, my daughter will ask if her brother has cancer and honestly, I have been avoiding the question...I don't remember answering her. I think I am afraid to use that word...I am afraid that once I confess it then my son will get worse...Does this make sense to anyone? I am also dreading that day when someone will use that word in front of my son... Any advice?*

David, Sandusky, OH.

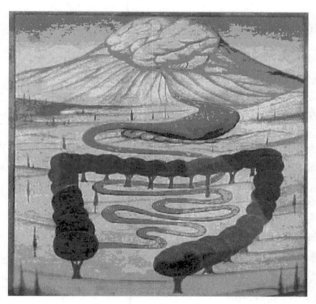

Figure 2-4 Mind Body Connection. Turkey 19th Century

So, although words like cancer can be upsetting, we can redirect our energy and use those same words to make informed choices about healing and life. The good news is that the brain is powerful enough to stop those uncomfortable feelings. How does our mind do this? You can learn how to have powerful, positive, internal conversations with yourself to make a shift in your way of thinking. (More on how we use our mind to feel better and promote healing in Chapter 18, Complementary, Alternative and other Therapies, in *Brain Tumors: Finding the Ark*.[1]

A personal example: When I was 14 years old, I swore at my mother because she grounded me for staying out too late. She made me repeat that swear word 150 times. By the 50th repetition, it became just a bunch of sounds and lost its meaning. Maybe you can try that with the word "cancer" or the name of your brain tumor. Repeat the word 25 or 50 times and see if it still feels the same. This might desensitize you to the emotional impact of the word. Why is this important? It may be difficult to ask a question about your tumor, share your feelings with someone, or search the Internet if the word ties you up in knots or makes you feel uncomfortable.

> We do not have to be prisoners of words like cancer.

CODE WORDS: WHAT DO THEY MEAN?

Words… words… words. They can help us or mystify us if we do not know the code. Here are some that you may hear around health care professionals. More appear in the Glossary.

- *Cyst*: a fluid filled sac. When not attached to a cancer, it is considered "benign." A benign cyst is different from a benign tumor. Cysts can sometimes be associated with a tumor.
- *Lesion*: a catch-all term for any tissue mass ("lump") in question.
- *Astrocyte*: a brain cell that provides support, structure, and nutrition to other brain cells.
- *Tumor* or *neoplasm*: a solid "anything" that should not be there, before or after it is actually diagnosed.
- *Cancer*: any tumor that has the potential to grow without treatment.
- *Benign cancer*: a tumor that tends to grow slowly, if it grows at all.
- *Malignant cancer*: a tumor that has grown or is growing, usually rapidly, and will not stop without some type of therapy.
- *Glioma*: a tumor from glial or astrocyte cells. Astrocytoma and glioma are interchangeable words in this book. There are a few gliomas that are called "benign", but they are more accurately named "low grade" (slow growing). High-grade gliomas are more malignant (faster growing).
- *Metastasis*: a tumor that spread from some other part of the body.

WHAT IS CANCER? HOW DID CANCER INVADE MY BODY?

To clarify what cancer is... and what it is not:
- Cancer happens when cells in the body lose control over their own growth and division, so they continue to multiply. Pretty soon, they form a lump that interferes with surrounding cells. Then, a symptom develops; something does not feel, act, or move as usual.
- Cancer is not infectious: it cannot be "caught" from someone else. People's mistaken belief that cancer can be contagious might explain why some people are uncomfortable visiting or being around those with a tumor. There is no evidence to date that brain tumors are linked to infections.
- In the last 10 years, scientists have uncovered some of the mechanisms that control the growth and death of cells. For example, each of our cells has two major "software" programs that tell it when to divide and when to die. These

"divide or die" programs are independent of one another and are contained in every cell in your body. Even in normal developing infants, some brain cells will divide until they have completed their functions at 18 to 24 months of age. At that time, the signal to die is activated and – *poof* – the cells are gone. That is normal.

- Cancer cells have lost control at both ends – the program to divide stays activated, and the program to stop dividing and enter "senescence" (dying) is inactivated. These changes can be caused by chance mutations (mistakes) in the DNA programs or exposure to toxins in the environment.

ARE ALL BRAIN TUMORS A TYPE OF CANCER?

THE QUICK ANSWER IS YES. BRAIN TUMORS ARE CANCER... MOST OF THE TIME

Some cancers grow quickly and become almost as large as a newborn baby in less than nine months. Others remain as small as a peanut for 20 years before they begin growing again. Both the type and location of the tumor are important to know in weighing your options. For example, meningioma, pituitary tumors, and craniopharyngiomas are often called benign, but they are treated like a cancer because of their potential to interfere with brain functions. Again, benign gliomas can grow and are better described as "low-grade."

> Not all brain tumors are cancerous.

IF SOME BRAIN TUMORS ARE NOT CANCERS, WHAT ARE THEY?

I've had patients who were told that they had a "brain tumor" (cancer - the "C" word) and "had the scans to prove it." Remember, MRI scans are just black and white and shades of gray on film or a computer screen. They alone cannot diagnose cancer. Some patients had a tumor that was actually composed of parasites, acquired from undercooked pork they had eaten. Other tumors consisted of blood or calcium deposits, plaques from multiple sclerosis, or abscesses from infections like sinusitis or a decayed tooth. Even disappearing "UBOs" (doctor-speak for

> Cancer cannot always be accurately diagnosed on an MRI scan alone

"unidentified bright objects") on an MRI scan have been called brain cancer. This is one reason why a biopsy should be performed to make sure *it* is cancer and not something else.

Robert G., the 66-year-old father-in-law of an internationally-recognized brain tumor specialist, had four months of headaches and then a seizure. In July 2002, a "brain tumor" was diagnosed by CT scan, and he was scheduled to have surgery, then radiation in three days. His son-in-law sent me the CT scans over the Internet for review. I felt that it did not look like a clear-cut case of cancer because of its unusual appearance and calcium deposits. I recommended a "watch and wait" approach or biopsy, but definitely, no radiation based on the scan. His doctors decided to operate and "it" was an old blood clot with calcium deposits- no cancer anywhere. Radiation or chemotherapy without a biopsy would have been an incorrect choice and could have been fatal.

Meningiomas, gangliogliomas, and juvenile pilocytic astrocytomas in the cerebellum are all tumors. But most are low grade, do not behave like cancers, and usually do not recur after complete removal.

IS IT A BRAIN TUMOR OR A TUMOR IN THE BRAIN? WHAT IS THE DIFFERENCE?

One of the most common questions on the Internet asks about the difference between primary and secondary brain tumors. A primary brain tumor starts from actual brain or surrounding cells. Most of these are in the family of *astrocytomas* or *gliomas.* (Figures 2-1, 2-2). Secondary brain tumors are referred to as *metastases* (mets) and have spread from other organs in the body. The latter are named by their tumor of origin: for example, breast, lung, colon carcinoma metastases, and so forth. (See Chapter 15.)

It is critical for you to know whether your tumor started in the brain or came from elsewhere (*metastasis*), because the treatment plan will be different. For example, about 15,000 of those 150,000 people diagnosed annually with brain tumors will learn for the first time that they have cancer elsewhere in the body as a result of their neurological symptoms. This happens frequently with lung cancer. They may also find that their brain tumor arose long after the primary tumor (in breast, ovary, or colon) was treated. This is actually a sign of success. Why? Because treatments have improved to the point where people are living long enough for tumor cells to travel to the brain and set up shop there.

> Primary tumors start in the head. Metastases come from elsewhere in the body.

WHAT ARE THE DIFFERENT TYPES OF PRIMARY BRAIN TUMORS?

We do not know precisely what causes a cancer to start growing (mutations and possibly environmental toxins play a role), but we do know which types of brain cells are involved.

Tumors from the *astrocytoma* family are derived from brain cells (glia or astrocytes) that protect, feed, and support neurons that, in turn, store and transmit information through electrical energy.

> Tumors are named by the cell types they come from.

Tumors from the *oligodendroglioma* family come from a special type of astrocyte that wraps around and provides electrical insulation for neurons. (See Chapter 10.)

Tumors derived from actual neurons are called *gangliogliomas* and *primitive neuroectodermal tumors* (PNET)s. (See Chapter 11.)

To add to the confusion, some tumors also are named by their location: *brain stem* gliomas, *cerebellar* astrocytomas, *pituitary* and *pineal region* tumors. Tumors from the coverings of the brain (meninges) are called *meningiomas*. (See Chapter 12.)

WHY DOES AN ADULT GET A TUMOR TYPICALLY FOUND IN CHILDREN?

Children and adults differ in the frequency with which they develop various kinds of brain tumors.[2] (Figures 2-1, 2-2) Many adults are confused when they hear that they have a tumor type that is more frequently seen in children. This is an uncommon, but not rare, occurrence. For example, medulloblastoma tumors occur most often between three to six years of age, but about 10 percent of all medulloblastomas occur in people age 18 or older.

Adult oncologists and neurosurgeons may be uncertain of the most recent and effective approaches for these kinds of tumors; therefore, consulting a pediatric oncologist or

> See www.yahoo.com , click on "connect" then "Groups" and search under "brain tumor".

a major brain tumor center can be helpful. Adult patients with medulloblastoma have responded to this knowledge gap with a grassroots initiative: a special chat group listserv on Yahoo! through which they can share useful information and first-hand experience. See www.yahoo.com and click "connect," then "groups".

DID I INHERIT A BRAIN TUMOR FROM MY PARENTS? CAN I GIVE IT TO MY CHILDREN?

We have talked about children's tumors occurring in grownups. But what is the possibility of giving a brain tumor to your child? What are the chances of that? Besides experiencing guilt about developing a brain tumor, many people wonder if their tumor is hereditary. Harriet, a patient of mine, once articulated this concern in a special way: "Can the genes that caused my glioblastoma tumor, and my mother's tumor, be passed on to my three daughters? Did I doom them to a fate like mine?" (Harriet is a family matriarch and geophysicist who has earthquake fault lines in California named after her.)

> 95% of brain tumors are NOT inherited or passed in the genes.

This question led to a discussion about genes, the beneficial and not so beneficial ones. There is indeed a possibility that a tendency toward cancer can be inherited, since some kinds of cancers run in families. Therefore, Harriet's daughters could seek *genetic counseling* to find out whether their mother's cancer was just bad luck or they are carriers of cancer susceptibility or tumor genes. Although Harriet may have been responsible for parenting her children, educating them, and developing their character, she was not to blame for carrying genes that cause illness, any more than she could control the genes that govern hair color or height. (See Chapter 24, Heredity and Other Causes of Brain Tumors, in *Brain Tumors-Finding the Ark*.[1])

> Genetic counseling can answer whether your brain tumor was inherited or not.

HOW SHOULD I THINK ABOUT STATISTICS FOR BRAIN TUMORS?

People die from brain tumors, yes. But many physicians, specialists and family doctors alike, use statistics to "write off" patients because they believe the survival rate is so low. This can be a self-fulfilling prophecy. You want to be with doctors who are positive and know what can be done and how to do it! Usually doctors like this can be found at major brain tumor centers. For example, "At Duke there is Hope" — is the motto of the Brain Tumor Center at Duke University.

While it is true that some types of brain tumors have low survival rates, not everyone with that tumor type will die of it. Statistics can be very misleading. I like the story of Stephen J. Gould who was a professor at Harvard University and wrote many bestselling books about natural science and the human condition. He, too, was faced with his own mortality after being diagnosed with a rare tumor, called mesothelioma. Gould's essay about cancer, "The Median Isn't the Message"[3] is one of the most helpful, wise, and humane pieces ever written about statistics. It challenges the idea that "just the statistics matter," and is a warning to physicians

who have the unfortunate habit of pronouncing death sentences on patients who face a poor prognosis. An excerpt follows:

> Prognoses are for groups of people. No doctor knows ahead of time who the survivors will be.

After my surgery in 1982, I asked my doctor what was the best technical literature on the cancer. She told me, with a touch of diplomacy, that there was nothing really worth reading. I soon realized why she had offered that humane advice: my cancer is incurable, with a median mortality of eight months.

The problem may be briefly stated: What does 'median mortality of eight months' signify? I suspect that most people, without training in statistics, would read such a statement as "I will probably be dead in eight months" – that very conclusion must be avoided, since it isn't so.

Stephen Gould.[3]

Some brain tumors are 100 per cent curable while there are one to five per cent of long-term survivors with even the absolute worst type of brain tumors. No doctor knows ahead of time who those survivors will be. It might as well be you.

WHAT FACTORS DETERMINE THE CHANCES FOR A CURE?

Statistics are great for populations, not individuals. One doctor's personal view or out-of-date knowledge may be his/ her statistic. There are, however, some general statements that seem to apply to groups of people, again, not individuals. For brain tumors, these are the observations that can affect chances of a cure:
1. Tumors can invade the brain tissue itself. This infiltration makes surgery more difficult.
2. Location is important. MRI scans determine location and tumor size, factors that affect the type of surgery, as well as how much tumor can be removed safely.
   a) Top or superficial areas (easier to remove) versus deep within the brain near critical structures (more difficult to remove).

b) Meningiomas usually can be separated from brain and completely removed.

c) "Eloquent" areas of the brain control language or motor function. Tumors in or near this area can be more difficult to remove.

d) Gliomas in the lower brain, called the *brain stem*, can be low grade, but they infiltrate and are at a critical crossing point where information travels between the brain and spinal cord. They may be accessible by needle biopsy only.

3. The tumor grade is based on how it looks under the microscope, not its size or location: from low (grade 1) to high grade, very malignant (grade 4).

4. Expertise of your neurosurgeon: This factor is partly under your control. A general neurosurgeon might not be as aggressive or knowledgeable about new techniques in brain tumor removal compared with an expert who removes 5 to 10 tumors each week.[4] Two recent studies now show that high-volume centers (that conduct more than 50 brain tumor surgeries per year) have better survival rates and fewer complications.[5,6]

These are the factors that statistics say affect survival. Betty has a very practical approach in dealing with her brain tumors:

Who knows when our time is up... so live each day to the fullest... Have dessert for breakfast!" If you tell yourself negative things over and over, you'll start believing it... so I surround myself with positive things: the sunshine in the morning, the birds, being with family, my girls and grandchildren... the dog lying in my lap. Each day is special. I started classes at the local college last quarter... anything to keep my mind off the fact that I have 4 tumors growing in my head.!!! I am not dismissing the tumors - but I decided to fill my life up with pleasant thoughts and positive people.

Betty, Laguna Hills, CA.

WHAT ROLE DO I HAVE IN THE TREATMENT DECISIONS AHEAD?

Now that you have more background about brain tumors, we should talk about decision-making. You will make the choice as to whether treatment should proceed... or not. For many patients, surgery is the obvious best choice, particularly when MRI scans confirm that surgery is possible and may restore your functions. It's important to ask about and carefully weigh the short- and long-term benefits and risks of the various treatments.

- You should be assured that your surgery can be done with a degree of risk that is acceptable to you. Rarely is the need for surgery an absolute emergency.
- You should have confidence and comfort from the knowledge that your surgeon operates on at least 25 to 50 people with tumors per year.
- Take your time to weigh all the factors. Questions to ask about your specific tumor can be found in Chapters 10-15, and in Chapter 5.

ADAM AND EVE IN THE GARDEN OF EDEN: WHAT DOES THIS HAVE TO DO WITH BRAIN TUMORS?

I end this chapter with reference to the first story of Genesis: Adam and Eve. I don't bring up the Book of Genesis to convert you to religion. It is just that different interpretations of the stories may have relevance to your ability to heal. These lessons have persisted for thousands of years and influenced our secular views on illness, life, and death. We may hold unconscious judgments about what is "correct" or "truth." I offer a perspective on these stories that may have a positive effect on your healing. It is up to you to decide whether or not my interpretation has value to you.

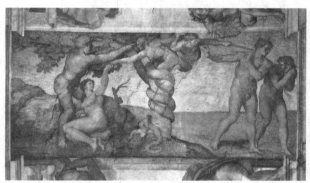

Figure 2-5 Sistine Chapel Ceiling. Adam and Eve Leaving the Garden

I want to discuss an action and a belief that make many people uncomfortable:
- Action: Challenging your doctor and bringing him/her information.
- Belief: My brain tumor – a punishment or curse?

Many of my family and friends don't question a doctor's word because they think it is disrespectful or he will be angry or not take good care of them. "Will I be rejected (punished) for seeking more knowledge about my tumor?" they ask. It is possible that some physicians will feel threatened by your knowledge and questions.

Adam and Eve were punished for taking the "fruit" – Knowledge of Good and Evil. The deity had reserved this awareness for himself. For the sin of challenging higher authority, by becoming conscious of the earthly world and losing their innocence, three consequences befell the pair: 1) they were expelled from blissful immortality

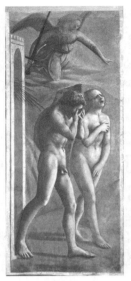

Figure 2-6 Masaccio. Adam and Eve. Leaving the Garden

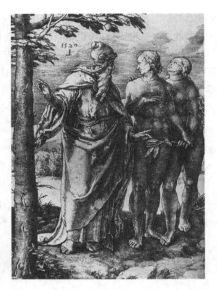

Figure 2-7 van Leyden. Adam and Eve Leaving the Garden

and the good life (as children) in the Garden, 2) they would suffer toil and pain, and finally, 3) they became "adults" and... mortal.

Is this really so different from what has happened to you? We always knew of our own mortality; it is just that a brain tumor makes us think about it more immediately. If challenging the doctor is going to make her/ him angry, and you fear his punishment, then its time to get another physician!

> Choosing your tumor as punishment or curse is an option, not necessarily an accepted truth.

As I noted in the Preface, many people tell me that they think of their lives before the tumor as Eden and afterward as the punishment. It isn't necessarily logical; it is just a feeling. But it turns out that there is more than just one interpretation of the expulsion as a punishment for questioning a higher authority. Great religious artists portrayed different interpretations of the "Fall" from Eden; so might you.

Almost everyone is familiar with the genius, Michelangelo, the Renaissance painter who was perhaps best remembered for his rendering of "The Creation" on the ceiling of the Sistine Chapel at the Vatican in Italy. One scene includes the banishment of Adam and Eve from the Garden of Eden in the presence of a condemning angel who is brandishing a sword at Adam's neck. (See Figure 2-5.) Less familiar is the work of Michaelangelo's role model who, 75 years before, created a fresco portraying a saddened but wiser Eve and Adam leaving their childhood in the Garden of Eden. In contrast to Michaelangelo's version, however, and like no other artist before, Mosaccio added rays of light (enlightenment) over Adam's right shoulder and a guardian angel with upturned sword accompanying the now more knowledgeable, yet mortal adults on their life's journey (Figure 2-6). Lucas van Leyden in Holland, at about the same time, portrayed a fatherly sage guiding the happy and wiser couple out of the Garden into adulthood. (Figure 2-7). There was no harsh punishment in these last two interpretations.

So what might this all mean? Choosing your tumor as punishment or curse is an option, not necessarily an accepted truth. By choosing to educate yourself about your condition, I do not believe that you will be punished, but rather, you will be rewarded with enlightenment and empowerment.

With an understanding of the basics, we move on to the next step on strategic gathering and organization of information for more effective decision-making.

Table 2-4 Internet Resources Basics About Brain Tumors

Basic information	http://www.cancerindex.org/medterm/medtm13.htm http://www.cancerindex.org/clinks2a.htm#0305
Glossary	http://www.neurosurgery.org/health/patient/answers.asp?D isorderID=51 http://www.neurosurgerytoday.org/what/glossary.asp www.virtualtrials.com http://www.sfn.org/baw/pdf/brainfacts.pdf
Brainstem anatomy	http://www.waiting.com/brainstem.html#anchor580032
On-Line Help book for anatomy, functions, and tumor information.	http://www.braintumour.ca/braintumour.nsf/eng/home (Canada) http://www.oncolink.com/types/article.cfm?c=2&s=4&ss=2 5&id=102
Chat group	www.yahoo.com ('contacts'- then 'Groups') http://www.braintrust.org/services/support/braintmr
Advocacy Groups	http://www.nabraintumor.org/members2.html

CHAPTER 3

Getting Organized —
The Key to Regaining Control

And the day came when the risk to remain tight in a bud
Was more painful than the risk it took to blossom.

Anais Nin. French-American Poet: 1903-1977

GETTING ORGANIZED

KEY PREPARATIONS FOR THE BATTLE AGAINST A BRAIN TUMOR

Creating the notebook

A medical dictionary

Separate file for all medical/insurance bills and correspondence

Planning not to get overwhelmed

⚷ Key search words

- organization
- second opinions
- notebooks
- keeping records
- clinical trials
- diary
- laboratory & scan reports
- support, friends and groups

KEY PREPARATIONS FOR THE BATTLE AGAINST A BRAIN TUMOR

It pays to be organized whether you are fixing a leaky faucet, meeting with your tax accountant, or getting your automobile's transmission repaired. The principle is the same in overcoming a brain tumor: organization of your information is the key. Through my experience with thousands of patients, I have found four activities that are essential for your success:

- Creating the notebook;
- Having a medical dictionary;
- Keeping medical related bills and insurance papers in one place; and
- Planning to not get overwhelmed.

STEP 1 – CREATING THE NOTEBOOK

Organizing your medical information is the first step in regaining control of a situation that might seem out of balance right now. It may sound silly but I suggest you follow the steps in making a medical notebook. Later, you can decide if it was good or bad advice. Having this data at your fingertips saves significant time and aggravation, because records are lost or not available when you most need them (like midnight in the emergency department). In the words of the poet Dylan Thomas[1], a notebook is your first step "to rage mightily against the dying of the light."

Materials I Need to Get Started

You need to obtain the following materials and assemble your notebook as soon as possible:

1. Three-ring, loose-leaf binder
2. 10 dividers, labeled as they appear in Sections 1-10 below (Table 3-1).
3. Notepad or loose-leaf paper, lined, three-hole-punched (for Section 6)
4. Two types of plastic storage sleeves 8.5" x 11", three-hole-punched One holds business cards (baseball trading card size) with 5 x 2 = 10 slots/ page. These can be found in office supply or drug stores in packages of 10 (e.g., Wilson-Jones #21471 "Business Card binder pages") (Section 1).

   The other is to hold several CD-ROM disks. (Section 4)

Table 3-1 Content of My Survivor's Notebook

Section 1.	Business Cards or "Who's who?"
Section 2.	Pathology Reports
Section 3.	Laboratory Reports and Blood Tests
Section 4.	MRI and CT Scan Reports
Section 5.	Second and Third Opinions
Section 6.	Questions and Answers at Doctor Visits
Section 7.	Medications: A Summary
Section 8.	Resources and References
Section 9.	Calendar
Section 10.	Summary of your medical and surgical history

Using My Notebook

Section 1 – Business cards or "Who's who"?

Business cards of doctors, consultants, health professionals, social workers, insurance companies, and case managers are easy to find when inserted into the 5 x 2 plastic slots. When you meet with a new professional, write the name and contact information in this section. If you obtain a business card, place it in the sleeve or case – no more searching under couches, through drawers, and in handbags for a name or phone number. Your time is too valuable for that.

Section 2 – Pathology reports

This is absolutely critical information. Many patients will have major brain surgery (costing thousands of dollars) to confirm a diagnosis and, hopefully, reverse damage caused by a tumor. Yet, they do not know what their pathology report actually said, nor do they have a record of it. Trust me: Taking hold of your own pathology report empowers you. It is about you; the report is yours, and its accuracy is essential for correct treatment.

> Accurate diagnosis of your tumor type is essential for correct treatment. Having the pathology report is key.

An analysis of brain tissue and final diagnosis by a pathologist can sometimes be controversial and unclear. Moreover, some oncologists will conduct treatment based on a verbal statement or written note by the patient, without ever confirming the diagnosis by personal review of the "tumor tissue slides." The following is a true story to illustrate the importance of having pathology reports in your possession:

In the Fall of 2000, James, a 36-year-old stockbroker from New York City, consulted us for a second opinion about a "very malignant, fatal tumor." He brought copies of dictated notes from his oncologist, who was based at a major New York medical center, along with records of his medical history, examinations, and tests. We did not feel, however, that his young age, history of seizures, and two years of headaches fit the diagnosis of glioblastoma multiforme. The pathology report read, "The tumor had flecks of calcium in it, as well as cysts, and not much swelling (edema), which is consistent with glioblastoma". Fortunately, James had his MRI scans (at home) and the actual tumor specimen was sent from the hospital for our review. With this data, it became abundantly clear that the general pathologist had over-interpreted the features of the tumor. James did not have a glioblastoma, but rather an oligodendroglioma, a tumor that is much more responsive to both chemotherapy and radiation... and consistent with a longer life.

Without the actual written pathology report for me to review, this young man may have been condemned to a dismal prognosis and needless, inappropriate therapy. The initiative he took to keep his own records saved his life. Doctors can help you make decisions... if they have the complete set of data on which to base their recommendations. (See Chapter 5: The Team; and Chapter 8: Traditional Diagnosis.)

Section 3 – Laboratory reports and blood tests
Why are you collecting these reports? Isn't the hospital or doctor supposed to do this for you? As if you don't already know, it isn't a perfect world. Having these records immediately available saves a lot of time in delays and mix-ups caused by the continual shuffling of your files. Reports can easily fall out from charts, be misfiled, and become lost. You can hand the doctors or nurses the critical information they need on the spot. Immediate access to the records within my patients' personal notebooks has spared them countless hours of waiting and even the need to have extra tests.

An example: When I calculate chemotherapy dosages each month for my patients, I must have their blood chemistry profiles to ensure that their bone marrow, liver, and kidneys can handle the medication. In order to calculate the proper dose of drug, I also need to know the levels of their complete blood count: red cells or hemoglobin (for carrying oxygen); white cells (for fighting infection); and platelets (for clotting). When results are not readily available, this requires a call to the lab, a wait until they locate the results, and then a delay while waiting to receive a FAX copy of the report. A Tracking Form to record your hospitalizations or clinic treatments is available, if you wish to use it. (See Table 3-3.)

Bottom line: Organizing your medical information = regaining control = power.

Section 4 – MRI and CT Scan reports

Each time you have a scan, obtain paper copies of the scan reports and actual images on film (or ideally on a computer disk, or CD-ROM) before you leave your doctor's office or the imaging laboratory. The CD-ROMs can be inserted into their plastic sleeves in this section of your notebook with the dictated reports.

Most centers will provide a CD-ROM that includes a software program called eFilm™ to enable you to view images on any computer with Microsoft Photoshop or a similar program.

Why do this? Having your own copy of films and reports makes getting second opinions and switching doctors much easier, faster, and cheaper. Hospitals and doctors' offices are notorious for misplacing things. A lost film means loss of your precious time and opportunity to get a copy of that film. In the brain tumor arena, these are the keys to high-quality care, an accurate diagnosis, and an effective treatment plan. The reports are your lifeline. Here is another real life example that shows why having your own copies of your reports at hand is essential:

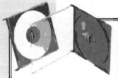

Most Centers provide MRI scan copies on CD-ROM.

Rosa, a vital and attractive 47-year-old, had dramatic shrinkage of her "atypical" brainstem tumor after receiving a new chemotherapy drug called Temodar on a clinical trial. A few months later, she developed weakness in her chest and facial muscles. My colleagues and I were not sure whether the change was due to a recent lowering of her steroid dose, low calcium levels, or recurrent tumor. We obtained an emergency MRI scan, but the previous scan from two months ago had been "misplaced" (read: lost) by the hospital x-ray file room, so we had no comparison film. Thankfully, Rosa's husband, Rudolfo, had been carrying her scans in the trunk of his car. Within 10 minutes, we knew that the tumor had not changed. The muscle weakness resulted from lowering her steroid dose too quickly.

If Rudolfo had not had the scans, we would have waited three days for copies. The family was spared an anxious weekend ruminating over worst-case scenarios. I cannot state emphatically enough how important it is to keep a file of your own records. And, by the way, many doctors (and centers) will review your MRI films without charge.

What if your doctors question your record keeping? You have a right to this information, although medical personnel may be skeptical about your request.

Simply reassure them that you trust them and you want to make sure that you have all the results in one place for the many consultants who you may need to see. Don't let any doctor, nurse, or assistant intimidate you.

Your scans and scan reports belong to you!

You can get these documents from the doctor who ordered the test or the radiologist who interpreted it. Your physician should not be upset by this. Speak up! Ask for your copies. You can place the written reports in your notebook in the order in which you had the MRIs done.

Section 5 – Second and third opinions
If you are comfortable with your current team, there is no pressure or reason to switch. In this section, you will file the following:
- Questions for the expert;
- His/her answers; and
- Copy of the dictated consultation.

Four reasons for getting second and third opinions
Remember: The treatment of brain tumors is an evolving field with a select number of experts around the country. Multiple opinions:
1. Confirm your diagnosis. At the least, it's important for you or your doctor to consult with a major brain tumor center, especially if your doctor sees fewer than 25 brain tumors per year.
2. Confirm that you are with a doctor you can trust or help you find one.
3. Can expand your treatment options.
4. Give you peace of mind later to know that you have left no stone unturned.

You don't have to be dissatisfied to ask for a second opinion.

Sample questions to ask the expert
Here are eight sample generic questions to ask the expert whom you consult for a second or third opinion. More detailed questions for each specialist can be found in Chapter 5: The Team – Doctors and Other Members; and in Chapter 6: Experts and Second Opinions.
1. What is my diagnosis?
2. What characteristics of my tumor lead you to arrive at this diagnosis?
3. If there is uncertainty about my diagnosis, are there any tests that could give you the information you need to be more definitive?
4. What are my treatment options?
5. What are the pros and cons of these options?
6. What would you do, if you were in my shoes?

7. Do you work closely with a team?

8. Whom would you recommend that I consult for another opinion?

Politics of second opinions

There are a few important pointers about the politics of getting multiple opinions. First, you do not need to apologize for this; it's your right! If questioned, you might say, "I'm getting several opinions in order to make the most informed decision possible about my treatment options." If a doctor gives you a hard time or shows an attitude problem, don't let it bother you. It's immaterial if doctors approve or disapprove of your decisions. Remember, you are out of the Garden of Eden already. Now is the time to search for knowledge to make your life better. In many ways, you have to think selfishly and follow your own instincts – no matter what other people say or think.

- Tell your primary physician that you are seeking a second and third opinion.
- He may be helpful in referrals or in interpreting any conflicting information.

Do you tell each doctor what the previous ones said? You want an independent view, so wait until each formulates his/ her opinion before asking how and why it might differ from others. (See Chapter 6: Experts and Second Opinions.)

Section 6 – Questions and answers

Put a ledger pad or lined notebook paper in this section. This is your journal or diary of medical or other healthcare visits, conferences or meetings.

You, or members of your support team, enter the questions that you would like to ask your doctor, so that you are prepared at the next opportunity.

Under each question, you or your companion write the answers that the doctor is giving while the conversations are taking place. You might have to elaborate on and complete those answers immediately following the conversation, once you have more time to sit and digest all that was exchanged. Record the answers as soon as you can because you won't remember everything later. But you will have clear and comprehensive notes to refer to and review whenever you need them. Sometimes, during medical appointments, the information flows so quickly that it's hard to remember it all. You may even want to tape record the meetings, if your doctor will allow it.

Bottom line: Write down important questions to ask; check them off as the meeting progresses. This should not be embarrassing. If your doctor is irritated, it is his problem, not yours.

It's easy to forget to ask critical questions during appointments with the doctor, particularly when you are nervous about these visits or your doctors are hurried. The following story demonstrates the value of keeping updated notes of questions and answers:

> Fred was a strapping 65-year-old clothes wholesaler from Santa Barbara who experienced a seizure on the golf course. Two weeks later, he had a CT scan in a local emergency room that showed a tumor. Fred was referred to the Neurosurgical Institute where he had a complete removal of a ganglioglioma, a benign tumor. A week after surgery, Fred had the skin staples on his incision removed. During that visit, the neurosurgeon informed me that the tumor was completely removed and the pathology reported a very low-grade tumor. Soon thereafter, I met with Fred and his family for one hour. We discussed the slight paralysis that remained after surgery and its chances for improvement, his scheduled return to work, and his ability to drive again.

Despite having had two appointments with his physicians, Fred neglected to ask whether the tumor was benign or malignant. He left the meeting thinking that because the subject was not discussed, the tumor must be malignant. In his mind, he would not have elected to receive any further therapy because he would die anyway. Two days later, I received a telephone call from Linda, his wife of 40 years, who asked, "Is it true that he was going to die?" It took an hour of conversation to find out how our communication was so mixed up.

This is a good example about "ass-umptions" – making an ass out of you and me. We, as physicians, and he, as the interested party, were both at fault. A single question, unasked and unanswered, can have an enduring negative impact.

Section 7 – Medications history

Knowing which medications and dosages you are taking, and when they started or stopped, can save your life. It also allows your doctor or future consultants to sort out any side effects you might be having.

Recent reports suggest that childhood and young adult survivors of cancer may not know the details of their medical history as they become older. This means they

> Know your medications and doses - it could save your life!

may not get the care and monitoring they require.[2] Keeping records is important for everyone to have available, even years later. (See Table 3-4 for template charts to record your medications, doses, who prescribed it, etc.)

Section 8 – Resources and references

On this journey to more knowledge, you will collect handouts, articles, phone numbers, websites and other useful resources. This section can be used to store such information in one place until it is needed.

Section 9 – Calendar

A small calendar in the medical notebook makes things technically easier. You can look back to when the last scan was done and write in when the next appointment is scheduled. It's also helpful for detailing when an insurance claim is being questioned, as companies often put the date, but not the reason for the claim.

Section 10 – Summary of (Brain Tumor) medical and surgical history

This is where you can keep your time-sequenced history of treatments and important events, as they occurred, in a medical summary that you can use when you meet a new physician or need to send your scans away for review. (See template Table 3-5.) A sample signature for e-mails is suggested in Table 3-6 and how to use it is described in Chapter 4: Searching the Web/ Internet.

Okay, the hard part about organizing the notebook is over. Now on to getting this "tumor thing" more under control.

STEP 2 – MEDICAL DICTIONARY AND OTHER BOOKS

Christine, the mother of a young adult with an astrocytoma, reminded me that a medical dictionary is a necessity. Dorland's is a classic. Used editions can be purchased on www.amazon.com from $11-22. Basic books about brain tumors are available from foundations like The Brain Tumor Society (BTS), American Brain Tumor Association (ABTA), and National Brain Tumor Foundation (NBTF). Their websites have a glossary and suggested books that can be helpful (also see the Glossary in this book). You can obtain a free copy of the dictionary distributed by the ABTA or view it online (Table 3-2). Call 1-800-886-2282 or e-mail info@abta.org . *100 Questions & Answers About Brain Tumors* also has useful information, a book available through the ABTA.[3]

STEP 3 – SEPARATE FILE FOR ALL MEDICAL/INSURANCE BILLS AND CORRESPONDENCE

> Insurance and hospital bills can be overwhelming. File them right away. Use tracking forms to stay sane.

Dealing with the health insurance can be overwhelming. For now, just file this information and you will learn more about bills, denials and appeals, and insurance later in Chapter 23: Managing Costs, Benefits and Your Healthcare with Insurance.[4] You can use the Medical Bill (Table 3-7) and Insurance Tracking Forms (Table 3-8) in this chapter to organize what is paid or owed.

STEP 4 – PLANNING **NOT** TO GET OVERWHELMED

A. Bring Someone With You to Your Medical Appointments

You may not be able to understand what your doctor says or remember what to ask, especially if you are recovering from surgery and your brain is swollen, or you are on steroids. Also, doctors are not always aware when they use medical terms or technical language that can confuse you. Your "buddy" can help in several ways:

> You can avoid being overwhelmed.

- Discuss and compare with you, after the appointment, what you heard the doctor say (and help you record good notes).
- Offer emotional support, if you need it.
- Ensure that all predetermined questions are asked...and answered to your satisfaction.
- Ask additional questions or ask for clarifications.
- Drive you, as it may not be safe for you to drive just yet.

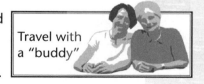

Travel with a "buddy"

So I started doing a status sheet of each of Steve's symptoms. It's still two pages long. But we cover each of the problems Steve is experiencing and it lets the doctors know everything that is happening with Steve. They kind of made fun of me at first, but now it has eliminated that initial visit with the nurse asking about Steve's symptoms. And it eliminates that problem that we were experiencing where the doctor comes in the room and asks, "How are things going?" Steve (his personality) would say, "Fine." And I (my personality) would go into a litany of complaints.

So I just do this status list now and it creates wonderful conversations that answer all our questions (I still keep a list of questions). It's sort

> Say YES to offers of help.

of like having an agenda for a meeting instead of a free for all. And the doctors now all have mentioned that they appreciate it.

Melodie, Seattle, WA

You've shown kindness to people over your lifetime; this is the time to ask for help with your needs. (See Chapter 5: The Team – Doctors and Other Members.)

B. Ask About Clinical Trials

For some types of brain tumors, there is the prospect of long-term survival. This progress has been made in part through clinical trials, which are experimental studies for new treatments. Clinical trials are the best way for you to get the latest, state-of-the-art treatments. Moreover, the only way to move closer to a cure is by participation. Studies have shown that people on clinical trials live longer than those people receiving conventional therapy for recurrent tumors. Over the last decade, such trials have given thousands of brain tumor patients access to the benefits of Temodar for gliomas, "PCV" combination chemotherapy for anaplastic astrocytoma and oligodendroglioma, and Gliadel for glioblastoma multiforme. To learn more about clinical trials, or to find one, see Chapter 21: Clinical Trials and Table 3-2.

Clinical trials mean hope.

C. Visit Internet Websites

Websites such as www.virtualtrials.com or the Brain Tumor Society at http://www.tbts.org/virtual_html/welcome.htm are excellent resources for patients with brain tumors. They offer everything from companionship to detailed treatment information, with discussion about specific brain tumor types. In addition to directly providing information, they also include links to other web page resources.

Remember, websites were started by people like you who said, "Hey, there has to be a better way to learn about this thing." One such individual is Dr. Al Musella, whose sister-in-law was diagnosed with a brain tumor about eight years ago. Instead of cursing the darkness of not enough information, he lit a candle to shed the light of knowledge around the world, creating www.virtualtrials.com. Visit the TBTS, NBTF, and ABTA sites to see how much information has been collected for your immediate use. Most of the hard work has already been done for you. (See Table 3-2.)

Use Internet for information & support.

D. Get in a Group

Support groups are essential for both treatment and recovery. In fact, studies show that people in these groups even live longer (more on this in Chapter 18: Complementary and Alternative therapy). Not only do groups provide comfort and understanding, but also they are a great source of information on treatments, nutrition, costs of care, newer therapies, things your doctor does not tell you, etc. They help you know that you are not alone. Groups take many forms, from formal meetings near home to informal chats on the Internet, and to national meetings of survivors. Here are some examples:

Join a Group.

Hi everyone: Felt the need to share our good news, too. My husband Garry just completed a 6th round of Temodar and had an MRI today. It shows "significant reduction in extent of the previously documented altered signal intensity with less enhancement and reduced mass effect when compared to MRI of 26 Jan. There is less enhancement of the splenium of the corpus callosum. Appearances indicate further response to therapy." Our oncologist was very pleased, and we are most excited.

It is one year on 28 April since we started on this dreadful journey. We know there is still a long road ahead. With good news like this, it helps us to remain positive. Best to everyone making this journey with us.

Louise w/o Garry, Temple, TX. Anaplastic oligo, radiation 2001, regrowth or radiation necrosis September 2001, six rounds Temodar.

Many local hospitals run cancer support groups. There may even be a brain tumor support group in your area. Look for Wellness Community meetings on the web. You can ask the social worker at your treatment center for location and time of meetings. (See Table 3-2.)

For most people, you are basically doing this yourself and nobody around you has any idea what you are going through. But at these meetings, everyone is in the same boat, and they all know what you are going through. You don't have to feel funny if you are bald, or have trouble talking or walking. It's so easy to meet people and start up a conversation with "strangers," because you already have so much in common.

Dan, Houston, TX

With Internet access and an e-mail account (you can sign up for a free account through search engines such as at Google.com's G-Mail, Yahoo.com or Hotmail.com), you can be in continual dialogue with a community of tens to thousands from around the world who understand what you are experiencing. (See Chapter 4.)

The following e-mail conversation describes an experience with Temodar for glioblastoma multiforme. Many people learned on the Internet that people who received radiation and Temodar together may have better survival. The jury is still out on the use of Temodar in glioblastoma multiforme, so this person represents a case study. It demonstrates the power of finding knowledge.

> *I would like to share Ted's progress using stereotactic radiation with Temodar 150mg daily following total visual resection of glioblastoma multiforme on 9/24/02. He showed changes on an MRI after the radiation and daily Temodar. A subsequent craniotomy found necrosis, not tumor. He continued with the Temodar monthly (now on cycle six). In May, he showed more changes and had a needle biopsy: pathology was gliosis (scar tissue). He also had some edema, both of which have cleared with Decadron. I guess my point is:- the combination of radiation, Temodar and aggressive follow-up by the medical team in West Virginia is keeping my husband working as a Dean of Students and football coach. This man coached a basketball game six days post-craniotomy; so who knows what fatigue is to him?*
>
> *Just knowing you all are out there and that you are on the other side of this fog we are walking through makes it more possible to take things one step at a time.*
>
> Jane, Morgantown, WV.

A warning about Internet chat groups or rooms: Consider using the web – and not chat groups – in the very beginning. The websites in this book contain information that has been validated by those responsible for the sites. The chat groups and listservs are "real time" conversations among people in all circumstances. Thus, it can be emotionally challenging at times to read about someone's opinion of a doctor, or his or her own suffering at that moment, especially if you are not ready to listen.

How do I contact a group? How do I take the first step? In Chapter 4, I will walk you through it step-by-step. If you cannot wait to become a member of an e-mail list of people from around the world who have experience with your type of brain tumor, you can go to www.virtualtrials.com and select the list(s) of your choice right now. There will be larger and smaller (25–1000) e-mail membership lists for brain tumors (general), brainstem tumors, pituitary tumors, medulloblastoma tumors, temozolomide, and much more. (See Chapter 4: Searching the Web/ Internet.)

E. Take It One Day at a Time

- Think in terms of taking your life one day at a time, until you begin to feel better.
- Don't worry about next month or even next week.
- Take a breather and listen to what Melinda, someone who has "been there", has to say.
  - Keep a diary.
  - Find something to rejoice and be glad about every day. I told my husband we could laugh or cry for whatever time he had, but I wanted to make happy... memories.
  - None of us is guaranteed tomorrow.

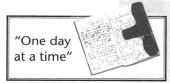

"One day at a time"

F. Ask Your Friends for Help

The following is advice from one caretaker spouse to another who expresses how overwhelmed he felt in taking care of his wife:

As far as trying to manage everything: Can you ask friends to help with groceries or some housecleaning, or any chores that simply could be done by others? People want to help and many of our friends find that is also a way for them to cope. I have stepped aside and swallowed my pride – more people watch our children than before; meals are prepared for us; our yard is maintained by a landscaper. One of my wife's very good friends comes over and housecleans once a week. It's too much to ask of someone to handle all of the responsibility, so try to delegate so you can stay strong! You will have your time in life to give back to those that give to you. Take care.

Scott, husband of Julie, parents of 2 girls,
Dawn, a 4 yr old w/Down Syndrome and
my 9 yr old Eva, also diagnosed w/GBM
12/01. Tacoma, WA

Read how relieved one spouse was after saying, "Yes, you can help":

In the past, I have been reluctant to accept help because I didn't want to impose on anyone. Then a friend of mine who recently underwent treatment for Lymphoma gave me a great piece of advice. He told me that many people would offer to help during this difficult time. The best thing I could do for Kate and myself was to practice saying the word yes. I guess I have finally practiced saying it enough, because I am actually starting to accept offers of help and even solicit help from family and close friends when really necessary.

Our neighbors would just do things for us without our knowledge like cut our grass or plant flowers in our garden. We had meals given to us for three months straight. People are so good when a tragedy strikes.

Rod, husband of Kate. Chicago, IL.

You now know the why and how of getting organized. In the next few chapters, you'll learn more about assessing your current medical team, your individual tumor, and the different options for therapy. Remember: There are always options.

Table 3-2 Internet Contact Resources for Getting Organized

Clinical Trials	http://clinicaltrials.gov/ct/gui http://www.cancer.org/docroot/ETO/ETO_6.asp www.virtualtrials.com
Support group	http://www.thewellnesscommunity.org
Dictionaries and Terminology	http://virtualtrials.com/dictionary.cfm http://www.mtdesk.com/d.shtml http://my.webmd.com/medical_information/drug_and_herb/ default.htm http://neurosurgery.mgh.harvard.edu/ABTA/diction.htm http://www.abta.org/buildingknowledge3.htm
The Brain Tumor Society (BTS)	www.tbts.org
American Brain Tumor Association (ABTA) e-mail	e-mail: info@abta.org http://www.abta.org

National Brain Tumor Foundation (NBTF)	http://www.braintumor.org
National Cancer Institute Information	http://cis.nci.nih.gov/

Table 3-3 Hospital Stay Tracking Form

Date Admitted	Date Discharged	Hospital Name	Reason for Admission	Admitting MD Notes:

Table 3-4 Medications Tracking Form

My Allergies:					
Pharmacy 1:			Phone number:		
Pharmacy 2:			Phone number:		
Date Started	Date stopped	Medication Name	Dose	Time given	Prescribed by Dr.___

Table 3-5 Sample Template – Brain Tumor History & Summary

Name : LAST _____ FIRST _____ AGE: _____ Male/ Female   Right /Left Handed

Address: _____ City _____ State _____ Zip _____   DOB: __/__/__

Family Contact: _____ Relationship: _____

My Phone: (Day)_____(Evening)_____(Fax)_____(Email)_____

Date Original Diagnosis/ Biopsy or No Biopsy? _____

Diagnosis/Pathology: _____Pathology Second opinion? Y/N_____

MAJOR SYMPTOMS/ DATES OF TUMOR PROGRESSION #1, #2

1._____   2._____   3._____   4._____

MY CURRENT DAILY LEVEL OF FUNCTIONING :   Karnofsky scale: ___ % or

Independent ☐   Needs assistance ☐   Dependent ☐

TREATMENTS/   DATE (s) PERFORMED

Surgery: Open biopsy ☐   Stereotactic biopsy ☐   Tumor Removal ☐

DATES   ___ / ___ / ___   ___ / ___ / ___   ___ / ___ / ___

Radiation therapy

External/Focused beam   ☐   dates/ Treatment Center_____

Whole brain   ☐   dates/ Treatment Center_____

Radiosurgery

X-knife ☐ _____ GammaKnife ☐ _____

Chemotherapy   Names and dates of therapies/drugs:

1. _____   _____   _____ _____

2. _____   _____   _____ _____

Clinical Trials   Y/N   ☐   If yes, please list trials, institution and dates:

3.

4. _____

Complementary Alternative therapies Y/N   ☐   Complementary Professionals?

If yes, please list with dates:_____

____ __ ____ ___ _____

Previous Recommendations?

5. _____

What Is/Are Your Most Important Question(s)?

Table 3-6 Three Sample Brief Histories for E-Mail Signature

- Diagnosed 1 Sep 02 with Stage IV NSCLC w/brain mets;
- WBR w/Temodar for 2 weeks; carboplatin and taxotere every three weeks for the lung tumor (19 rounds).
- Since 1-03, 800 mg of Celebrex daily. Increased mass and contrast on brain MRIs (at site of the original 3-x-4-cm lesion), along with recurring neurological symptoms, prompted
- Awake craniotomy 3 Oct 03.
- Radiation necrosis debulked; Gliasite balloon inserted because "a few live cancer cells" were also found.
- Still trying to wean from decadron.
- On a break from chemo since late December.
- January 2004, preparatory to start second-line therapy.

- Lloyd Hartzsmith, Columbus, OH diag 8/98 Oligo II, Left Parietal lobe near midline Surgery 8/98 Partial Brain radiation 9/98 31 rads
- Dilantin 100mg + Phenytek 300 mg daily Celexa for depression 12/01 It's back? 3/02 Biopsy- Oligo III/Astro III Tumor size of an egg 4/02 Started Temodar and Zofran
- 10/02 Down to nickel size - Whoo Hoo! 9/03 Completed 19 rounds Temodar. No change since 10/02 Taken off Temodar- 11/03 MRI 4-5 new spots - Back on Temodar

---

10/27/02 Seizure, MRI shows small (1cm) lesion, right frontal lobe. cyst suspected. Started Dilantin

11/05/02 D/C Dilantin due to rash, started Depakote

02/04/03 2nd MRI - dramatic increase in size of lesion - 5 cm

02/14/03 Craniotomy, 95-99 percent resection, no deficits, Biopsy confirms GBM

03/06/03 D/C Depakote due to rash, started Tegretol

03/28/03 Started concurrent Rad and low dose Temodar (daily for 30 days)

05/18/03 Admitted for 10 days, double Pneumonia, Neutropenia, WBC 800

06/24/03 Started Temodar, 5days/mo for 6 mo.

06/25/03 3rd MRI - Tumor stable

07/12/03 Married at Lake Jane, Acadia National Park

10/08/03 4th MRI - Slight regression

11/30/03 Temodar concluded

01/25/04 5th MRI - Major Regression in Tumor size!

04/25/04 Problems with Nausea, and Ataxia noted

05/07/04 6th MRI - Tumor found in brain stem, admitted for dehydration

Table 3-7 Medical Bill Tracking Form:
Notes:

Date	Provider	Service Hospital dates	Charges	Insurance payment	We owe	Date paid

Notes:

Table 3-8 Insurance Coverage and Funding Sources
Insurance Company Policy Number Contact Person Address Phone
Insurance Company Policy Number Contact Person Address Phone
Insurance Company Policy Number Contact Person Address Phone
SSI Supplemental Security Income Contact Person Address Phone
MediGap Insurance & Number Contact Person Address Phone
Notes:

CHAPTER 4

Searching the WEB and Internet

The Brain Tumor list has taught me a great deal about life, about living, and most of all about dying. We all know that our lives will be affected almost daily by such things as fatigue, memory loss, confusion, seizures, etc. But we share, with our Internet members the feelings and the losses. We are advocates for each other. We each need the power of purpose.

Gladys, a NJ Lady

Key search words

- internet
- treatment choices
- URL
- web indexes
- search engine

- browser
- www
- brain tumor sites
- chat rooms
- websites

- jump sites
- ISP
- hyperlinks
- chat groups
- searches

The following 8 pages are intended for those who have managed not to become involved in the Internet so far. If you are already Internet savvy, you may want to skip to page 77.

THE INTERNET – WHAT IS IT?

> World Wide Web – all websites & e-mail from anywhere in the world that is publicly accessible through a computer.

The Internet is a network of linked computers that transmits information from files and documents over telephone lines or cable. Every personal computer, cell phone, or other device that people use to look at websites or exchange e-mail is all part of the Internet. The "World Wide Web" refers to information, such as websites and e-mail from anywhere in the world, that is publicly accessible through computers. Once you have accessed the information, you are connected or "online."

There are three basic tools that enable you to get from your computer to the World Wide Web:

THE INTERNET SERVICE PROVIDER (ISP)

This is the highway from your computer to the outside world. You pay a provider such as AOL™, EarthLink™, Roadrunner™, or MSN™ etc. for access to this "on-ramp" to the World Wide Web.

THE BROWSER

A *browser* is a software program (or the "taxi") that takes you along the highway to the World Wide Web to find websites that contain documents, graphics, sound, movies, games, chat rooms, and more. Two common browsers are Netscape and Internet Explorer. Your browser helps you *link* or travel to pages on websites around the world.

THE SEARCH ENGINE

The *search engine* is the guidance system in your taxi that "crawls" on the web highways and finds specific information using "keyword" searches. It can search for cover titles of books or documents, a Uniform Resource Locator (URL) which is the web address, location codes, or full text. (See Table 4-2 below for a list of popular search engines.)

> For WWW access, you need an Internet Service Provider (ISP) a "browser" and a "search engine"

71

HOW DO I MAKE THE INTERNET WORK FOR ME?

I Am Overwhelmed by Too Much Information

Do these suggestions from relatives and friends sound familiar?
- Use only holistic medicine and eat macrobiotic foods.
- Find an expert or major center to get your treatment.
- Try other treatments. A guy I know with your type of tumor was cured!
- Enroll in a clinical trial.
- Use acupuncture and yoga.
- My father's neurosurgeon is the best neurosurgeon in the state.

On the one hand, information is power. On the other hand, you may find yourself frozen by the vast and overwhelming amount of medical information on the Internet. You are going to read many articles. You are going to meet people who have miracles to sell for the small price of your house or your first-born child.

> If you feel overwhelmed, ask someone whom you trust to help you "surf the net."

But how do you remain sane and use what is important to answer questions about your own specific problem? How do you distinguish between good and bad advice? How do you manage all the information on this journey?

You may also feel physically incapable of handling an Internet search at the present time. That is okay too. If you have just recovered from surgery or are in the middle of radiation, then it might be stressful to start researching your own tumor. In that case, ask someone whom you trust to help. Or divide the task and designate someone in your circle to help wade through the majority of the information, eliminating the irrelevant, and allowing you to review the findings. This will reduce your feelings of being overwhelmed.

Remember that the original purpose of this book is to empower you and equip you with relevant, critical knowledge about options. (Table 4-1) My physician Assistant colleague, D. Heimer, once summed up the answer with the acronym "K-O-P-E":

Knowledge + Options + Positivity = Empowerment

Table 4-1 Choices You Can Find on the Internet

- Health information to help guide traditional treatment decisions = **Knowledge**
- Second and third opinions from experts = **Options**
- A clinical trial or other treatment options = **Positivity**
- Complementary and alternative therapies and support = **Empowerment**

As part of the decision-making process, people often seek answers to important questions on the Internet, especially when they are unsuccessful in obtaining such information from their physicians. After you find these answers on the Internet, you must next resolve this series of questions:

- How do I evaluate the information I find?
- Why didn't my doctor tell me about these options?
- Will my doctor be upset with me for sharing the information that I have found and may want to try?

You may have some concerns about doing an Internet search. For instance, many people are worried about offending their doctor by doing so. To this, I respond that

> Many people may feel awkward about offending their doctor by doing their own research. There is no reason to be concerned about this.

there is no reason to feel awkward about this; it does not negate your current treatment program and you can inform your doctor that you are leaving no stone unturned. It also means that you and the "medical professionals" are starting to work as a *team*. You are now asking your physician for help in understanding material, rather than blindly following recommendations.

PERFORMING AN INTERNET SEARCH

For those of you who have not gone online previously, the task is not as daunting as it seems. A friend or a local librarian may be able to get you started and show you how to search for sites. And if you do not have access to the Internet, your local library can provide access. For a nominal fee of $2-5 an hour, some coffee shops (Internet Café, CyberCafe) and copy centers such as Kinko's provide access too. The American Brain Tumor Association (www.abta.org) publishes a resource called "The Brain Tumor Survivor's Guide to the Internet" that is available through their site or by calling 847-827-9910. There are websites that will define the tech lingo for you, too (Table 4-6). So, let's start:

Step 1. Go to Your Browser.

- Start up your computer.
- Make sure that your modem is on and connected to a telephone line (unless you are always connected by cable).
- If you have a dial-up connection, click on your ISP (AOL, EarthLink etc.) icon on your screen. This will connect your computer to the Internet. This generally takes between 15 and 60 seconds.
- If you have cable, you are always connected. Just click the browser icon on your screen.
- Once connected, you will see the home page of your web browser. This is the page that shows each time you go "on-line." You can change the home page to any site of your choice.
- Depending upon the speed of your modem (dial-up telephone line or cable), and complexity of the home page that you are accessing, the time to load a page can range from seconds to several minutes.

Step 2. Use the Browser to Launch Your Search Engine.

- Choose one of the *search engines* (Table 4-2).
- Some browsers enable you to select a search engine by merely typing the name of the search engine into the search *window* of the browser.
- "Ask Jeeves™" is perhaps the easiest search engine to use, if you are unfamiliar with the Internet. Type in the search engine address (URL) such as www.ask.com or http://www.ask.com into your browser (Internet Explorer or Netscape). Click on "Go" or "Search." Or press "Enter." (With many recent browsers you will not have to start with http://)
- The search engine comes up. (Figure 4-1)

Internet Search: 1) Connect to a search engine with your browser 2) Type in key words. 3) On your Results page, click on hyperlinks or type the URL.

Table 4-2 Search Engines for Brain Tumor Information

Engine	Address (URL)
AskJeeves	http://www.ask.com
Excite	http://www.excite.com/
Google	http://www.google.com
HotBot	http://www.hotbot.com/
InfoSeek	http://www.infoseek.com/
Lycos	http://www.lycos.com/
MSN Search	http://search.msn.com
WebCrawler	http://www.webcrawler.com/
Yahoo!	http://www.yahoo.com/

Step 3. Enter Keywords to Select the Topic Area to Be Searched.

- I will use AskJeeves as an example. Type in a question such as *Can you tell me about brain tumors,* or the key search word(s) *glioma* **or** *hydrocephalus* into the search window of the engine (*"Ask"* rectangle). Press "Enter" or click *"Ask."* This will take you to information sites. (A list of key search words appears on the first page of each chapter in this book.)
- For example, if you type brain tumor trial in the Ask rectangle of AskJeeves on the Greetings page (Figure 4-1) and click on "Ask," you will get the results as shown on Figure 4-2.

Note that what appears is the "general information on" option on "Where can I learn about brain | general information on ▼ |
tumors". If you point to the down-arrow tip on the side of the box, you could choose as your search options "symptoms of," "diagnosis of" or "treatments for," which will give you very different results.

- A different search engine, like Google can come up with quite different results. Try one or two search engines to see which works best for you.
- For other search engines, type in the web address (also called a URL), or click an underlined link (address), like http://www.tekmom.com/buzzwords/zdurl.html, or select a website from the browser toolbar.[1] Some websites will lead you to a host of other useful sites. For example, the following Australian

brain tumor site has many additional helpful URLs: http://www.snog.org.au/brochures.htm.

Why do sites come up in a particular order?

Generally, it takes money and savvy computer engineering to get a particular website to pop up first among a long list of other sites during a search using any of the search engines. Sites that have paid "Ask Jeeves" or other search engines to advertise will come up first. As a case in point, note that "4uherb" and "vinyl-chloride-lawsuits" websites come up on top before virtual trials or The Brain Tumor Society websites. At the bottom of the search, the numbered boxes show the number of pages of sites that you retrieved from this search. Sometimes, useful sites are listed a few pages away from the first page, so it is a good idea to scroll through several pages to get a sense of what is available.

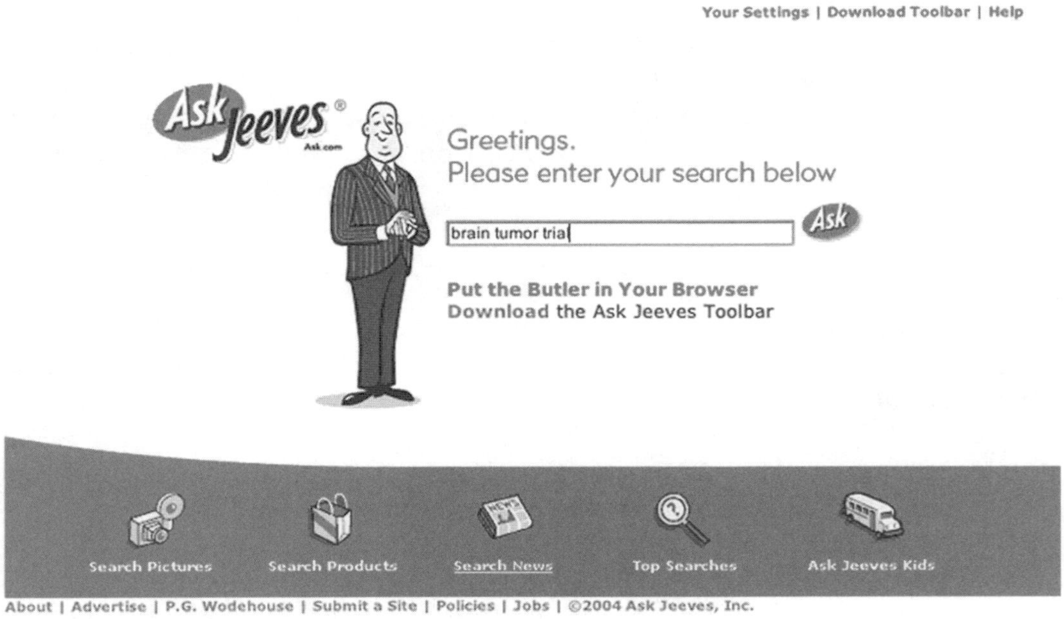

Your Settings | Download Toolbar | Help

Ask Jeeves ®
Ask.com

Greetings.
Please enter your search below

brain tumor trial

Ask

Put the Butler in Your Browser
Download the Ask Jeeves Toolbar

Search Pictures   Search Products   Search News   Top Searches   Ask Jeeves Kids

About | Advertise | P.G. Wodehouse | Submit a Site | Policies | Jobs | ©2004 Ask Jeeves, Inc.

Figure 4-1 The Greetings page on your screen when you connect to ASKJEEVES.

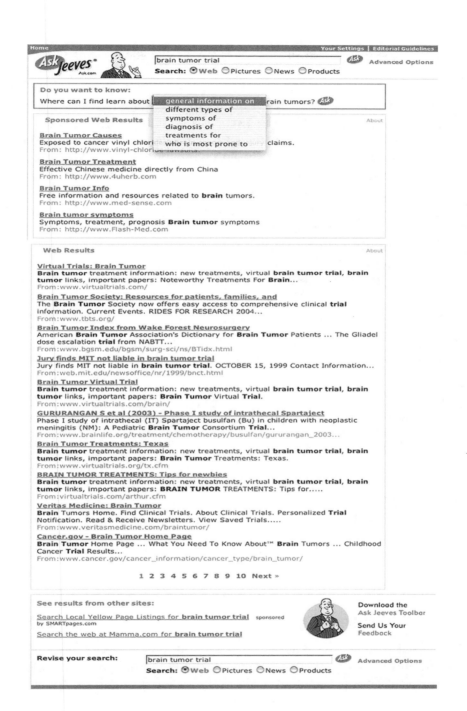

Figure 4-2 The page one of search results from "brain tumor trial" in ASKJEEVES.

Step 4. Fine Tune Your Search

- Use descriptive words or names as you search. *Tumor* will gather too much information. *Brain tumor* or *brain tumor treatments* is more definitive, at least initially. Try specific tumors such as *glioma, oligodendroglioma, astrocytoma,* or other specific conditions such as *hydrocephalus, metastasis,* or *neurofibromatosis* (NF-1, NF1). Watch your spelling when entering key words or phrases.
- If too many sites are found, try adding to your first word *AND mutism* or *AND radiation* or *AND chemotherapy* to the tumor name. To get more specific references, you can combine words like *melanoma* AND *brain metastasis*. This is called "building your search." This trick will make your search yield fewer, but more specific sites.
- AskJeeves does this for you when you click "diagnosis of" or "treatments for"
- Below are sites where you can obtain non-commercial, basic information:

Table 4-3 Helpful Brain Tumor Websites

American Brain Tumor Association (ABTA)	http://www.abta.org
Brain Cancer Links for Self Sufficiency	http://www.cancerlinks.org/brain.html
Brain Tumor Society (BTS)	http://www.tbts.org
Cancer Information Network	http://www.cancerlinksusa.com/brain/
Clinical Trials and Noteworthy Treatments	http://www.virtualtrials.com
MD Anderson Cancer Center	http://www.mdanderson.org/ departments/braintumor/
New Approaches to Brain Tumor Therapy	http://www.nabtt.org
National Brain Tumor Foundation (NBTF)	http://www.braintumor.org
National Cancer Institute	http://www.cancer.gov
WebMD (commercial)	http://www.webmd.com

Step 5. Access the Important Sites

The Basic Method

Now that you've navigated the web and found some sites, you're probably wondering how to use things like <u>hyperlinks</u>, <u>jump sites</u>, <u>web indexes</u> and <u>chat groups</u> that connect with sites that other people may have spoken about. These are the shortcuts to find what you need.

For example, to get to the Brain Tumor Society, type into your browser the complete URL for Brain Tumor Society (www.tbts.org). Then click the "Go" button or press "Enter" on your keyboard. The site's home page will then appear. When a URL is underlined, in bold or another color, you may click on it or type the address into your browser window, but you do not need to underline it.

You must know and type accurately the exact address in order to get there. One letter off or a period or parenthesis at the end of the address, and you will get nothing! Newer browsers compensate for some errors (allowing you to omit "http//" at the beginning of a URL, for example). Some URLs are too complicated for a browser to correct.

Once you are on a site, select the subject of your interest by clicking on the appropriate word, phrase, or icon. The information will then appear on the screen.

Hyperlinks

Hyperlinks are direct connections to a specific site. Usually the words or topic items are in bold and appear different in color. When you click on these bold or colored words, you are taken to another web page. You can click on the hyperlink www.tbts.org site, and it will transport you instantly to dozens of other helpful sites. If you are reading this text online, click on this hyperlink to a meningioma support group: http://health.groups.yahoo.com/group/meningioma.

Jump Sites

Jump sites contain collections of hyperlinked, special-interest sites (akin to pages of information on specific topics). For instance, if you click on the ABC^2 site, you will find a choice of several topics and over 80 sites. Click on one that interests you, and it will "jump" you to another site where the information is located:

Web Index

Web indexes contain more comprehensive and diverse collections of resources. If you're on the web and are not sure where to go, head to the nearest web index:
* While logged on to the web, type http://www.yahoo.com in your browser's URL entry field.
* Press ENTER (the return key) or click GO. This will take you to a popular Web index. (Yahoo! is also a search engine.)
* Underneath the Yahoo! logo, you will see a

A Web Index is the "Yellow Pages" of brain tumor resources.

blank search entry form, as well as hyperlinks (also known as "hotlinks") to site categories.

- Type one or more words for information you'd like to locate on the web: "brain tumor," for example.
- After a few seconds, Yahoo! will give you thousands of "hotlinks" matching your search criteria. The more specific you are, the more selective and relevant the hotlinks will be.
- Click on each link until you reach a site that matches your interests. I typed in "meningioma" and found 10 pages of helpful links.

CHAT ROOMS AND GROUPS: ARE THEY HELPFUL?

Chat rooms allow you to communicate with people in real time, just like talking to a group of people at a party. You enter a "room" and every time you write a message, everyone in the room sees it instantly. Chatting online allows you to meet and speak with other individuals who have interests similar to yours.

A listserv allows you to post messages and exchange written information.

A "listserv" is a site that allows you to *post* a message on a bulletin board and wait for an answer, which can be immediate or days later. If many people participate, there will be a sequential "string" of questions and answers. Each underline is a "hyperlink" to the text of the message. Below is an example of such a string:

Chat groups allow you to meet & speak in real time with others who have similar interests.

Weight gain...anyone know anything about this??? – Jan , Thu Mar 25 03:17

- weight gain – Don, Fri Mar 26 06:04
  - jan/weight gain – marjorie, Thu Mar 25 07:27
  - weight gain – Renee, Thu Mar 25 19:36
    - weight gain – vaj123, Fri Mar 26 04:31
      - weight gain – Robyn, Sat Mar 27 18:38

To Find a Chat Room or Group:

- While logged on to the web, type http://www.yahoo.com in your browser's URL entry field. This will take you to Yahoo! http://www.yahoo.com. Many people also use Google, since it is designed to give results which are prioritized on the basis of popularity.
- Click on the "Groups" hotlink, which is to the right of the "Connect" line.

- Go to "Health and Wellness" or type in your specific tumor and see if there are groups for your tumor type. Below are other examples of "chat rooms" for brain tumor support (Table 4-4).
- In using listservs, many people find that using a non-identifying "signature" is helpful to avoid having to type it each time (Chapter 3, Table 3-6). To do this: If you use Outlook, under <Tools> then <Options> then <Mail Format>, you can set up one or more signatures to include your relevant information. Many folks on the listservs can help you.

> Be careful about how much personal, identifiable information you make known on public sites.

Table 4-4 Chat Room & Listservs & Group Sites on the WEB

American Brain Tumor Association	http://www.abta.org/supportgroups2.htm
Brain Tumor Society	http://www.tbts.org
National Brain Tumor Foundation	http://www.braintumor.org/patient_info/ connecting_and_coping
National Cancer Institute	http://cancer.gov/cancerinfo/support
Virtual Trials chat room	http://virtualtrials.com/chat1.cfm

"I am so grateful for the Internet. The most important thing I have learned from these lists is how to take care of our loved one. Doctors and nurses know their professional stuff, but it's the spouses on the lists who suggest clever ways of dealing with constipation, rash, heat/cold, how to swallow pills, etc. Isn't it amazing... people from all over the world are able to communicate and learn from each other without ever meeting."

Lucille. London, England.

- Explore these chat rooms and use them for support, advice, and coping. Be prepared for the raw stuff in the beginning, though. You will be exposed to many successful outcomes, and some not-so-successful ones. Many people's stories may echo similarities to your situation, but keep your focus. You must be wise and realize that not all the questionable or negative outcomes will happen to you.
- There are two dark sides to the Internet in any chat room:
  - There is always a chance that someone in the room is not telling the truth.
  - Motives for what people say in the rooms may be questionable. It is not uncommon for someone who needs investors to try the chat rooms to drum up business. Never give out your full name, address, or phone number to someone in the chat room.

- If you see something interesting, discuss it on one of the lists. You may learn of new options, better treatments, and clinical trials through these chat rooms. However, just to be sure, you should discuss the advice that you obtain here with your healthcare team.

HOW DO I EVALUATE THE TRUTHFULNESS OF DIFFERENT WEBSITES?

Once you start looking for information and open the door, you will be deluged. This wealth of information is a double-edged sword. Much of it is meant for medical professionals, some is purely subjective, a portion is unreliable, and some is plain dangerous. Furthermore, reading about a therapy that was a "cure" for one person and hazard for another can be confusing. Unfortunately, there is no surefire way to control false or misleading claims on health-related Internet sites, so be cautious about using the Internet to diagnose or treat yourself. The general rule of thumb in using the Internet is to do the following:

- Use common sense.
- Discuss your Internet findings with your doctor before taking action. You might handle this as you would with any health information that you obtain from more traditional sources (newspapers, magazines, television, etc.).

FIVE QUESTIONS TO ASK ABOUT CANCER INFORMATION WEBSITES[2]:

1. **What entity is responsible for the site?** Government agencies (web addresses that end with ".gov"), universities (".edu"), and reputable organizations (".org") usually contain more reliable information.
2. **Is it a commercial (".com") site?** Many commercial sites are hyping a product or are designed to sell you something, although some commercial sites do provide useful information. Try to distinguish between promotion, advertising, and serious content within any commercial site. This can be difficult as an increasing number of legitimate organizations include ads on behalf of their sponsors. Also, remember that many sites have paid to be listed near the top of a search, so that commercial sites will be prominently placed above governmental, educational, or organizational sites. For example, on page two of a Yahoo! search for brain tumors, two "sponsored" (paid) commercial sites appear at the top:

> To evaluate information sites, follow the 5 question rule.

- Alternative for Brain Tumors "Brain tumors are a special case. Specifically, we recommend a judicial use of our Protocol; it does work, almost too well. See how we have gently helped hundreds like you."
- Herbal Solutions for Brain Cancer "Foyo herb applies traditional Chinese medicine to treat benign and malignant brain tumors. Free online consultation offered."
- There has been no independent verification of the effectiveness of these products. Buyers beware!

3. **What are the credentials of the individual(s) posting the information?** Is it posted by someone with medical expertise? Are persons with science or medical expertise consultants or advisors to the site? Are information sources listed? Is the site kept up-to-date?

4. **Does the site feature outlandish claims and testimonials?** If a product or treatment seems too good to be true, it probably is.
5. **Can you contact the site for more information?** Reputable sites provide an e-mail address for a person who is responsible for the site. The response that you receive will provide a clue as to the site's reliability.

TIP-OFFS TO RIP-OFFS

New health frauds pop up all the time, but the promoters use the same old tricks to gain your trust and get your money. According to the Food and Drug Administration, here are some red flags:
- Claims that the product works by a secret formula. (Legitimate scientists share their knowledge so peers can review their data.)
- Advertising for this product can only be found in the back pages of magazines, as newspaper advertisements in the format of news stories, by telemarketing or direct mail, or 30-minute "infomercials" done in talk show format. (Bona fide treatments are reported first in medical journals.)
- Claims that the product is an amazing or miraculous breakthrough. (Real medical breakthroughs are few and far between.)
- Promises of a quick, painless, guaranteed cure. (Unlikely when treating brain tumors)
- Testimonials from satisfied customers. (These "customers" may never have had the disease that the product is supposed to cure; they may have been paid advocates, or they may never even have existed!)

Talking With My Doctor About My Research

Gather your family, friends, and advocates to brainstorm and think critically about the sources and their authenticity. Choose the treatments that you are interested in discussing further with your medical team. Then ask the team what they would advise for your individual case. Together, develop an action plan.

Table 4-5 Medical Decision-Making and the Internet

1. Read about the best possible approaches to your condition on Internet sites and in written resources.

2. Get help from those closest to you in conducting Internet searches. Have friends, family, and advocates help you in this process.

3. Evaluate web pages critically, and question the source. Be on the lookout for exaggerated claims and aggressive advertising.

4. Recognize the difference between commercial/ personal web pages and governmental/ educational centers of excellence.

5. Get your doctor's opinion on the options that sound best to you.

6. Always ask the doctor what she or he would do in your circumstance and how you should take care of yourself.

7. Ask yourself, "Are my prejudices stopping me from making smart decisions?"

We are all biased by our experiences, education, and cultural attitudes – doctors included. Sometimes, those biases are valuable. Other times they can be limiting. Ask questions!

Table 4-6 Internet Resources for Surfing the Web

Type of Resource	Website
Internet definitions	http://www.boutell.com/newfaq/basic.html http://wings.avkids.com/SPIT/glossary.html
"The Brain Tumor Survivor's Guide to the Internet"	www.abta.org or call 847-827-9910
Tech "buzz" words	www.tekmom.com/buzzwords
Dependable search engines	http://www.ask.com http://www.excite.com http://www.google.com http://www.infoseek.com http://www.lycos.com http://www.webcrawler.com
American Brain Tumor Association	www.abta.org
Brain Cancer Links for Self Sufficiency	http://www.cancerlinks.org/brain.html
Brain Tumor Society (TBTS)	http://www.tbts.org
Cancer Information Network	http://www.cancerlinksusa.com/brain/
Clinical Trials and Noteworthy Treatments for Brain Tumors	http://www.virtualtrials.com
MD Anderson Cancer Center	http://www.mdanderson.org
National Brain Tumor Foundation (NBTF)	http://www.braintumor.orgv
National Cancer Institute	http://www.cancer.gov
WebMD (commercial)	http://www.webmd.com
Lists of Groups (30+)	http://virtualtrials.com/lists.cfm

CHAPTER 5

The Team – Doctors and Other Members

Challenge your physicians to respond to the opinions of their colleagues as well as to your own concerns, so that all of the issues are clear to you or someone you can rely on. Only then will you be armed with the resources necessary to make a decision in the absence of consensus.

Neal Levitan, brain tumor survivor. Executive Director, Brain Tumor Society.

DOCTORS AND OTHER TEAM MEMBERS

MULTIDISCIPLINARY TEAM

MY MEDICAL TEAM – WHAT ARE THEIR ROLES?

Partner or caregiver
Primary care physician (family doctor)
Neurosurgeon
Neuroradiologist
Neuropathologist
Radiation Oncologist
Oncologist or Neurooncologist
Neurologist
Social worker or case manager
Pharmacist
Rehabilitation specialist (Physiatrist, Occupational Therapist, Physical
    Therapist, Speech Therapist)
Neuropsychologist, Psychologist, Psychiatrist
Endocrinologist
Ophthalmologist
Dentist
Nurse
Tumor Board

Key search words

- caregiver
- primary
- neurosurgeon
- oncologist
- neurologist
- pharmacist
- psychologist
- ophthalmologist
  (eye doctor)

- care-partner
- doctor
- neuropathologist
- neurooncologist
- endocrinologist
- rehabilitation specialist
- neuropsychologist
- dentist

- medical team
- specialist
- radiation oncologist
- social worker
- case manager
- physiatrist
- psychiatrist
- team evaluation

THE MULTIDISCIPLINARY TEAM

Let us start with an outline of the professional players, in addition to the caregiver, who will have major roles at different points in your care. I will describe their roles and relationship to each other. After diagnosis of a brain tumor, medical care instantly becomes complex:

- Unfamiliar doctors and other professionals;
- Different hospitals and medical centers; and
- Conflicting opinions about how to treat you.

This can be confusing for someone who has been in relatively good health and has seen mainly the internist, pediatrician, or family medicine doctor for all his or her medical needs.

The reality is that no one doctor has all the skills needed to care for a patient with a brain tumor. You need to have faith in and be able to rely on your team. This *team* is a collection of specialists and caregivers in various fields (See Table 5-1) that, when working together, can tend to and address all your needs. You can evaluate your team by the ease of communication that takes place between you and the team members. If the different specialists are not working together or your questions remain unanswered, you should contact one of the major brain tumor centers, which offer a team approach as part of their service.

A partial listing of major brain tumor centers in the United States, Canada, and elsewhere can be found in Chapter 7, Tables 7-7, 7-8 and 7-9, throughout these books and on the Brain Tumor Society and www.virtualtrials.com websites.

Table 5-1 Your Multidisciplinary Brain Tumor Team

1. Partner or Caregiver	10. Pharmacist
2. Primary Care Physician	11. Rehabilitation Specialists: Physiatrist, OT, PT, Speech, others)
3. Neurosurgeon	12. Neuropsychologist, Psychologist, Psychiatrist
4. Neuroradiologist	13. Endocrinologist
5. Neuropathologist	14. Ophthalmologist (eye doctor)
6. Radiation Oncologist	15. Dentist
7. Oncologist or Neurooncologist	16. Nurses
8. Neurologist	17. Tumor Board
9. Social Worker and Case Manager	

MY MEDICAL TEAM – WHAT ARE THEIR ROLES?

1. PARTNER OR CAREGIVER

Some of you might wonder why I place caregiver ahead of medical personnel. What is a caregiver anyway? How or when does he or she contribute to your care?

Having practiced oncology for more than 25 years, I have concluded that the caregiver is the most important, yet unrecognized member of the team. Despite seeing 10-20 patients a day, it took me a long time to appreciate the caregivers' role in the success, or sometimes failure, of my efforts. I did not acknowledge them enough and other physicians might not as well. Little seems to work well without your special someone there. You can always find more doctors, nurses and specialists, but a caregiver is not so easy to find.[1]

> "The caregiver is the most important, yet unrecognized member of the team."

Table 5-2 Caregiver: Primary Roles & Responsibilities

1. Calls the doctor on your behalf, if you cannot do so.
2. Helps decide if a visit to the emergency room or doctor is needed.
3. Drives and accompanies you to rehabilitation and doctors' offices.
4. Reviews notes and records from doctor visits.
5. Keeps materials organized in your notebook. (see Chapter 3.)
6. Comforts you when you feel lousy, with talk, medications, or a hot bath.
7. Knows about and helps you with intimate details of your life like constipation, nausea, and so forth.
8. Pays the bills and balances the checkbook, if you cannot do it.
9. Screens phone calls for you when you do not wish to talk.
10. Contacts the extended family and friends with progress reports.
11. Performs Internet or library searches for new approaches to treatment.
12. Troubleshoots when the doctors are not communicating with you.
13. And a whole lot more…

The caregiver can be one or more important persons: a spouse, significant other, parent, child, or friend who can be with you, especially at crucial moments. The following two vignettes illustrate how different life can be with and without caregivers:

Melanie is a successful 45-year-old, single businesswoman who fought breast cancer for many years, when she developed a metastasis to the brain. She always came by herself to see me and seemed to carry all the responsibility for her illness; there appeared to be no one to ask for help or discuss what went on in our conversations. She understood and remembered possibly half of what we discussed. I would ask about family or friends to discuss some difficult choices. She said, "I don't want to burden anyone with my problems. Besides I really don't have anyone."

Bob was a 60-ish biker who looked like a shiny-headed "Mr. Clean" and lived in the desert part of Southern California. I learned a lot from Bob. He was back on his Harley-Davidson going to breakfast with his buddies at the local hangout in Lancaster 60 hours after having his glioblastoma tumor removed! Bob was always on time for his visits, accompanied by either two daughters, friends and/or his girlfriend and former wife (two different people!). He was highly functional until the last week of a two-plus year battle. One or more significant people in his life stayed at home with him every night of his last five months of life, just in case he would need them. They volunteered lots of information about how he was pursuing his life, tolerating or experiencing side-effects with medication changes. They asked pertinent questions…but only when his memory would slip. There was humor and serious talk. He was surrounded by people who cared for him, loved him, and fought for him every step of the way.

My secretary, Michele, offered some of her concise, no nonsense wisdom, after observing how many of my other patients and their caregivers followed different pathways over time. "You die like you live," she said. "You act like a decent human being most of the time, and good things come back to you." "Act like an S.O.B., and who wants to be with you?"

Bottom line: Appreciate the caregivers in your life who help you through this difficult journey. As trying and emotionally intense as the process of dealing with cancer can be, it can also be an uplifting and gratifying experience:

> *My job as a caregiver has been the greatest job and the finest privilege I have experienced. We need to recognize more clearly that in dealing with health, the 'caregiver' has a crucial role. Doctors and nurses are in no way positioned to understand a patient wholly, and we must never expect that of them. We would improve the effectiveness of the health system enormously if 'caring'*

Bottom line: You need to appreciate the caregivers in your life who help you through this difficult journey.

91

became a natural part of education…and …a general acceptance of personal responsibility for health.

Daniel, Melbourne Australia.
in an e-mail about his wife who had a brain tumor

You can sustain significant stress in caring for someone who not only has cancer, but also exhibits personality changes and memory loss. Dr. E. Farace, of the University of Virginia, gave caregivers 10 weekly sessions of counseling using a short manual on how to combat stress. She found that this instruction benefited quality of life and reduced stress not only for the caregiver, but for the person with the brain tumor, too![2] Perhaps this manual and other helpful books would help your caregiver.[3,4] More information for caregivers is available at the caregiver support site at www.webmd.com. (See Table 5-28.).

Being a caregiver is both rewarding and stressful. There are resources for helping caregivers.

Stress, however, is a normal part of the caregiver's experience, as illustrated in the e-mail below:

"Jill… You are SO allowed to moan whenever you need to. This is the hardest thing I (and I'm sure most of us) have ever gone through. Although I know we as the caregivers can never understand what our loved one is going through with their brain tumor, our loved ones can't possibly understand what we go through. It is so hard to watch them go through the treatments and wait in anticipation for the results of any tests. Through it all we are expected to be the strong one. Our friends and family can try to help, but these [on-line] people truly understand what you are going through."

Helen, Macon GA.

I saw the following quote a while ago and think it belongs here: "Never miss an opportunity to say 'I love you'." You don't need a grave illness to tell the people who you love how important they are to you and what pleasure they have given you. Waiting for the end of life to say these things diminishes the value of the words that we all want to hear.

2. PRIMARY CARE PHYSICIAN (FAMILY DOCTOR)

Your *primary care physician* is usually the person who you first consulted when symptoms began and he or she started you on the road to the diagnosis of a brain or spinal cord tumor. Most primary care doctors only see two to five patients with brain tumors in their lifetime of practice; this is a rare event for them. However, if you have a good relationship with your primary care doctor, he or she may become a critical link in your care. Why? With so many specialists seeing just a small part of who you are, the "whole you" can get lost. Your primary care doctor will orchestrate the coordination of all members of your team and can explain what the different opinions and options mean for you.

> You don't need illness to tell people how important they are to you.

Your primary physician can often see the big picture:

> *"We have been fortunate to have a wonderful general practitioner who has been the central core to our entire brain tumor journey. Some areas of the United States are not fortunate enough to have the money or location to make a brain tumor center be accessible, but sometimes it's the local doctor that makes all the difference in the world. I don't think that we are second guessing a specialist's prescription by talking to him or simply making a decision a day later. We are giving ourselves a moment to listen to ourselves and weigh the differences. We all need to step back from this terrible situation we're in and look 'in' instead of 'out.' "*

Jeanne, spouse to Richard, Idaho Falls, ID

Table 5-3 Primary Doctor: Roles & Responsibilities

1. Translates to you what other doctors may not have effectively communicated.
2. Advocates for more or less aggressive therapy, depending upon your wishes.
3. Cares for medical problems that the specialists do not recognize or treat.
4. Manages urgent problems that are not clearly the responsibility of specialists.
5. Treats side effects of medications and other therapies.
6. Recommends specific consultants for second or third opinions, if necessary.

These are important and major roles. In many HMOs, you must obtain the initial referral from your primary doctor, or the specialist's fees will not be covered under your plan. (See Chapter 23, Managing Costs, Benefits and Insurance Companies.)

You have an obligation and responsibility to give clear direction to your primary physician with regard to how you want him or her to function. It is true that some generalists are intimidated by specialists or step out of the picture when a serious, life- threatening illness presents itself. Notwithstanding, I have been impressed

> Your primary care doctor- a critical link so the "whole you" does not get lost.

with how many primary doctors enjoy and accept this crucial role, which directly benefits the patient.

3. NEUROSURGEON

The *neurosurgeon* is usually the first treatment doctor you'll meet after your diagnosis. Often you will meet with the neurosurgeon in the emergency room or at an urgent referral visit, once the scan shows a tumor. It's totally normal to be concerned and frightened at the prospect of your neurosurgeon opening up your head, handling your brain, and traversing part of it to get to the tumor. This should generate a lot of questions, but these are often forgotten in a tense, urgent setting.

Table 5-4 The Neurosurgeon: Roles & Responsibilities

1. Assesses the need, benefits, alternatives, and risks of surgery.
2. Recommends the type of surgery (closed, open) for diagnostic and treatment purposes.
3. Organizes the surgical team, if other specialists are needed, like a head and neck surgeon or endovascular surgeon for embolizing tumors before surgery.
4. Advises you on chances of recovery from any problems caused by the tumor or surgery.
5. Proposes surgery-related therapies that may help fight the tumor, including: Radiosurgery, Gliadel chemotherapy wafer implants during surgery, GliaSite implant of radioactive therapy, Reservoirs for later treatments.
6. Safely performs the surgery to biopsy or remove the tumor.
7. Manages your after-surgery care so the next specialist can proceed safely with therapy.
8. Ensures that your incisions have healed and are free of infection.
9. Prescribes medications to reduce or treat complications from the surgery or tumor by prescribing replacement hormones.
10. Monitors your response to steroids and adjusts the dosage to the lowest possible amount.
11. Works with your other doctors to ensure that the diagnosis is correct, assessing your response to treatments, and referring you to other specialists, as needed.
12. Your neurosurgeon may take a less active role after your incision has healed and you have recovered from the effects of surgery. He will be available as questions arise, second surgery, etc.

How Do I Choose My Neurosurgeon?

The best answer: carefully. There are many areas of specialization within neuro-surgery, including brain and spinal cord tumors, vascular (aneurysms, stroke treatment, and prevention), pain, spinal disc disease and pediatric neurosurgery, to name a few. Many, if not most, neurosurgeons are essentially generalists. Each operates on fewer than five tumor patients a year in a practice mostly devoted to repairing spinal disc problems, nerve injuries, and the like. This experience directly affects you. A general neurosurgeon might not be as aggressive or knowledgeable about new techniques in brain tumor removal compared with an expert who removes 5 to 10 tumors each week.[5]

We know that the more tumor that is safely removed, the longer the patient will live.[6] Two recent studies indicate that high volume centers (those that conduct more than 50 brain tumor surgeries per year) have better survival rates and fewer complications.[7,8] The mortality rate was 2 per cent at high-volume centers and 5 per cent at low-volume hospitals. The average length of stay in high-volume centers was seven versus nine days in low-volume hospitals. My colleague, Professor Leland Albright at the University of Pittsburgh, and I reported on an analysis of neurosurgical specialization and the amount of tumor removal in children. We found that pediatric neurosurgeons, compared with general neurosurgeons, removed more tumor tissue in children without sacrificing safety.[9] Making a choice to see a specialist in brain tumors allows you to benefit from these latest approaches.

Fewer than 100 Neuro-surgeons in the US specialize in brain tumors.

A checklist has been provided for you to use when you visit each specialist. (See Table 5-5.)

Table 5-5 What to Ask the Neurosurgeon Before Surgery

1. Can the MRI findings be due to any other causes?
2. Is it a primary brain tumor or metastasis?
3. Where exactly is my brain tumor? How far does it extend?
4. Does its location explain my symptoms?
5. Which of my functions are at risk when you operate in this area?
6. Are there any special pre-operative tests that will help minimize these risks? (Functional MRI)
7. What could be done to reduce my risk and improve my outcome? (Intra-operative MRI, image guidance systems, awake brain mapping, etc.)
8. Is this surgery only a biopsy, or is it an aggressive tumor removal?

9. What will be my quality of life after surgery?

10. How many tumors in this specific area of the brain do you treat yearly?

11. Are any of your patients on clinical trials? How many and which trials?

12. What is your operative mortality rate? (How many patients die within one month of surgery?) It should be at or less than one per cent for brain tumor surgeries.

13. Is there another surgeon who has more experience with my kind of tumor that you would recommend? Should he or she assist you on my case?

14. How long will I be in the hospital?

15. Will I receive a post-operative MRI brain scan within three days after surgery? (Most experienced surgeons perform these MRI scans to check their work.)

The responses and completeness of your neurosurgeon's answers to these questions should make you comfortable enough to entrust your life to this person.

Table 5-6 What to Ask the Neurosurgeon After Surgery

1. Any of the questions in Table 5-5 that were not asked or answered.

2. How much tumor was removed? How much remains? What did the post-op MRI show?

3. What specific problems can I expect from the tumor and the surgery?

4. What did you see during the operation that was not evident on the MRI or CT scan?

5. What is the name and grade of the tumor?

6. Are there other special tests that should be done on the tumor specimen (electron microscopy, 1p/19q , gene array testing?

7. Should the tumor be sent for a second pathology opinion? (See Chapter 8: Diagnosis.)

8. Which other team members will you or my family doctor recommend that I see?

9. Can I have a copy of the surgery report, pathology report, and MRI scan reports?

What If My Tumor Cannot Be Completely Resected (Removed)?

If tumor remains after the surgery, then you should consider getting a second opinion with another neurosurgeon at a different center to see if more tumor could be removed safely. Once you have copies of the pre- and post-operative MRI scans, you can send them to other centers. That way, you can receive a preliminary opinion on whether it would be useful to seek consultation or consent to additional surgery.

What Do I Say to My Doctor If He or She Discourages Me From Obtaining Another Consultation for My Brain Tumor?

Two top neurosurgeons, whom I respect, commented here. Both said that your neurosurgeon, even if he or she is a recognized specialist in brain tumor surgery, should support your request to obtain a second opinion and should be willing to recommend another neurosurgeon that he or she trusts to offer another opinion.

> A less than complete tumor removal is a good reason for getting a second opinion.

Let your doctor know that you appreciate his or her care, but that you need the peace of mind that would come from getting another viewpoint before proceeding. If the clinician makes you feel guilty or threatens to refuse to take you back as a patient, then this was not a good match for you in the first place. You should move on to someone you can trust and who supports your right to make decisions about your own care.

I dwell on this point since the length of survival can be intimately linked with the amount of tumor remaining after surgery. Second opinions are discussed in Chapter 6: Experts and Second opinions.

4. NEURORADIOLOGIST

This physician is a specialist in all imaging procedures of the nervous system. This includes interpreting CT, MRI, MR-Spect, PET, and sometimes Thallium-Spect scans. It's unlikely that you'll meet or talk directly with this doctor, although he or she will send a report to your physicians. Brain tumors, surgery, radiation, and chemotherapy can all produce unusual findings on brain scans compared with other parts of the body. Thus, what appears to be tumor to a general radiologist can be read as *necrosis* (dead tissue) by a neuroradiologist. This is another reason why your scans should be reviewed by a neuroradiology specialist. I have translated (IN CAPS) some of the terms that you may find in your reports, as in the one below.

> Your Neurosurgeon should support your decision to get a second opinion.

Magnetic Resonance Imaging: Brain with/without contrast (DYE) and stealth protocol *(PRE SURGICAL or Radiosurgery LOCALIZATION)*

Indication: Glioblastoma Multiforme. This study is performed after radiotherapy.

Procedure: T1 (<u>TYPE OF ENERGY RELEASE AFFECTING DETECTION OF WATER</u>) weighted sagittal (<u>SIDE VIEW</u>) spin echo imaging was used for the localizer sequence (<u>CUTS ON FIRST PICTURE SHOWING ANGLE-LOCATION OF SCAN ON HEAD</u>). This was followed by high resolution axial Flair (<u>DESIGNED TO BRING OUT FEATURES OF TUMOR AND NORMAL BRAIN</u>) and fast spin echo T2 weighted (<u>TYPE OF SLOW ENERGY RELEASE</u>) sequences. Conventional T1 weighted spin echo imaging was performed before and after intravenous contrast (<u>DYE TO DETECT BLOOD-BRAIN BARRIER DISRUPTION</u>) administration.

Findings: There has been progression of the patient's right parietal tumor since the postoperative MRI of 8/29/02. The antero-posterior (<u>FRONT TO BACK</u>) dimension has increased from approximately 3 to 4 cm. The width has increased from 2 to approximately 2.8 cm. The rostral caudal (<u>LOWER BACK SIDE</u>) dimension is increased from approximately 2.6 to 3.8 cm. Of more significant note is thick rim enhancement (<u>BRIGHT AREA OF DYE</u>) representing progression from the thin postoperative rim enhancement of the 8/29/02 exam. In addition, there is thick enhancement along the surgical tract to the right parietal calvarium (<u>PART OF SKULL</u>). The T1 unenhanced images do not show abnormal signal to indicate subacute (OLDER) hemorrhage. There is evidence for hemosiderin (<u>OLD BLOOD PRODUCT</u>) deposition on T2 images. The medial (<u>TOWARD CENTER</u>) margin of the mass abuts the falx (<u>MEMBRANE SEPARATING LEFT OR RIGHT SIDE</u>). I do not see contra-lateral (OTHER SIDE) hemispheric enhancement. The ventricles remain normal in size. The basilar cisterns (<u>PLACES WHERE CEREBROSPINAL FLUID FLOWS</u>) are patent (<u>OPEN</u>)). There is vasogenic edema (<u>SWELLING</u>) and gliosis surrounding the tumor. These findings have moderately increased, however, there is no midline shift today.

Impression: 1. There has been significant progression of right parietal tumor since the postoperative MRI of 8/29/02 discussed above; 2. Thin section post contrast images obtained via the stealth protocol for radiotherapy.

Staging and Neuroradiology

After correct diagnosis, the next important part of the initial cancer evaluation is staging. This is the summation of all tests that determine the extent or spread of cancer – where it is and where it isn't. Surgical findings and scans (CT, MRI, and sometimes PET) are major components in this process.

When we conducted our international study of *medulloblastoma*,[10] we found that some general radiologists had made incorrect interpretations of scans, noting tumor spread in the spine. This error often occurred in the reading of scans taken in the first few weeks after surgery. Most neuroradiologists know that blood from surgery can look like tumor on MRI and CT spine scans. Thus, to the less trained eye, blood can be mistaken for tumor! This is another reason to ask questions and seek the opinion of a neuroradiologist.

Table 5-7 What to Ask the Doctor Receiving the MRI Scan Report

1. Were both unenhanced and contrast-enhanced (CT and MRI) scans performed? If not, why not? Some tumors are more obvious after contrast. Ask this question to the neurosurgeon, neurologist or oncologist.
2. Are your conclusions and findings unequivocal? Could they be due to other causes?
3. Were my previous scans available for comparison?
4. Did the (neuro) radiologist know whether or not I was on steroids? Steroids can reduce the contrast-enhancement of a tumor.
5. Were the scan results reviewed by a neuroradiologist, and did he or she agree?
6. If the questions above are not clearly answered, then a second opinion is warranted.

5. NEUROPATHOLOGIST

Chances are, you will never meet the *neuropathologist* who analyzed the tissue that your neurosurgeon removed under the microscope. Without his or her opinion, no treatment is possible. You should obtain a copy of the signed pathology report, naming the type and grade of your tumor, and put it in your notebook. (See Chapter 3: Getting Organized, and Chapter 8: Traditional Approaches to Diagnosis.)

> Staging: the summation of surgical findings and scans.

You, your primary doctor, and specialist should read the pathology report, which should be clearly marked that it came from a neuropathologist. If there is any doubt about the diagnosis, then your actual tumor slides should be sent to an expert for a second opinion. This is especially true if the original report was signed by a general pathologist, not a specialist in neuropathology. The following three questions need to be addressed and resolved as soon as the diagnosis is made:

1. Is the diagnosis unequivocal? Could it be something else?
2. Was it on a small biopsy or a large piece of tumor? (If it was a small sample, then the important portion of the tumor may have been missed.)
3. Was it reviewed by a neuropathologist, and did he or she agree?

If the questions above are not clearly answered, then a second opinion is warranted.

6. RADIATION ONCOLOGIST

After biopsy, tumor removal, or recurrence of tumor, you may be referred for radiation therapy.

Table 5-8 Radiation Oncologist: Roles & Responsibilities

1. Assesses the need for radiation, its expected benefits and risks.
2. Recommends the type of radiation, dose, and administration protocol.
3. Administers radiation to the tumor, accurately and safely.
4. Recommends newer types of radiation therapy to fight the tumor, like radiosurgery or radioactive Gliasite® implantation.
5. Advises you on recovery from problems that may be caused by the radiation.
6. Manages complications attributable to radiation.
7. Monitors your post-radiation skin condition (redness or burn); treats skin infection.
8. Prescribes medications to reduce or treat complications stemming from radiation.
9. Monitors your response to radiation, administering steroids like (dexamethasone) and adjusting the dosage to taper you off quickly and safely.
10. Works with your other doctors to ensure that the diagnosis is correct and assesses your response to treatment.

Often the *radiation oncologist* will not be an active participant once you have completed the course of radiation therapy and are free of short-term after-effects. Some radiation oncologists, however, continue to follow their patients for many years.

Newer radiation techniques are intended to minimize the serious side effects, especially to the normal brain. Research in the past few years has brought to light the types of problems that affect the long-term survivors. Unlike chemotherapy, where the side effects of low blood counts or infections usually are temporary, brain irradiation can cause permanent and major problems to what is known in the computer world as your "central processing unit".

Two to three months after radiation treatment, memory and attention problems may continue to worsen. Although these functions can recover, it can take up to two years to fully recover from the short-term effects – and then long-term effects may arise two to 10 years after radiation.[11] It's important to ask questions before beginning therapy, so you can understand the possible tradeoffs in quality of life that you may face in exchange for prolonging life through radiation therapy.[12,13]

> There are many types and forms of radiation: traditional, radiosurgery, implants, infusions.

Marie speaks of the effects of tumor and radiation on her husband's short-term memory and judgment in an e-mail to another spouse:

"Michael had a lot of these problems and also was very intelligent. The doctor told us these problems stemmed from a "host" of things such as the tumor itself, irradiation, and medication. Michael never fully regained his remarkable intelligence, and this caused him so much pain, as he was quite aware he had deficits. I used to "test" him, until finally he was aggravated by the "tests" and asked me to stop, as all it did was remind him of, as he put it, "how stupid he is." This disease can be really ugly and cruel. Even with all we had been through I still find that I truly hate this inanimate disease for what it robbed "us" of and most importantly, what it robbed him of."

Marie, wife of Michael. Indianapolis, IN

Table 5-9 What to Ask Your Radiation Oncologist Before Treatment

1. Where is my brain tumor? What functions could it affect?
2. What is the name and grade of my tumor?
3. Which of my functions are at risk when you irradiate this area?
4. What are the short-term effects? How soon will I get over them?
5. What are the long-term effects? Will these be permanent or will I recover? If so, in what time?
6. How much irradiation will my frontal lobes receive? What will be the effect of this?
7. How likely am I to lose memory function?
8. What kind of quality of life will I have after radiation? Will I be able to dress myself?

9. What activities of daily living might I be unable to do, if I live six to 12 months: Going to the toilet? Making a cup of coffee? Answering the phone? Getting out of bed?

10. How many tumors of the brain do you treat each year? Twenty-five or more?

11. Are any of your patients enrolled in clinical trials? How many?

12. Am I eligible for a clinical trial?

13. Is there another radiation oncologist who has more experience with cases like mine that you would recommend?

14. Which other team members do you recommend that I see after radiation treatment?

15. Which medical needs, problems, or medication adjustments will you be in charge of?

16. Will you communicate with my primary doctor or oncologist to define your area of treatment responsibility (such as fever, constipation, mental changes, or headache)?

17. Can I have a copy of the radiation consultation, MRI planning pictures and MRI scan reports for my notebook, after radiation has been completed?

7. ONCOLOGIST OR NEUROONCOLOGIST?

After biopsy, tumor removal, or recurrence of tumor, you may be referred to either a (neuro) oncologist or oncologist specialist. The referral will depend upon how your physician's office or center works and who is employed there. For example, if your center offers a treatment that involves a form of combined chemotherapy and radiation therapy, you may be asked to consult a radiation oncologist and (neuro) oncologist. Patients with brain tumors who receive any type of chemotherapy or immunotherapy should be cared for by an oncologist or neurooncologist.

What is the difference in the training of these specialists, and how does it affect me? An oncologist has received both internal medicine and oncology training for two to three more years and treats all types of cancer. A neurooncologist can have basic training as an oncologist, neurologist, or neurosurgeon with an additional year or two of training specifically in Neurooncology. Both types of specialists are familiar with administering chemotherapy. Those with a cancer (oncology) background usually will be more familiar with intensive and aggressive forms of chemotherapy because they have specialized in this area. Those with a neurology background will be more familiar with diagnosis and therapy for seizures. For these reasons, you may want to get a second opinion and recommendations from a neurooncologist that your home team can implement. This way you can have the best of both worlds.

Before starting chemotherapy, it's important to ask questions about things such as possible side effects and the expected benefit from chemotherapy. As with radiation therapy, it is important that you understand that *sometimes* the tradeoff for longer life is a significant reduction in quality of life.

> Patients receiving any chemotherapy or immunotherapy should be cared for by an oncologist or neurooncologist.

Table 5-10 The Neurooncologist or Oncologist: Roles & Responsibilities

1. Works with your other doctors to ensure that the diagnosis is correct.
2. Assesses the need for and administers chemotherapy, immunotherapy, and blood support (transfusions, growth factors; discusses expected benefits, side effects, and treatment of side effects).
3. Advises you on chances of recovery from any problems caused by therapy.
4. Recommends drugs, their dose, and the length of time to administer them.
5. Suggests newer types of chemotherapy (such as Gliadel for gliomas, high dose methotrexate for germinomas, or Rituximab for lymphomas).
6. Monitors your response to therapy with blood tests and follow-up scans.
7. Advises on need for blood product support and bone marrow stimulating hormones.
8. Administers steroids and adjusts the dosage to alleviate symptoms of brain swelling.
9. Follows your condition with your primary doctor after other specialists have completed their service.
10. Evaluates the need for aggressive treatment of distressing symptoms such as pain, fatigue, constipation, or infection.
11. Discusses and enrolls you in clinical trials for newly-diagnosed or recurrent tumors.
12. Works as a key member of your team to provide you with comprehensive care:
    - Assesses caregiver needs, stressors, and resources.
    - Identifies the need for physical therapy, occupational therapy, or speech therapy.
    - Discusses end of life care preferences, hospice alternatives, and so on, should this become necessary.

The following questions might make you may feel uncomfortable. Ask yourself, "do the questions or the possible answers make me feel uneasy?" Don't be afraid to ask these questions, and they will indirectly make you feel stronger. They are designed to bolster your confidence in your treating physician. No more, no less.

Table 5-11 What to Ask Your Neurooncologist or Oncologist Before Treatment Begins

1. Where is my brain tumor? What functions could it affect?
2. What is the name and grade of the tumor?
3. Are any functions at risk due to side effects of chemo- or experimental therapy?
4. What is the latest recommended treatment for my type of tumor? How recently has this therapy been made available?
5. Which activities of daily living will likely be affected by therapy?
6. What will I be unable to do: Take a bath? Dress myself? Go to the toilet? Make a cup of coffee? Answer the phone? Get out of bed? Be sure to list functions of importance to you.
7. What are specific side effects of the therapy that you recommend? Do you have written handouts describing these?
8. How many people with brain tumors do you treat each year? More than 25?
9. Are any of your patients enrolled in clinical trials? How many?
10. Am I eligible for a clinical trial with you or elsewhere? Which one(s)?
11. Is there another (neuro) oncologist that you would recommend who has more experience with cases like mine?
12. Which other team members do you recommend that I see now or after therapy?
13. Will you be taking care of my medical needs, problems, and medication adjustments, or will my primary doctor or neurologist do this?
14. Will you communicate with my primary doctor to delineate which problems (such as fever, constipation, or headache) are in your domain of responsibility?
15. May I have a copy of your consultation and scan reports for my notebook?

8. NEUROLOGIST

The *neurologist* specializes in diagnosis and treatment of diseases involving the nervous system. These can include stroke, headaches, Alzheimer's, multiple sclerosis, hereditary diseases (such as neurofibromatosis or tuberous sclerosis), and seizures. Most neurologists, however, have little background in treatment of nervous system tumors, except those who take additional training.

Patients may want to have a neurologist on their team. Why? It can be difficult to diagnose and treat seizures in the presence of a tumor. Often one or more drugs are needed to control seizures, and these can affect chemotherapy levels in the blood and vice versa. Sorting out live from dead tumor after therapy can also be difficult. Most neurologists work closely with neurosurgeons, oncologists and radiation oncologists to deliver excellent care.

Table 5-12 The Neurologist: Roles & Responsibilities

1. Works with your other doctors to ensure that the diagnosis is correct.
2. Assesses the need for anti-seizure drugs; explains expected benefits, side effects.
3. Administers medications and understands their interactions with chemotherapy.
4. Recommends drugs, their dosage, length of time over which to administer them.
5. Monitors your blood levels to assess effectiveness, toxicity, and seizure frequency.
6. Advises you on the chances of recovery from any problems caused by therapy.
7. Manages complications attributable to therapy (for example, gum growth, sleepiness).
8. Monitors your response to the therapy with blood tests and follow up scans.
9. Administers steroids, like dexamethasone, and adjusts the dosage to alleviate symptoms of brain swelling.
10. Assesses and treats distressing symptoms, such as headache or mental changes.

Answers to the questions below will help you assess the neurologist's participation in your care. The reason for repetition and overlap of questions among the different specialists is that one doctor might explain the process better than another or have a different opinion.

Table 5-13 What to Ask Your Neurologist Before Treatment Begins

1. What is the name and grade of the tumor?
2. Where is my brain tumor? Which of my neurological functions are affected?
3. How will I recognize a seizure? What should I do about them immediately?
4. Are any of my functions at risk due to anti-seizure or other prescription medications?
5. Are there specific side effects of the recommended therapy? Can I have written handouts describing these?
6. Which activities of daily living will be affected by therapy?
7. What will I be unable to do: Take a bath? Dress myself? Go to the toilet? Make a cup of coffee? Answer the phone? Get out of bed?
8. How many tumors of this type do you treat each year? More than 25?
9. For which of my specific medical needs, follow-up, or medication adjustments will you be responsible? Who will monitor the scans?
10. Will you communicate with my primary doctor to define which problems (fever, constipation, headache, and so forth) are in your domain of responsibility?

11. Are any of your patients on clinical trials? How many?

12. Am I eligible for a clinical trial here or elsewhere? Which one(s)?

13. Is there another neurologist that you would recommend who has more experience with cases like mine?

14. Which other team members do you recommend that I see now? After therapy?

15. Can I have a copy of the neurology notes and MRI scan reports for my notebook?

What Type of Problems Can a Neurologist Solve?

James has recently developed very odd behavior on Temodar. He is incredibly hyper and does things almost obsessively. He has confusion and short-term memory loss. He also has severe balance problems (presented recently) and is a real danger to himself as he keeps buzzing around trying to do things and falling over. Last night, he kept trying to get out of bed and fell over three times. Now he is asleep, but only after a sleeping pill.

James has had progression of his disease on several occasions over the two years since he recurred. He was never symptomatic until very recently. This change in mental health has been very rapid and his medical team is trying to rule out any possibilities of side effects from current medications. He is being weaned off Amitriptyline, Oramorph, hyoscine patch, and Zofran™. Could these symptoms be due to drugs, recurrent tumor, overly rapid tapering of decadron infection?

May, mom to James, Pocatello, ID

All are possible. A neurologist working with the other doctors would be helpful in sorting out the answers to May's questions.

9. SOCIAL WORKER AND CASE MANAGER

Whereas most treatments will be directed by people who do things *to* you, your *social worker* will do things *for* you. What does this mean? Every professional knows that your experience of having a brain tumor can be overwhelming and incapacitating, both in and out of the hospital. How do you continue from where you were before the diagnosis or start putting your life back together? This is the person to whom you should turn – a source of information, support, advocacy. The social worker usually has a master's degree in social work (M.S.W.), is hired by the hospital to assist you, and does not charge for his or her services.

Always ask to see a social worker during hospitalization. Initially he or she will perform a "needs and resource assessment." This means the social worker focuses on how you (and your family) are functioning psychologically, socially, and in the hospital setting. The social worker also takes into account the financial impact of your medical diagnosis. Out of this assessment, he or she can identify needs, provide information, and suggest referrals.

A *case manager* is a person assigned by your health insurance program to provide assistance when a complicated case needs a lot of coordination between agencies or specialists. If you need particular services after discharge, the person who normally handles this is the case manager (usually a registered nurse assigned to each area in the hospital) or a representative from the needed service (such as a liaison for a home health or equipment company).

> Your social worker will do things for you. Always ask to see him/her when in hospital.

The case manager's job is also to keep the insurance people updated as to your progress during hospitalization and expected length of stay. The social worker and case manager work together and are generally well-informed about government insurance program coverage, like Medicare and Medicaid, and viatical settlements, and can explain these to you.[15]

> Case manager- goes to bat for you; cuts down on red tape; interfaces with insurance company on your behalf.

A viatical settlement offers a terminally ill person a percentage of their life insurance policy's face value in cash. In consideration for delivering a cash payment to the policyholder and paying the premiums, the viatical settlement company collects the face value of the policy if the policyholder dies.

Make sure you know the social worker who is responsible for your care both in and out of the hospital. Put this contact information in your notebook (Chapter 3).

Table 5-14 The Social Worker: Roles & Responsibilities

1. Develops a comprehensive psycho-social assessment of you and your family unit.
2. Provides psychological support to you and the extended family.
3. Reviews insurance information and policies, and ensures that you are receiving your benefits.
4. Advises you, along with the case manager, on which services are covered under your plan.
5. Informs you of local, state, federal financial programs & services for which you are eligible.

6. Links you with appropriate support groups for your type of tumor.

7. Helps clarify and prioritize needs and assists with problem-solving.

8. Provides referrals to community resources and identifies services specific to your needs.

9. Provides contacts for local and nationwide transportation services to transport you to your treatment centers.

10. Helps you identify a "point person" to handle communication among doctors and family.

11. Talks with all members of your treatment team, on your behalf, to assess how much of the current and overall plan you understand, so you are not lost or confused in the process.

Table 5-15 What to Ask Your Social Worker and Case Manager

1. What will *not* be covered by my policy? For what will I be financially responsible?

2. Can you provide assistance in talking with my family about coping with this illness?

3. Can you provide practical guidelines to me for coping with anxiety or depression?

4. Can you help with referrals for inpatient and outpatient rehabilitation services?

5. How will you help in coordinating hospital discharge-planning for home care? (This involves all doctors and nurses who are caring for you.) Preparations for home equipment, visiting nurses, extra home help. Financial assistance programs, such as types of disability, and waiting periods. Other services you might need

6. Can you help in deciding who the family "point person" will be to handle questions?

7. Do you offer help in reviewing the need for a living will, advance directives, or a viatical insurance settlement?

8. Which resources for financial aid, transportation, and support are available at the treatment center in my city, in the state or nationwide?

How useful is a case manager?

The following are comments from people who accepted case manager assistance or were requested to use it by their HMO or insurance company:

- "It is nice to know that you have someone on the inside. This person is ready to go to bat for you and get the things that you or your child need from the company."

- "One person handles your case when you have questions. It really cuts down on red tape and telephone tag... not to mention not having to repeat yourself 100 times... made getting things he needed much easier and also more personal."

- "One insurance employee is up to date on your condition and can provide you, the nurses, and doctors with a number and a person to call to expedite approval for care. Should cut through the red tape or at least reduce it a bit."
- "My insurance has asked me if I would like to have my daughter Marcia put in their case management program. Three items I asked before getting involved:
  - Can you back out if it turns out not to work for you?
  - Can you switch to another case manager if there is a personality conflict with the assigned manager?
  - Can you get a copy of the policy explaining how this will change your situation? In other words, what benefit is there to you for choosing this program?

An example of how a case manager can accomplish a difficult task and overcome bureaucratic hurdles follows:

Our oncologist gave us a prescription for a motorized hospital bed and bedside table. The insurance company initially refused but having a case manager made a world of difference for Michael! We got the bed within three days after she got into action! The head of his bed is elevated at about 30 degrees (relieves pressure in his head... no headaches!). I can raise the foot of the bed and that greatly reduces the swelling! He can also use the rails to help turn over and he sleeps much better... so do I. The bed and table were completely covered by insurance and the table makes it easy to sit Michael wherever he wants to eat (in bed, on the bed, sofa, or chair.). Hope this helps some of you!

Georgette. Palm Springs, CA

10. PHARMACIST

This professional has responsibility for your safety and ensures that your medications are correct in name, number, dosage, and manner of administration. He or she plays a key part when you are home and needing emergency medications at 1:00 A.M. (headache, seizure, constipation) and helps with insurance company approvals and ordering special medicines like Temodar™. This person is key in maintaining your lifeline and medication safety. (See Chapters 9 and 19.)

11. REHABILITATION SPECIALISTS (PHYSIATRIST, OCCUPATIONAL THERAPIST (OT), PHYSICAL THERAPIST (PT), SPEECH THERAPIST)

If you have no deficits or problems in strength, movement, communication, or mental function after surgery, then chances are you will not need rehabilitation. However, if you or your family note changes, then these need to be brought to a doctor's attention. Post-surgical referrals for rehabilitation are often made by the neurosurgeon or primary physician. Usually the initial diagnosis and treatment team will notice these changes and set up a rehabilitation consultation. If they do not, definitely ask for one. You should be able to receive this level of care at a major brain tumor center.

A *physiatrist* (not a psychiatrist - the two are often confused) is an M.D. who has special expertise in Rehabilitation Medicine. He or she usually coordinates all services and prescribes medications. The physiatrist leads the rehab team, which includes:

- Occupational therapy (OT) for coordination, eating, and communication problems
- Speech therapy for speech-related problems
- Physical therapy (PT) for movement, lifting, and paralysis-related problems
- Neuropsychology for estimating mental function and perceptual problems
- Psychiatry or psychology for emotional issues

> A Physiatrist coordinates the Rehab Team. Not all Centers have one.

The team will meet and plan a program of inpatient therapy for a set duration (about two to eight weeks) or an outpatient program to be completed at home with or without regular visits to a rehabilitation center. The physiatrist can be your "primary" doctor during an inpatient rehabilitation stay.

Table 5-16 The Physiatrist and Rehabilitation Team: Roles & Responsibilities

1. Works with your other doctors to understand your medical condition and problems.
2. Performs a physical evaluation to identify your strengths and weaknesses in activities of daily living, mobility, eating, mental abilities, speech, understanding, ability to communicate.
3. Advises on progress and chances of recovery based on the initial assessment.
4. Recommends devices or medications to aid in rehabilitation: chairs, lifts, braces, muscle relaxants, medications for alertness or sleep, constipation, feeding tubes for nutrition.
5. Manages complications attributable to therapy.
6. Monitors your response to rehabilitation with charts, therapist reports, and blood tests.
7. Assesses and treats distressing symptoms, such as pain, constipation, and infections
8. Monitors steroids or anti-seizure medications continued by the neurologist or neurosurgeon.

Even ordinary functions can become difficult after surgery: eating, drinking, recognizing family, movement and emotions. A stroke or other complication also can occur that is not directly related to the tumor or its therapy. Medications may be responsible for poor concentration or weakness. Management of these symptoms requires a team approach which includes your physiatrist. The questions below ultimately define

> The Rehab Team has several members: Occupational therapy (OT), Speech therapy, Physical therapy (PT), Neuropsychology, and Psychiatry or psychology.

responsibility for each member of your rehab team based on your specific issues.

Table 5-17 Important Questions to Ask Your Rehabilitation Team Before the Program Begins

1. Do my brain tumor and surgery explain the changes in function that I have?
2. What is the plan for my rehabilitation? Who is responsible for monitoring it?
3. Which activities of daily living will be improved by therapy?
4. Are any of my functions at risk of becoming worse? Which ones might improve? Taking a bath? Dressing myself? Going to the toilet unassisted? Making a cup of coffee? Answering the phone? Getting out of bed?
5. What would happen if I did not receive rehabilitation?
6. What is the latest recommended treatment for my problems? How recent is it?
7. Are there (side) effects of the therapy that you are recommending? Can I have written handouts describing these?
8. How many people with my problem do you treat each year? More than 25?

9. Are any of your patients on clinical trials? How many?

10. Am I eligible to receive care at another rehabilitation center that has more experience with my type of problem?

11. Which other team members do you recommend that I see now? After therapy?

12. Will you coordinate my rehabilitation therapy as an outpatient? If not, who will?

13. Will you be taking care of my medical needs, problems, and other medication adjustments, or will my primary doctor or neurologist do this?

14. Will you communicate with my primary doctor to define which problems (such as mobility, fever, constipation, or headache) are in your domain of responsibility?

15. Can I have a copy of the rehabilitation consultation, tests that I have completed, and reports for my notebook?

Finances and Rehabilitation

A word of caution: Talk with your social worker or physician about which rehab services will, and will not, be covered under your insurance policy. Sometimes insurance will pay one facility but not another. Before you start rehabilitation, read the fine print; call the insurance company, and ask if it can explain in plain language which coverage you do have. Do not assume anything! Ask for confirmation in writing, with a fax or letter.

The rehab team can help you with tools and products for home use to make your life easier. I have seen dramatic, positive changes with rehabilitation, from infants to people 100 years of age. This improves quality of living, an area that should not be overlooked or forgotten. Much helpful information is also available on the web (Table 5-28).

12. NEUROPSYCHOLOGIST, PSYCHOLOGIST AND PSYCHIATRIST

Neuropsychologists, psychologists and psychiatrists are often part of the neuro-oncology or rehab team and offer valuable service. Unfortunately, misconceptions about "psychology" can interfere with proper assessment and treatment of normal reactions to all you have experienced. The long-held idea that psychology is the realm of maladjustment or "being crazy" is no longer true in a medical setting. Psychological help has three major goals:
- Helping people cope with their illness
- Structuring their lives so that they can get the most out of their treatment
- Aiding them to improve and maintain quality of life

Behaviors that suggest a need for psychological assessment and intervention are described in this section, as well as what can be expected from mental health professionals.

You have undergone probably the most frightening, overwhelming life event anyone could experience. Give yourself some slack! You have had a neurosurgeon tinkering with your brain; you received radiation and medications that you never knew existed. You are recovering and things may not seem quite right. You might be experiencing one or more of the following problems:
- Being absent-minded or easily distracted
- Stumbling over some words or forgetting words you ought to know
- Feeling down, depressed, or angry in ways that you do not understand or cannot control
- Crying more easily than usual
- Staring at the television endlessly without understanding what you see

The brain only has so many ways that it can respond to injury. Many of these problems can be identified and solved with the right help.

The *neuropsychologist* has obtained a doctoral degree (Ph.D.) and has the skills to select, administer, and interpret standard tests that evaluate the way that the brain performs everyday functions. The neuropsychological assessment reveals which functions are disrupted and where your strengths lie. Examples include the following:
- Executive function is based in the frontal lobes – this is your ability to initiate and organize complex tasks like brushing your teeth, planning a dinner, or walking from home to the shopping center.
- Word finding is located in the temporal lobes – this function enables you to choose the right word to express an emotion or name an object.
- Vision is governed in the occipital lobes – what you actually *see* is recognized in the back of the brain.
- Fine motor movement is regulated in separate sections of the cerebellum and brainstem – this includes picking up a pen or writing.

The *neuropsychologist* can evaluate your strengths and weaknesses, suggest compensatory strategies to capitalize upon your strengths, and provide information to the rehab team on specific areas needing work. For example, you may process *hearing* words better than *seeing* them.

It is important to remember that a neuropsychologist is also a regular clinical psychologist (described next) with an additional two to four years of training in how the brain influences behavior. Thus, your neuropsychologist can do things like discriminate medical or biological effects from life changes. For example, when our patients report memory problems, the neuropsychologist can help discern whether the problem is depression (which is easily treated) or memory problems related to medication or tumor changes (which require different treatments). He or she deduces this from a combination of your performance on special tests and an understanding of your overall life.

> The neuropsychologist evaluate your brain's strengths and weakness.

Table 5-18 The Neuropsychologist: Roles & Responsibilities

1. Assesses your current quality of life and finds out what bothers you most.
2. Assesses your condition; administers "paper and pencil" tests to see how your brain pathways are working.
3. Communicates to your doctors the findings that directly affect your safety and quality of life. You must give permission to share this information.
4. Advises you on the chances of recovery from your problems.
5. Recommends approaches to help you improve your quality of life.
6. Makes referrals for treating psychological symptoms such as depression or anxiety.
7. Monitors your response to the therapy with repeat testing, if needed.
8. Works with your primary doctor after other specialists have completed their service.
9. For adults, develops a return-to-work plan, determines if special accommodations in the work environment are needed, and/ or provides documentation to back up a disability claim.
10. For children, develops an Independent Educational Program (IEP) to assist the school district and teachers in determining the best ways to instruct and test.[14]

The neuropsychologist is not licensed to prescribe medications, but he/ she can make medication recommendations to your physicians.

Testing can benefit you in many ways. For example, a good neuropsychological evaluation can spare the patient a lot of heartache:

> The *cardiologist* with an oligodendroglioma was "fine" after surgery and radiation therapy, was back at work, driving... except he broke off his relationship of five years with his girlfriend, was terse with his patients, and made medically incompetent decisions, according to his colleagues. He

had neuropsychological testing and no deficit was found. The conclusion was that this behavior was probably a result of an overly rapid tapering of steroids and reflected brain inflammation as a result of radiation, which would be reversible with a reintroduction of steroids.

Table 5-19 What to Ask Your Neuropsychologist Before the Assessment

1. How much will the assessment (testing) cost? Is it covered by my insurance?
2. Where is my brain tumor? Which problems are due to the tumor?
3. Are my symptoms due to side effects of therapy or medications? Which ones?
4. What are the latest recommended treatments for my types of problems?
5. Do I have any visual problems that could affect my safety (e.g. a blind side)?
6. What are my strong points, and what are my weaker areas?
7. When and what findings will you communicate to my primary doctor?
8. For children: Will you send an individual educational plan (IEP) to my child's school? Will I receive it first?
9. Can I have a copy of the consultation and test results for my notebook?

A *psychologist* has a doctorate degree (Ph.D.) in Psychology and experience in helping people cope with emotional stress. They do not make a moral or value judgment about the type of problem that you have. They do, however, try to understand the stresses in your environment, including your family setting, in order to help you feel better and be more in control. The psychologist will ask you about your current function, learn about your treatment regimen, and make suggestions for improving your overall quality of life. This may be discussed in a one-time consultation or be handled over several sessions. Please note that your psychologist cannot prescribe medications for you because he/she is not a medical doctor.

> Psychological help is not recommended because you are "crazy." It is to cope with illness, to improve and maintain quality of life.

The spouse of a cancer patient offers her perspective on when to seek counseling:

> *Counseling is a personal thing and all depends on one's personality. Not everyone benefits from it. Some people seem to handle stress better than others do and can get themselves through the rough times. I, too, have a husband with glioblastoma multiforme, and he is doing quite well. At this point, I don't feel as though I would really benefit from counseling. We take each day as it comes*

and appreciate today. I think you will know if the time comes when you can no longer handle the stress on your own, and you will seek it out at that time.

June, spouse to Donald, Las Vegas, NV

Table 5-20 The Psychologist: Roles & Responsibilities

1. Assesses your anxiety and depression levels and helps you to understand the uncomfortable or distressing feelings that keep you from enjoying your life.
2. Advises you about treating symptoms such as pain, depression, and anxiety.
3. Counsels you on how to cope better with your illness and its effects on your life.
4. Works with your doctors using the information that you give permission to share.
5. Advises you on the chances of recovery from your problems.
6. Monitors your response to therapy.
7. Works with your primary doctor after other specialists have completed their service.

Table 5-21 Questions to Ask Your Psychologist

1. How much will the therapy cost? How much is covered under my insurance?
2. Where is my brain tumor? What functions could it affect?
3. What is your approach to helping me?
4. Over how many weeks will we need to meet for counseling?
5. Are my symptoms due to effects or side effects of therapy?
6. What is the latest recommended treatment for my symptoms?
7. Which other team members do you recommend that I see now? After therapy?
8. What and when will you communicate with my primary doctor?
9. Can I have a copy of the consultation for my notebook?

Another spouse talks about difficulties that she and her husband faced; it's possible that a better team with psychological advice would have helped them find a solution more quickly:

My husband also has anaplastic astrocytoma and has the weird personality changes you described. These are the things doctors don't tell us. Another group member had the observation about steroids, which I completely agree with. While he was on steroids, I prayed for the day that I would see his teeth again - just a little smile would do! He yelled at me, our kids, did mean things totally out of character and threatened to leave since "his opinion didn't count around here" and so on… It dramatically improved once he got off steroids. He is closer to his normal self now, more than ever, since the diagnosis.

Lucy, spouse of Gordon, Naples FL

A Psychiatrist has a doctoral degree in Medicine (M.D.). He or she has experience in diagnosis and treatment of mental problems. As medical doctors, they can prescribe medications to help make your symptoms more controllable and manageable.

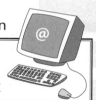

A useful website that defines mental health terminology
www.therapistfinder.net/glossary

Psychiatrists deal with tumor-related mental problems that could require drug therapy such as violent outbursts or psychotic symptoms involving visual or auditory hallucinations. Psychologists are often more helpful with common behavioral problems, such as coping, anxiety, and depression. Through the rehabilitation team, you can arrange to consult a psychiatrist (or psychologist or neuropsychologist), even if you are not referred to one. Here is a report from a satisfied customer:

Celexa helped me get up and running when I was extremely depressed after the surgery. I seemed to tolerate it well, notwithstanding that I was on Tegretol™ and probably tapering off Decadron at that time. I may also have been on a drug to control stomach acid, but I don't remember for sure. Anyway, it really helped with the depression and had seemingly no adverse side affects.

Arnold, Albany, NY

Table 5-22 The Psychiatrist: Roles & Responsibilities

1. Assesses your mental health and helps you to understand the uncomfortable or distressing feelings that keep you from enjoying life.
2. Assesses your condition and advises you about using medications to treat symptoms such as severe depression, paranoid feelings, or drug abuse.
3. Prescribes medications to help your mental functioning.
4. Works with your doctors and communicates the findings… that you give permission to share.
5. Advises you on the chances of recovery from your problems.
6. Monitors your response to therapy by interview and/or blood tests.

An online chat group veteran benefited greatly from seeking psychiatric help early in the process:

As someone who went through a major depression when I first was diagnosed with a brain metastasis, I knew I needed help. My problem was finding the right psychiatrist to help me, but once I did, the change was dramatic. Before that, I had no feeling of need for counseling, and I was doing fine on my own. Lots of people 'push' support groups and other types of 'help' but they are not right for everyone.

Helen, monitor of an online chat group. New York City, NY

Table 5-23 What to Ask Your Psychiatrist Before Treatment Begins

1. How much will therapy cost? How much is covered under my insurance plan?
2. Where is my brain tumor? What functions could it affect?
3. What is your approach to help me?
4. Over how many weeks and how frequently will we need to meet?
5. What is the latest recommended treatment for my symptoms?
6. Which medications will you prescribe? What are the side effects of each one?
7. Can I have written guidelines for taking and monitoring the drug's side effects
8. Are any of my symptoms due to side effects of therapy? Which?
9. Which other team members do recommend that I see now? After therapy?
10. What and when will you communicate with my primary doctor?
11. Can I have a copy of your consultation for my notebook?

13. ENDOCRINOLOGIST

An *endocrinologist* is a medical specialist for diseases of the glands that secrete hormones. The glands include the pituitary, thymus, adrenal, pancreas, ovaries and testicles, pineal, and thyroid (Figure 5-1). Most people with brain tumors will not have glandular problems requiring an endocrinologist. However, surgery or radiation therapy to the upper spine, or area around the pituitary gland, can cause damage.

The hypothalamus and the pituitary, the latter also known as the "master gland," control secretion by sending messenger molecules to other glands in the body. Two common problems associated with pituitary failure are *hypothyroidism* and *water*

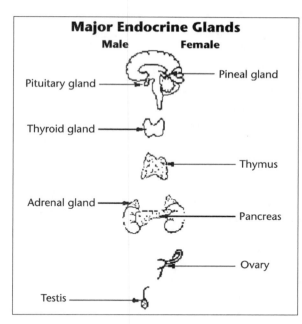

Figure 5-1 The major endocrine glands

diabetes. The former is due either to the inability of the pituitary gland to stimulate the thyroid (TSH) or direct damage to the thyroid gland in the neck. Symptoms are weight gain, tiredness, hair loss, and thickening of the skin.

Water diabetes is caused by damage to the rear part of the pituitary gland which results in low secretion of the hormone ADH, whose function is to signal the kidney to save water. A person can easily become dehydrated without ADH. Other gland-related problems can occur as well; for example, damage to the pituitary or adrenal gland results in underproduction of the anti-inflammatory stress hormone, cortisol. The latter is critical; without it, infection or surgery could be fatal. Anyone having hormonal problems, such as sugar diabetes, or who is having radiation or surgery to the head or neck should have an endocrine consultation. (See Tables 5-24 and 5-25.)

Table 5-24 The Endocrinologist: Roles & Responsibilities

1. Works with your other doctors to understand your medical condition and problems.
2. Completes a physical evaluation and testing of how your endocrine glands are working; recommends hormone supplements, if necessary.
3. Prescribes and adjusts replacement doses of hormones.
4. Advises you on progress and chances of recovery from the problems found at the initial assessment.
5. Monitors your response to therapy by examination and blood counts.
6. Monitors appropriate steroid dosage and its effects with neurology or neurosurgery.

Table 5-25 What to Ask Your Endocrine Specialist

1. Do my brain tumor and surgery explain my changes in endocrine function?
2. What is your plan for me?
3. Which of my gland functions are at risk of becoming worse?
4. What would happen if I did not take the medications?
5. What activities of daily living will be improved by therapy?
6. Are there specific (side) effects of the therapy that you recommend? Can I have written handouts describing these?
7. Can any of the medications cause my cancer to grow?
8. How many people with my type of problem do you see yearly?
9. Are any of your patients enrolled in clinical trials? How many?
10. Am I eligible to receive care at another center that has more experience?
11. Will you be taking care of my medical needs, problems, and other medication adjustments, or will my primary doctor or oncologist do this?
12. Will you communicate to my primary doctor which problems are in your domain of responsibility?
13. Can I have a copy of the endocrine consultation and test results for my notebook?

14. Ophthalmologist (Eye Doctor)

This is the medically trained doctor who has an M.D. degree with specialization in the diagnosis of eye conditions, eye surgery, and field of vision testing. Not every brain tumor patient will need this specialist. (See Tables 5-26 and 5-27.)

Based on an evaluation, the ophthalmologist can modify treatment with tumors of the optic nerve in neurofibromatosis NF-1. Here, the visual field exam is critical for determining when to operate or when to administer radiation, if the tumor is not evidently changing on an MRI scan. The ophthalmologist can also advise on cataracts from radiation therapy or eye infections like herpes simplex or zoster.

Table 5-26 The Ophthalmologist: Roles & Responsibilities

1. Performs visual field examinations to confirm improvement or loss of sight from tumor effects on the retina, optic nerves, cornea, lens or brain
2. Corroborates suspicions from the other doctors, such as increased pressure in the eye or head, possible bleeding in the eye, or viral infection
3. Performs operations on the eye, optic nerve and bony orbit

Table 5-27 What to Ask the Ophthalmologist

1. What does my routine eye exam show?
2. What does my visual field show about my tumor condition? Where is there loss?
3. Do I have any cataracts in my lens?
4. How do I compensate for the visual loss in that field? Special lenses, glasses?
5. Will you communicate your findings to my doctors?
6. Do you have a record of my examination that I can keep for my notebook?

15. DENTIST

The *dentist* is often overlooked by both the layperson and the treating physicians. My awareness was piqued when Marjorie, wife of Arnold who received head and neck radiation, told me that her husband suffered terribly from radiation-induced cavities! Anyone who is about to get chemotherapy or head radiation should visit the dentist ASAP, as a minor gum infection (gingivitis) or cavity can mean a big infection when immunity is compromised by therapy. Regular follow up for cleaning, exams etc. would also be important.

> Dentists: Visit yours before starting chemotherapy or radiation.

16. NURSES

Nursing is a basic part of any diagnostic plan or treatment you will experience. *Floor nurses* care for you in the hospital. *Specialty nurses* in the clinics – Radiology, Oncology, Neurosurgery – to name a few, attend to your needs and advise on helpful strategies and give medications. More descriptions appear in Chapter 7: The Referral Hospital or Academic Center.

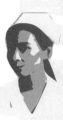

17. THE TUMOR BOARD

It is a great advantage to have your case presented at a *tumor board* meeting. Why? At what other time could all your treating physicians be together to focus on and discuss *your* case with all the pertinent information available? This setting also enables physicians not associated with the treatment team to offer their expertise. It's like getting 10 to 15 consults at no charge – Free consultations! This is a requirement for hospitals to maintain their accreditation by the Hospital Joint Commission. (See also Chapter 6: Experts and Getting a Second Opinion.)

This chapter was designed to familiarize you with the various professionals you'll meet and who may care for you. Now it's time to move on to Chapter 6 to find out if you need a second opinion or to learn more about diagnosis and specific treatment options.

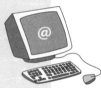

Table 5-28 Internet Resources for the Team

Caregiver resource	http://media.seniorconnection.org/?doc=booklist.inc
Caregiver support (e-mail to enroll)	http://my.webmd.com/medcast_channel_toc/ 4041?z=1621_4041 http://www.braintrust.org/services/support othergroups/ btcaregivers-captain@braintrust.org (e-mail to enroll)
Rehabilitation devices	http://www.makoa.org/cmpyinfo.htm
Viatical insurance information	http://viatical-expert.net (See also Chapter 25)
Psychology terms; finding a therapist	http://www.therapistfinder.net/glossary/

CHAPTER 6

Experts and Second Opinions

Don't defy the diagnosis; try to defy the verdict.

Norman Cousins

8━ **Key search words**
- experts
- team
- tumor necrosis
- specialists
- scan reviews
- treatment
- second opinions
- tumor board

I thought long and hard about where to put this chapter. It could have been placed in the middle or near the end of the book, but I decided to place it closer to the beginning because having a brain tumor is an urgent matter. Your survival depends on the expertise of the Team in whom you entrust your care.

This chapter will help you decide if you need a second opinion, show you how to find an expert, and prepare you for the actual meeting. It will also explain how to quickly assess your current doctors for their strengths and weaknesses. It should be read together with Chapter 7: Academic Centers, University Hospitals, and Institutes – Where You Go for a Second Opinion.

The reality of having a brain tumor is that no single doctor can possess the knowledge to address all your needs. For instance:

> Without an accurate diagnosis, it is almost impossible to begin.

- An experienced neurosurgeon is absolutely critical to the surgical part of your care.
- A neurologist diagnoses and treats seizures or distinguishes tumor symptoms from side effects of medication.
- A radiation oncologist can determine if radiation is needed. And, if so, what type to give, and how best to aim the radiation beams with a high degree of accuracy.

- A neurooncologist might help you decide upon and administer the best treatment options: combinations of chemotherapy, immunotherapy, and radiation.
- A neuropsychologist can test and diagnose your strengths and weaknesses to help you develop strategies to accommodate parts of the brain that have been injured temporarily or permanently.

The concept of a medical team is revisited throughout the book. More information on the specific players can be found in Chapter 5: Doctors and Other Team Members.

> A specialist covers just one area of medicine.

DO I NEED AN EXPERT?

You may be very satisfied with your current doctors. But there are a few questions that you might ask yourself.

What Is the Difference Between a Specialist, an Expert, and a Second Opinion?

A specialist covers just one area of medicine, such as Neurosurgery, Internal Medicine, or Pediatrics. A specialist may not necessarily be an expert in a specific area, however. An expert is more knowledgeable about a specific area like brain tumors. A second opinion is what you seek from an expert. For example, if you have had surgery, but part of the brain tumor remains, you would want to ask an expert neurosurgeon in brain tumors about removing the rest of the tumor. You would not ask a medical oncologist or radiation oncologist for his/ her judgment, since it is a surgical decision. You can find specialized neurosurgical centers that have a reputation for being aggressive. Alternatively, if you have a question about chemotherapy or an experimental therapy, you can look for a major center that has different experts who can give input, since a combined approach might be needed.

> A specialist may not be an expert in your specific area of need.

The example below is an actual question that was sent to the www.virtualtrials.com website. Why does the patient's wife have to ask this question on the Internet, if her spouse is getting expert care from her team? Does she trust her doctors?

Question: "My husband has had complete disappearance of his anaplastic astrocytoma tumor with Temodar. But now he has enhancement on MRI. Is it radiation necrosis? Can this large enhancement area hurt him if there is no sign of the recurrent tumor? He has minimal short-term memory deficits, a few aura-type seizures, and slight difficulty with word associations."

My answer: This is an interesting and challenging dilemma to solve that requires input from members of your team. Tests, such as the MR-Spect and Thallium-Spect, often can distinguish the difference between live and dead tumor. Also, dead tumor may sometimes need to be removed surgically. In addition, steroids can affect the results of biopsies and MRI scans. It is time to talk with your treating doctor.

How to Decide if a Second Opinion or Particular Expert Is Needed?

How do you choose whom to consult? The answers depend upon what you want… and expect. In this battle with your brain tumor, accurate diagnosis is essential to your care. Without this, it is almost impossible to begin. Read about Karen's experience and what happened when the diagnosis was misinterpreted.

By all means get second opinions concerning surgery and pathology! My daughter's original diagnosis was AA3 in June 2001. After surgery with 100 percent resection, she received radiation and ten rounds of chemotherapy. We discovered, after moving to another town, that she had been misdiagnosed and actually had a JPA, a low-grade tumor that needs no further treatments after a 100 percent resection. Not saying that is your situation of course, but if I had my time to go over again, a 2nd opinion would be a must!! Good luck!

Karen, Hilton Head, SC

Medical humanitarian and writer Norman Cousins spoke of the use of humor in his own successful battle with arthritis of the spine. He said "Don't defy the diagnosis; try to defy the verdict."

My wish is that you defy both the diagnosis *and* the verdict! First, make sure that the diagnosis is correct, then obtain the knowledge that you need in order to play a positive role in determining the "verdict." To accomplish this you will need some expert assistance.

WHAT DOES AN EXPERT OFFER ME?

The same question could be asked about cars. If you have a Volvo, you probably don't take it to a Ford dealer for repair? Both are automobiles, and both dealerships could fix the problem. However, it would take a Ford technician longer to do the job because the Volvo has unique computer components in critical locations and other unfamiliar features, such as metric measurements instead of feet and inches. Like a computer, the brain, your "central processing unit," is critical to your "operating system." There is less margin for error and a shorter time to act. Doctors who are highly familiar with the unique features of the brain, its danger zones, its responses to therapy, and the range of new therapies available, can act more skillfully, safely and quickly. For example, a 2.5 cm (one-inch) breast tumor can exist for years before diagnosis, but it usually does not affect day-to-day function. Conversely, in the brain, a one-half-inch tumor can cause a stroke or memory loss if it is not removed or resected properly.

> An expert is more knowledgeable about a specific area, like brain tumors.

The other major way in which an expert can help is in the reassurance that she or he can give as a result of knowledge and experience, if you ask the right questions.

> A second opinion is what you seek from an expert.

127

The following e-mail, sent to an Internet brain tumor chat room shows a caring, responsible person who feels desperate because his mother's doctors are not offering hope or alternatives.

Hello, I desperately need advice on how to proceed with my mom's glioblastoma multiforme treatments. On Thursday, she had her first MRI since her craniotomy. During surgery, Gliadel wafers were inserted. She took Temodar (7 days a week/ 6 weeks) and radiation therapy at the same time (5 days a week). Today, she got the results of her MRI back. They are not good...

Her tumor increased in size, and I need advice on how to proceed. She had her craniotomy done at General Hospital and the doctors are now telling her that any form of radiation treatment is no longer an option (including stereotactic radiosurgery) and that another course of Temodar is her only choice. On Thursday, she and my dad will meet with Dr. M. I will also attend the consultation.

Which treatments can I propose to the doctor? I have heard of good results with Temodar in combination with other drugs such as CPT-11 and Accutane®. What about stereotactic radiosurgery, GammaKnife, X-Knife? Any advice is GREATLY appreciated. My mom told me this morning that she will try anything...

Doug, Sacramento, CA

After posting a "help," Doug received 10 responses in one day. Five examples follow:
1. Hi Doug - When we were in your shoes, the doctor stopped Temodar altogether and hit the tumor with CPT-11 every two weeks. This bought us six more months. Mary
2. When you go, bring the last two sets of MRIs with you. Very rarely did the doctors agree on size of tumor or even on progression versus stability. Your mom had Gliadel, which causes changes around the tumor cavity. Ask about fractionated stereotactic radiosurgery, high dose tamoxifen, thalidomide, or blood brain barrier disruption. Marvin
3. You are going to the closest major medical center I would have recommended. While they are not known for brain tumor research as much as other cancers, it is an excellent medical center. I think your family should be blunt with Dr. M. You want her to take a fresh look at everything, and she should be aggressive in treatment suggestions. The feeling at the "big" centers is that combinations are more effective and no more toxic nor hard on the patient than temozolomide alone. Lloyd

4. I don't know if it would make sense, but you might want complementary nutritional support. Dr J. is a nutritionist who specializes in brain tumor patients and nutritional supplements that may help and are not likely to cause harm. You may want to discuss this with Dr. M. Additional information on www.virtualtrials.com Bob.

5. "WOW - I feel like we are living parallel lives. We didn't detect much hope from our local doctors. So, Cyndi got on the phone with the University of California, San Francisco that day, and she and my uncle flew out to San Francisco. She will begin treatment tomorrow on a clinical trial program followed by a second surgery. Go where doctors see hundreds of these cases a year, not just a few. "NEVER give up! Take your mother's health into your own hands. You will become the doctor to some degree. Doctors often do not appreciate lay persons having input or asking about their treatment. You'll be amazed at how doctors become obstacles to one's own survival at times! We do not find this "attitude" at the major centers. Plus, they exude hope and positivity. I also suggest two books: Surviving "Terminal" Cancer by Dr. Ben Williams (diagnosed with a glioblastoma multiforme in 1995 and currently cancer free!) and There's No Place like Hope: a Guide to Beating Cancer in Mind-Sized Bits by Vickie Girard. There's no way we are going to let her go. We're fighting this thing all the way!" Amy.

I do not advocate getting medical consultations from the lay public. The Internet community has made positive suggestions that Doug can use in consultation with his mother's physicians for her benefit. The Internet should provide information and support so you are equipped and motivated to ask your questions. But never consider the Internet and its content as a substitute for your medical team. Remember this when you read about the role of the "caregiver" in Chapter 5: Doctors and Other Team Members.

CAN SELECTING A PARTICULAR SPECIALIST AFFECT MY SURVIVAL?

In the brain tumor world, this decision can be a matter of life or death. Most people simply assume that their physicians (or auto mechanics) are competent. They may be right, but unfortunately, that's not always true. All professionals, from hair stylists to doctors, have differing levels of skill. Knowledge about different brain tumors is no different. You want to be sure that you are in the most expert hands possible. Remember, it is not the institution you go to that is responsible for your care, but your physicians within it. You could be at the most prestigious institute for brain tumors and still encounter incompetent or less experienced physicians.

Let's start with the neurosurgeon. Over the past seven to 10 years, it has become apparent that survival for both adults and children with brain tumors depends upon the amount of tumor that remains after surgery. The Children's Cancer Group (now called COG, Children's Oncology Group) completed a series of trials for ependymomas, medulloblastomas, and astrocytomas (I was the principal investigator for the main trial). For each group, survival at five years was improved...if the surgeon left no more than ¼ teaspoonfuls (1.5 cc) of tumor. The difference between having leftover tumor and no tumor was astounding.[1] Twenty-five per cent more children with medulloblastoma were alive five years later... if the surgeon performed a nearly complete resection! The same principle was generally true for newly diagnosed and recurrent gliomas in adults. The experience of your neurosurgeon is critical, because surgeons who operate more frequently tend to leave less tumor behind.

> The experience of your neurosurgeon is critical.

Dr. Raymond Sawaya, Chief of Neurosurgery at MD Anderson in Texas, had the following comment:

> *It is better to receive a second opinion prior to beginning any treatment. Sometimes a patient is told that the tumor is inoperable, when the local physician says it's "too risky." We recently conducted a study of 80 people who came to M. D. Anderson for second opinions. We found that at least one-third of these patients had been diagnosed inaccurately. Many had been told that their tumors were inoperable when in fact we were able to remove the tumors in three out of four of the patients.[2]*

I once heard a neurosurgeon at a major university hospital refuse to obtain CT scans after surgery, because "they could be misleading." Clearly, this neurosurgeon had not wanted his patients to know the truth about how much tumor had actually been removed. Fortunately, this practice is almost unheard of today. With modern MRI imaging, the standard of care is to obtain an MRI scan after surgery.

In short, both the skill and experience of the neurosurgeon is critical. Let's do the math. If we take the 30,000 primary brain tumors that occur each year in the United States and divide them by the 4,500 active neurosurgeons in this country, this equates to about six patients per surgeon per year. But in reality, a small number of neurosurgeons at major centers in the United States perform the majority of brain tumor operations (50 to 200 per center), and they have better outcomes.[3] I ask, would you prefer to be operated on by a surgeon who performs one to two tumor resections each week, or only two each year?

Pathologist

The actual tissue diagnosis is made by a pathologist. Brain tumors represent a great challenge for accuracy, even to experts in Neuropathology. On our recent clinical trial for highly malignant astrocytomas, we found that almost 25

> Has your tumor been reviewed by a neuropathologist for its accuracy? This can be life saving.

per cent of patients who were enrolled in the trial were actually found to have low-grade tumors when later reviewed by a panel of experts.[4] Even then, there were disagreements among the reviewer neuropathologists. So, has your tumor been reviewed by a neuropathologist? If not, it can be life saving to ask for such a review.

Radiation Oncologist

The same issue of experience can be said for radiation therapy. In a study for the Children's Cancer Group performed about 10 years ago, we found that in about 15 per cent of 400 cases, the aim of the radiation beam was not only inaccurate, but it also missed parts of the brain tumor! Recurrence is more likely to happen in this circumstance. Experience, care, and expertise counts in radiation therapy, too.

Oncologist and Neurooncologist

Evidence for the importance of selecting specialists in Oncology and Neurooncology is more indirect. Patients with recurrent tumors treated in early Phase 1 or 2 experimental chemotherapy protocols lived longer than those treated by their physicians' personal choice of therapy. This occurred despite no shrinkage of tumor for most patients on the trials. Most likely, the longevity effect was due to more careful monitoring, thus improving the basic clinical care.[5]

I am reminded again about the story of Adam and Eve being evicted from the Garden of Eden because they took from the tree of Knowledge of Good and Evil. We all face mortality; but we do have a choice of whether to use the knowledge available to us in order to improve upon the quality and length of our life on Earth. It is up to you to decide how much information you want to access.

DO I SEEK ANOTHER OPINION ONLY WHEN I HAVE A PROBLEM WITH MY CURRENT CARE?

No. Seeking another opinion does not mean that you have not been getting good care or that you do not trust your physician. It is to ensure that you will continue to get the best and most up-to-date choices for your treatment.

HOW DO I ASSESS MY CURRENT TEAM?

This is actually a complicated question with a three-minute solution. First, read the following posting on a brain tumor list server and see how this father might answer the checklist regarding his adult son's treatment team. Then, answer the 20-question checklist about your current care (Table 6-1).

> Seeking a second opinion does not mean that you mistrust your physician.

Does anyone know of a support group for brain tumor patients in North Carolina? I talked to my daughter tonight about my stepson Carlos, who is having problems with nausea and can't keep anything down. The tumor in his brainstem is on the "nausea button." When he was diagnosed, the kids were in Blacksburg, Virginia. Carlos went to a Dr. in Winston-Salem on the recommendation of his grandfather. Surgery was performed by a Dr. who said after the surgery that the tumor was removed and that he would "be fine." His MRI three months later showed that the brainstem tumor was still there. He was referred to Wake Forest for oncology.

The main problem is that Carlos really doesn't have a team of doctors working with him. There is no internist, just specialists. He went to a doctor near where he lives... but the doctor wouldn't take him as a patient because of his problems. The nausea has gotten worse since he started and finished radiation in October. The kid needs nourishment and as long as he keeps throwing everything up, he's not going to get it. What he needs most right now is a doctor who can treat his nausea.

Father of Carlos, Houston, TX.

> Seeking another opinion is to ensure that you get the best and most up-to-date choices.

132

Table 6-1 20-Point Checklist to Assess My Team & Care

General	YES	NO
1. Do I know which doctor is in charge of my care?		
2. Am I informed about my illness in a way that suits my need to know?		
3. Do my doctors take time to answer all my questions?		
4. Do my doctors communicate well with each other, so I do not need to play the role of "go-between" or fill in my own gaps of understanding?		
5. Am I comfortable with and do I have confidence in my doctors?		
About my Diagnosis	YES	NO
6. Have I been told the name and grade of my tumor, where it is located, and why I have my symptoms?		
7. How secure is the tissue diagnosis? Is its accuracy unquestionable?		
8. Have I been shown the pre- and post-operative CT or MRI scans, so that I understand the problem and treatment plan?		
9. If I ask for a second opinion, will my doctor refer or recommend me to an unbiased outside doctor?		
Treatment		
10. How many patients with brain tumors do the neurosurgeon, radiation therapist, and oncologist personally treat each year? More than 25?		
11. How much tumor can be removed? Did the neurosurgeon discuss how this might affect my prognosis?		
12. If the tumor is inoperable at this institution, can it be removed more completely at another center? Am I told where?		
13. Have the benefits, possible side effects, and risks of surgery been discussed with me?		
14. Have I been informed about how my activities of normal daily living may be affected by treatment?		
15. Do my doctor and medical center specialize in this type of tumor?		
16. Am I informed of the benefits, long-term side effects, or risks of radiation, chemotherapy, or other treatments?		
17. Is my care being given or directed by an expert in brain tumors?		
18. Have I been told what will happen if I do nothing?		
19. Has my case been presented to the hospital tumor board?		
20. Does my team offer clinical trials for my type of tumor?		

If the NO column has more checks than you are comfortable with (I would be concerned with two or more), then perhaps you should consider a second or even third opinion. This does not mean that you are deserting your current doctor or team. It means you are uncovering all possible avenues for healing and longer life. In this way, you will be more prepared to make strategic choices in the treatment process.

HOW COULD A SECOND OPINION CHANGE MY TREATMENT?

Neurooncologists, including myself, are often asked to render an opinion about whether a "tumor" on the MRI scan is dead tissue or live cancer. Those trained and familiar with problems unique to treatment of cancer in the nervous system can assist you. Many neurooncologists have seen patients who were told that their tumor had returned, only to discover that it was actually "necrosis" or dead tissue that looked like tumor on the scan. The treatment for recurrent tumor is quite different from that of dead tumor!

A recent e-mail "progress report" to an Internet chat group describes the process and outcome of a second opinion for a complicated but not unusual course.

> Ricardo has a glioblastoma multiforme grade IV that was diagnosed on 6/10/2000. He had surgery on 7/2/2000 followed by 33 rounds of radiation treatments with 100 mg. of Temodar daily (during radiation) completed on 9/23, and then he finished one round of Temodar on the 5/28 day cycle. The local radiologist stated that the tumor was larger than in August and there was 'evidence of hemorrhaging.' I wanted to be more aggressive and asked Ricardo's oncologist about a "cocktail," maybe Celebrex™ with Temodar. He wanted to wait because of the 'hemorrhaging.'

> I decided to go to MD Anderson (MDA) for a second opinion, as I had received many positive comments about MDA from 'group' members. Ricardo's oncologist gave his 'blessing.' MDA was troubling because they told us something completely different from local specialists!

> The oncologist at MDA met with us for about 90 minutes and said 'If it ain't broke, don't fix it.' He explained that from the MRI films of Oct 14 and Nov. 14, he could not tell recurrence from necrosis (dead brain tissue) and scar tissue. He said, 'Whatever it is, it is STABLE.' He said that their radiologists are 'among the best in the world,' and they are only right 80 percent of the time in

telling necrosis from tumor recurrence. The only way to tell would be by biopsy (surgery). He did not recommend this.

I asked about 'clinical trials.' He stated that no trials or cocktails would be available to patients who do not have clearly defined tumor. We are going with the local oncologist's recommendation, Temodar. The trip to MDA was positive in that the MRIs are stable and might be showing necrosis or scar tissue. It was disappointing for two reasons:

1. MDA cannot tell the difference between necrosis or tumor recurrence from the MRIs. The local radiologist and radiation oncologist have been telling us that it is tumor recurrence. They never suggested that it might only be necrosis or scar tissue. To me this is a major problem. I am inclined to believe MDA.

2. We went to MDA hoping to get into a clinical trial or at least be prescribed a cocktail of Temodar and Celebrex, Accutane or ??, as I am pretty sure Ricardo has not been cured. To leave with 'If it ain't broke, don't fix it was disappointing.' "Maybe my expectations were too high - this is a long battle with constant highs and lows.

Miriam (w/o Ricardo, GBM Grade IV. Austin TX.

Your plans after the second opinion could be affected in at least three ways:

1. Your current assessment and treatment plans are confirmed. Now, you have reassurance and peace of mind. You stay with your current team.
2. You get new treatments or courses of action to follow, which your current doctors can implement for you. The following are five possible scenarios:
   - Have no further therapy and wait.
   - Begin a clinical trial given by your current doctors. Make occasional visits to the referral center.

   > **A second opinion gives 3 options:** • Current treatment plans are confirmed. • Get new treatments. Your current doctors implement them. • Switch to the new team.

   - Change medications to minimize side effects, such as pain and nausea, with your current treatment plan.
   - Add conformal radiation (after completing traditional radiation) to "boost" the tumor area, as recent data indicate this may increase survival.
   - Change chemotherapy drugs.
3. You have more confidence in the new team and switch for this stage in your care. This may happen because the Phase 1 or 2 studies that interest you are

only conducted at the referral site. New therapies are often tested in a limited number of institutions as a pilot study, such as the immunotherapy trial that my colleagues and I conducted at Cedars-Sinai Medical Center in Los Angeles. Our trial required processing of tumor tissue at the time of surgery to make a patient-specific vaccine. Its later administration and follow-up required a Clinical Research Center, only found at larger medical centers. After the study is completed, patients often return to their former physician teams for care.

The following Internet exchange illustrates how treatment approach, quality of life, and longevity can be changed by a second opinion:

> **Question:** My father has a brain tumor…two cm on the right side and halfway between the ear and forehead. The biopsy showed "some malignancy." He is a healthy 88-year old man. The doctor is recommending six weeks of radiotherapy. Any comments or other information that I can give him?

> **Answer:** This is an interesting question and an increasingly common problem, as people are living longer and adult children must make important decisions about the quality of life….and death of their parents. First, do not accept "malignancy." You deserve to know exactly what type of tumor it is. Without this knowledge, NO therapy should be considered. There is a big difference between a meningioma, which can be stable for a long time, and a malignant astrocytoma, that progresses without treatment.

Depending upon an individual's wishes regarding quality of life, we have at times recommended no therapy at all, only supportive care. Knowing the exact diagnosis and patient's wishes should be the first consideration in determining appropriate care. You need more information. Ask your doctor to consult experts at a major medical center that has experience in this area.

At the 2001 Neurooncology Society conference it was reported that people more than 70 years of age with malignant astrocytomas responded well to treatment with Temodar, administered by pill. The survival of those taking Temodar was similar to the group who received three to six weeks of radiation therapy; they had fewer side effects.[6]

Comment: Most 88 year-olds do not tolerate radiation therapy, especially to the frontal lobes. They often develop accelerated dementia and rapidly become non-functional in a manner similar to Alzheimer's disease. Therefore, this is a challenging situation. Having this case presented to experts, as well as to a tumor board could serve both the individual's and family's best interests.

WHAT IS AN MRI OR CT SCAN REVIEW? HOW CAN I GET ONE?

In order to attract you as a patient, many brain tumor centers will review your MRI scans gratis, in other words, *free*, without charge. This is not a trick; you can benefit from this.

A brain tumor center offers an MRI scan review and suggests alternatives for further care as an incentive for you to ask for a consultation and then have your care administered there. In our program at Cedars-Sinai Medical Center, about 10 per cent of people whose MRI scans we reviewed from out of state or country eventually had surgery at Cedars-Sinai. Thus, 90 per cent of the people who submitted scans were rendered a free "educational opinion" (unlike a "consultation," involving an official doctor-patient relationship), which helped them to understand options and receive better care.

"Educational opinion" protects an institution and its physicians from possible legal sanctions and malpractice suits. Unfortunately, no good deed goes unpunished. Many centers have stopped providing this service or have begun charging fees for "scan reviews," because of additional legal ramifications. Several websites list institutions that provide "educational opinions." (See Table 6-3.)

Many centers will request a short history (on their form or in your own way) and copies of the actual scans (on film or CD-ROM) (See Chapter 3, Tables 3-5 and 3-6.). Be brief. Unless specifically asked, avoid the temptation to send volumes of records and reports. Usually, they won't be read.

> Scan reviews offer a free or inexpensive way to get a second opinion.

HOW DO I FIND AN EXPERT OR TREATMENT CENTER?

RESOURCES FOR FINDING CENTERS

Ten years ago, it was difficult to find out who and where the experts were located. Economics and the Internet have combined to change this in the consumer's favor. How? Hospitals and experts need to pay their bills in an increasingly competitive environment. They have become "consumer friendly" and advertise in magazines and on the Internet to expand their clientele. Many helpful Internet sites contain advertising from major centers; one click and you are there!

Foundations like The Brain Tumor Society (BTS) and American Brain Tumor Association (ABTA) have lists of major referral centers in or near your area, accessible by phone, mail, or the Internet. When searching for clinical trials for specific tumors, extensive listings can be found on www.nci.gov and www.virtualtrials.com. You can contact the physicians in charge of the studies and obtain a consultation to find out if the studies are appropriate for you. (See Table 6-3.) There is a list of pediatric and adult brain tumor centers worldwide that have membership in the Society for Neurooncology (SNO) in Chapter 7, Tables 7-7, 7-8, 7-9.

> Foundations can help you find experts.

The consumer now has access to websites like those of the National Brain Tumor Foundation (NBTF), which provide information on estimated number of cases *seen* per year by specialty program and state. This is not the same as number of cases *treated*, but it is an indicator of expertise with brain tumors. Major centers, located throughout the country, are at most a four- to six-hour drive or a one-hour flight.

WHAT PREPARATIONS SHOULD I MAKE BEFORE SEEKING A SECOND OPINION?

It pays to be prepared. Follow the steps in Table 6-2 below for getting the most out of the expert, second opinion. As the e-mail reprinted below demonstrates, even the best preparations can go awry:

First off, anyone going for a second opinion - especially out of town - make sure that you have the last two MRI films (they are by far the most important). To make a long story short, the MRI envelope said Nov. 14, but the actual film inside was the Oct.14 MRI. I thought that I had double-checked, but I missed it. When the nurse informed us of the problem, I was more than a little upset. I phoned the MRI place, and they guided the MD Anderson oncologist to their webpage, where he was able to view the Nov. 14 MRI film! Moral Of The Story: Check the MRI Films Inside the MRI Envelope!

Miriam (w/o Ricardo, GBM Grade IV, Austin TX

Table 6-2 Eight-point preparation for the second opinion

1. Phone, e-mail, or write to the expert or assistant. Ask what to bring.
   This allows time to gather all information from hospital & physicians before you leave.

2. Ask if the actual pathology slides will be reviewed there before making recommendations. If the answer is "No," then you may want to ask, "why not?"

3. Make use of records you have organized (per Chapter 3). Bring all your data.

4. Before leaving:
   - Ask for copies of your original and latest scans on a CD-ROM disk with the program to view scans. They are a lot easier to transport this way.
   - Contact your insurance/HMO plan to find out what is covered and how to get the consultation authorized.

5. List all questions that you want answered by the expert. Put this list in second opinion section of your notebook. Check off as answered.

6. Include items to which you answered "No" in the 20-Point Checklist to Assess My Team & Care. Other questions might include:
   - Do you agree with my current assessment & treatment? Why, or why not?
   - If not, what are the advantages /disadvantages of your treatment plan(s)?
   - If additional surgery is recommended, who will actually be performing it?
   - Are there any side effects to your suggestions that I should know about?

7. What will my personal financial obligations be?
   (Get these in writing from financial personnel, not the doctor.)

8. If you do forget a scan, call your MRI center:
   Ask if your scan can be posted on their website or e-mailed as a "jpg"
   image to the physician you are visiting. This might salvage a less-than-use-ful trip.

WHAT ARE THE HIDDEN COSTS IN GETTING A SECOND OPINION?

There may be several costs in getting a second opinion. The actual doctor's fee is only one of these. For example, a consultation at a university or large clinic might include a "facility fee." This is a charge that the center administers in order to pay for their space and operating expenses; it often comes as a surprise to those seeking a consultation.

HOW DO I OBTAIN A SECOND OPINION WITHIN MY CURRENT HEALTHCARE SYSTEM?

WHAT IS A TUMOR BOARD, AND HOW CAN IT HELP ME?

Most hospitals have at least one Tumor Board. This is a group of doctors, nurses, administrators, psychologists, and other interested professionals who gather regularly for an hour or so to discuss recent cases. Their meetings begin with a formal written history that details how the diagnosis was made, pertinent examinations, surgical results, laboratory findings, and scan reports. Test results are usually presented by experts in specific areas. The neuroradiologist will present findings from MRI scans; the neurosurgeon will discuss surgical outcomes, observations, and diagnostic impressions. The pathologist will project a sample of tissue onto a large screen or through a microscope and discuss the different diagnostic possibilities and how he or she arrived at a final diagnosis. The social worker or psychologist may offer insights on the patient and his family's strengths and weaknesses. Lastly, the oncologist and radiotherapist will give their rationale for therapy. This is sometimes a lively and controversial part of the conference.

A Tumor Board presentation is like getting 10-15 consults at no charge.

It is a great advantage for patients to have their case presented at a Tumor Board meeting. Why? At what other time could all treating physicians be together to focus on and discuss a case with all the pertinent information available? This setting also enables physicians not associated with the treatment team to offer their expertise. It's like getting 10 to 15 consults at no charge. This is a requirement in order for hospitals to maintain their accreditation by the Hospital Joint Commission. So ask your physician about this.

If your hospital does not have a Tumor Board, obtain a second opinion and consult with doctors who practice at a hospital that does have one. This is another way that you can benefit from the collective expertise of a hospital without leaving your current team. Recommendations can only be as good as the experience of those present, however. If brain tumors are infrequently seen at a hospital, or a team is not aware of the newest options, then their recommendations can only be mediocre.

How Do You Assess a Tumor Board?

Ask the hospital administration or Pathology Department for the following information:
- A list of its Tumor Board members.
- If any of the members are experts in brain tumors.
- If any members regularly publish their results and experience in recognized journals.

This information can be obtained by phone or found in the annual report of any hospital or cancer center. These reports are public documents.

What if My Neurosurgeon Discourages Me From Obtaining a Second Opinion?

Remember, getting second opinions satisfies your own need to know that no stone has gone unturned; seeking a second opinion is not due to mistrust. Actually, obtaining a second opinion has become such a standard practice that there are relatively few obstacles. Many centers willingly will perform a "scan review" for individuals who seek second opinions. You can easily find the names of such centers by contacting brain tumor organizations, the list in Chapter 7, or websites in this book.

My own thought is that we may, in the past, have taken the lesson of Adam and Eve too literally and tended to view "knowledge" as not for us, inappropriate, or limiting. On the contrary, lack of knowledge may do us more harm than good. We cannot change our mortality… but we can acquire the knowledge to delay it. What is your choice?

How Do I Get Expert Care From My Prepaid Health Plan or HMO?

From my experience, few HMOs or health plans offer well-coordinated, well-supported, or high-level expertise in the treatment of brain tumors. They manage common diseases, like diabetes

> HMOs have dedicated and skilled Neurooncology professionals who get little attention or notice for their expertise.

and heart disease, much better than brain cancer. Frankly, they lack the motivation to provide expertise in narrow specialty areas such as Neurooncology, which costs money and resources. Having said that, however, there are often dedicated and skilled healthcare professionals in these groups who get little attention or notice for their expertise. It is your challenge to seek them out and tell them how much you appreciate their service. How do you find them?

1. Use the eight-point checklist for preparing to seek a second opinion. (Table 6-2).
2. Ask your primary doctor which physicians have the most experience with brain tumors. Ask for a specific referral to them. Tell them after you meet them why you chose them.
3. Ask your primary doctor to serve as the team leader to consolidate your treatment and interpret what the specialists are saying.
4. Collect and organize your medical information. (See Chapter 3: Getting Organized.)
5. Share the results of your research with the experts and ask them to comment on what is applicable to you.
6. If a treatment is not available to you in your HMO, ask why?
   • Is the treatment's effectiveness unproven?
   • Is the cost too prohibitive to be justified?

If it is the latter, then you have a strong argument against the denial of your care. Regardless, petition the *ombudsman* (an impartial person within the organization whose function is to resolve such matters) as instructed in the section below on challenging a denial. Or contact an ombudsman through brain tumor foundations. (See Table 6-3.)

> Petition the ombudsman (an impartial person within the organization who resolves denial of care issues) in an HMO to contest a denial.

Can I Obtain a Second Opinion in an HMO or Kaiser Plan?

The answer is yes… and no. Yes, because usually the plan will allow you to see another physician in the same department as your current physician. Will you get a different opinion? My experience with patients who have come from these plans is that the answer is more than likely, "No." Do doctors not want to disagree? Are they succumbing to financial pressures? Are physicians of similar mind and training? Your guess is as good as mine.

Bottom line: Prepare before going for a second opinion.

In a prepaid health plan, like an HMO, the contract between you and the organization is that you will only use physicians in their "network." But the expertise you need might not be in their network. What do you do then? (See Chapter 23: Managing Costs, Benefits and Health Care with Insurance, HMOs and More.[7])

What are your alternatives? I have had several patients who have written letters, discussed the complexity of their case with an ombudsman, and have been persistent "squeaky wheels." They have had their plan pay for an outside consultation at a specialty center, often at a university hospital. You can use the five-point outline below for your challenge letter. Your plan will not tell you this is possible, but you have nothing to lose (and all to gain).

FIVE-POINT LETTER TO CHALLENGE DENIALS

1. Write a detailed letter to the highest administrative official in the network, explaining the life or death situation that you face.
2. Let him/ her know the urgent time frame you face. Request an answer within 7 to 10 days.
3. Detail reasons that you want the consultation (such as results of your web, newspaper or magazine research that indicates a consultation is necessary; informal consultations; or that the expert surgeon or clinical trial is not available in your network).
4. Explain consequences of the expertise being unavailable or not meeting your needs.
5. If that is not successful, then you may be better off going outside your network. Pay the cost of the consultation and argue about it later, based on the information that you receive from the consultation.

CONCLUSION

No one said that this process was going to be easy. My desire is that your efforts to get a needed second opinion are successful, and that it leads you to a place of comfort with your treatments. In the other chapters, you will learn how to use your skills to surf the Internet and find more detailed information about your illness, complications, and new treatments, which only 10 years ago were off-limits to patients. In the next chapter, I explore the local rules and procedures at the academic center or university hospital – what I call High Tech U (HTU).

Table 6-3 Internet Resources for Experts/Second Opinions

Organization/ Resource	Website/ Contact
Brain Tumor Center Locations	http://www.braintumor.org/patient_info/surviving/ treatment_center_database/state.asp or www.braintumor.org (click on services/ treatment)
General information	www.virtualtrials.com
Brain Tumor Society (TBTS) American Brain Tumor Association (ABTA) National Brain Tumor Foundation (NBTF)	www.tbts.org www.abta.org http://braintumor.org
Scan Reviews, Educational opinions	http://www.virtualtrials.com/btcenters.cfm
Clinical trials	http://clinicaltrials.gov/ct http://cancer.duke.edu/btc/Treatment/ClinicalTrials.asp www.virtualtrials.com www.nci.gov http://acor.org
Ombudsman Program (adult) National Coalition for Cancer Survivorship Advocacy for second opinion	http://www.nci.nih.gov/clinicaltrials/understanding/ insurance-coverage/page3 http://www.canceradvocacy.org/programs/ toolbox.aspx (Telephone: 1-877-866-5748) http://www.patientadvocate.org/resources.php
Child Related Help for Second opinions	
Parents of Children with Cancer Support Group	http://www.cancercare.org/CancerCareServices/
Ombudsman Program (HMO, Insurance Advocacy)	http://www.childhoodbraintumor.org/ombuds.html http://www.cancernetwork.com/journals/oncology/ o9602j.htm
Questions to Ask (child)	http://www.pbtfus.org/PatientResources/Questions/ page1.htm
General Child information	www.virtualtrials.com http://www.btfgainc.org/index.asp
E-mail Online Support Groups to Find Centers	
Patient Groups (child)	http://health.groups.yahoo.com/group/ Pediatricbraintumors/
Pediatric Brain Tumor Online Support Group	E-mail: pediatricbraintumors-subscribe@yahoogroups .com

Medulloblastoma Online Support Group	E-mail: medulloblastoma-owner@yahoogroups.com
Optic-Glioma Online Group	E-mail: optic-glioma-subscribe@yahoogroups.com
Hypothalamic Hamartoma Online Support Group	E-mail: rwdavis@logan.net Website: http://www.hhugs.com http://www.hhugs.com Meetings held: online, ongoing

CHAPTER 7

Academic Centers, University Hospitals & Institutes – Where You Go for a Second Opinion

Hope is an invaluable asset to all of us in coping with illness, as well as with the frustration of not being able to identify a single best treatment option. And hope becomes even more vital when affirmation as to the most appropriate measures for managing your disease does not exist.

Neal Levitan, Executive Director, Brain Tumor Society

Key search words

- referral center
- teaching hospital
- house staff
- tertiary care
- late effects
- academic center
- university hospital
- residents
- miscommunication
- radiation
- transportation
- professor
- fellows
- communication
- pain

I could have entitled this chapter, "Keeping Sane." Why? When you are referred to a brain tumor treatment center for special consultation, worries about your health may now be compounded by distress from unfamiliar surroundings and an entirely different set of institutional rules. Large institutions have their own policies, procedures, language, and buzz words that can be new and intimidating at first. (See also Chapter 6: Experts and Second Opinions, that describes the experts who can be found at these centers.)

DESCRIPTION OF A CENTER OR UNIVERSITY HOSPITAL

Any office or hospital can call itself a center. Of importance to you is the range of the comprehensive services and expertise offered by any particular center. An academic center is usually a medical school. Most often, it will have a University Hospital attached to it, where care is actually

> Any office or hospital can call itself a Center.

delivered by the professors. An institute (e.g., Barrows Institute in Phoenix, AZ) or clinic (e.g., Cleveland Clinic in Cleveland, Ohio) can be a hospital or outpatient treatment center. Choose a physician at a center that sees at least 50 to100 patients yearly with brain tumors. Web links can help you to find a local brain tumor center in your vicinity (Table 7-6). I have also compiled a list of centers worldwide that are represented by at least one member in the Society for Neurooncology, (See Tables 7-7, 7-8, and 7-9). They are listed as Pediatric only, Adult only, and combined Adult-Pediatric Programs.

Most centers with representatives in the Society are university-affiliated *teaching hospitals*. Hospitals cannot call themselves *teaching hospitals* unless they have a nationally approved educational program for Nursing or Medicine. The supervising doctors at any given teaching hospital are professors. If the teaching hospital is located off-campus in a neighboring area, its staff of physicians will have had their credentials screened by the medical school with which it is affiliated. Most children's hospitals, many large private medical centers, and some Veterans Administration Hospitals in the U.S. and Canada are off-campus teaching hospitals that are affiliated with a university medical school.

Throughout this chapter I will use the term *brain tumor center* to refer to centers that see at

> Teaching hospital or Center attached to a University assures a high level of oversight & competency.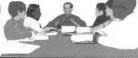

least 50 to 100 patients per year, whether or not they are teaching hospitals.

Bottom line: Look for a brain tumor center that sees at least 50 to 100 patients per year *and* is a teaching hospital. If you can't find a center that has both characteristics, then experience with large numbers of patients is most important.

PREPARING FOR THE VISIT TO A MAJOR BRAIN TUMOR CENTER FOR A CONSULTATION

You have assessed your current treatment team and institution using the 20-question checklist in Chapter 6: Experts and Second Opinions, Table 6-1. Based on this assessment, you have decided to get a second opinion or have at least some of your care at a teaching hospital. Before leaving, you have assembled:

- An organizational notebook (Chapter 3).
- A complete set of records.
- MRI or CT scans.
- A list of costs that your insurance plan will cover (Chapter 23). This list can be obtained in advance from the referral center.
- Transportation arrangements.
- Lodging arrangements.

There are different ways to arrange local and air transport assistance at reduced rates or no charge. Usually, the hospital social worker will know about these resources, but it will not hurt for you to check them out as well (See Table 7-6).

The staff in a consultant's office can advise you of discounted lodging rates for hospital visitors. Hotel websites online are also helpful. Several organizations provide assistance in finding places to stay. Internet veterans can start at the "Hospitality Hotline," see http://www.nahhh.org and Tables 7-6 for websites offering transportation and lodging connections.

> Preparation for your second opinions before leaving is key.

WHAT TO EXPECT AND NOT TO EXPECT AT A MAJOR BRAIN TUMOR CENTER

Most large centers have made serious attempts to deliver a more personalized service in the current competitive marketplace. However, the following scenarios are not uncommon:

- Your trusted physician refers you to a well-known medical center at "High Tech University" (HTU), or you decide to go on your own.
- When you arrive, you have difficulty finding a place to park. Tension builds. You wonder, "How is a sick person supposed to walk this far to see the doctor?"
- You go to the admissions office and wait in line for what seems like forever. The clerk asks, "What is your name?" "What insurance do you have?" before

asking, "How are you?" You now have a three-hour wait before you are seen or your bed will be ready.

- Within a very short time you will need to:
  - Sign your name giving consent for treatments or procedures from which you could benefit… or die.
  - Understand medical terms that confuse even many physicians.
  - Decide who is in charge of your care when you have consulted five doctors.
  - Realize that HTU is a business with a staff that is in great demand but short on supply. You, the customer, may not feel like a top priority.

Unfortunately, this is the reality of today's *tertiary care medicine* – a fancy name for specialized medical care that can only be given in centers that treat particular illnesses with advanced equipment and personnel skilled in using it. While you will benefit from expertise found at these tertiary care centers, you must know the rules of the game in order to receive optimal care.

The role of this Center is different from that of your primary care provider – they have huge demands as experts for a broad geographical area and as such have to focus on the illness, and not the person. The Center is also trying to be there for the person, so there will be advocates for the *whole you*, somewhere. With this understanding, you can still derive the best from the doctors and the other services at HTU. Knowing this upfront has importance, so you aren't intimidated about asking questions of the experts.

WHY ARE SOME PEOPLE FRUSTRATED WITH THE CARE THAT THEY RECEIVE AT A REFERRAL CENTER?

Perhaps you still yearn for the compassion and concern that we've seen in the *Dr. Kildare* movies of the 30s and *Marcus Welby MD* television shows of the 70s. Your sense of loss may be exacerbated in that medical care today is better represented by television shows such as *ER* and *Scrubs*, in which the flaws and personal dilemmas of the physicians take precedence over the effects of their sometimes-heroic deeds on you, the patient.

Most people still hold the fundamental belief that you get what you pay for. But regardless of what you have paid for a diagnostic test or comprehensive office visit, genuine empathy, reassurance, or a healing touch from the doctor is often missing.

> We all want to know that our fears about illness and pain are understood.

All of us have a story to tell behind our illness. And fears multiply and change into demons in that dark space in your mind. You do not only want to know what and where the *disease* is located, but you want to know that your fears and pain are understood by others, including your physician.[1]

Unfortunately, Marcus Welby, MD of 2004 is frenetically trying to pay his office expenses and make a living. He sees more patients and is paid less for each one. In the process of delivering medical care, he has lost some of the human connection because its value can be neither billed nor reimbursed by the insurance company.

THE "INSIDE" RULES AT MAJOR BRAIN TUMOR CENTERS

Calendar Safety: Avoid the Middle "J" Months

One under-recognized issue for patient care and safety in a teaching hospital is the time of year. In fact, June and July can be problematic months for patient care. This is because the new interns, residents and fellows all start at the end of June and beginning of July. Most hospitals try to stagger the change of service, so a completely new crew does not start on the same day or week; this is not uniform. If you can help it, avoid being an inpatient at a teaching institution for anything elective during these times.

> June and July are when new residents & interns start at teaching hospitals.

"Change of Service"

Another time of possible lapse in patient care is during a "change of service" when the house staff or fellows switch to another rotation. A new group takes time to familiarize themselves with its patients' histories and patterns of care. You must be vigilant during these times to ensure that your care is not derailed in the transition.

For both of the above situations, knowledge of your own treatment plans, medications, and test results is your insurance policy against unintentional errors. Being prepared means you are both taking control and sharing responsibility.

Responsibility for Diagnosis and Treatment (It Isn't Always Your Doctor!)

The center is a bit different from a smaller private hospital. Not only will you have a team of specialists, but each of them, as professors, will also have their own

Bottom line: Your "warm and fuzzy" needs are real, but they may not get attention at HTU. For them, you need to rely on friends, nurses, social workers, but perhaps not your doctor.

team of trainees – from fellows to interns and students. Thus, delivering expert and comprehensive care to you is actually performed by these people under the direction of the professor. (See more under fellow below.)

Table 7-1 Clinical Care Responsibility Ladder at a Teaching Institution

Position	Role
M.D. Professor	Consultant or expert who has ultimate responsibility for your care.
M.D. Fellow	Fully qualified physician receiving specialized training, working closely with a professor.
M.D. Resident	PL-2-5. Physician member of the hospital house staff, who is responsible for day-to-day care. Supervised by fellow and professor.
M.D. Intern	PL-1. First year physician who just completed medical school and is supervised by a resident.
Nurse Specialist and Practitioner (CNP)	Clinical nurse specialist has expertise in specialty areas and works with physicians on a hospital team. A Certified nurse practitioner (CNP) works independently under the supervision of a professor and can examine patients and prescribe medications.
Physician Assistant (PA)	Has expertise in a specialty area and works with physician on a hospital team. Responsibilities are similar to CNP above.

THE "PECKING ORDER" AT HIGH TECH UNIVERSITY – TITLES AND ROLES OF PROFESSIONALS

THE PROFESSORS OR "ATTENDINGS"

The professorial consultants, also called attending physicians (attendings), are at the top of the ladder for responsibility. They are accountable to you for your care at the brain tumor center

> The Professor or Attending Physician is ultimately responsible for your care.

that includes a teaching hospital. As you will find out, however, the attendings are not necessarily the ones to get the job done. They are appointed at a level that matches their experience. An *Assistant Professor* has been on the staff less than seven years, an *Associate Professor* for seven to 14 years, and a *Professor* for 14 years or more. Promotion from one level to another depends upon the number of research publications or recognition of particular expertise or teaching service. Being older does not guarantee that the doctor is more capable. At some universities, professors

> Your may have a Team of specialists and a Team of house staff caring for you.

may be promoted based on their research accomplishments rather than their clinical care expertise or bedside manner.

THE FELLOW

The fellow is a graduate physician who has completed medical school, and residency training in an area of specialty such as internal medicine, pediatrics, or neurosurgery. He or she is now taking subspecialty training to become an expert in a more focused area, such as Neuroradiology for those who have completed a radiology residency, or Neurooncology for those who have completed an Oncology Fellowship. These younger doctors are motivated to become the best in their field with this additional one to four years of training. The fellow is the professor's *right hand man*.

> The Fellow is your key "go to" person working under the Attending.

At a teaching hospital, the fellow answers to the attending physician (professor) and is responsible for overseeing your care. He or she is the person to whom the residents will ask questions about dosages of drugs, medical conditions, ordering of tests, and plans for care. The fellow may also be responsible for special procedures or major portions of your surgery. These committed, skilled individuals are there to learn under the guidance of attending physicians. They are not there as an excuse for attending physicians to avoid visiting you! Fellows can be your most valuable contact persons, with a direct line to the attending's ear.

From a practical viewpoint, the competency of your fellow can make all the difference in the quality of your stay. Communication between the attending physician and the family rests with the fellow. Here is an example from my own experience:

> David was a model of most fellows under my supervision. He had great communication skills and led daily rounds in addition to "nudging" me and other attendings to meet families and discuss results of tests. He supervised the residents well, was there to answer their questions, and made sure that they were always up-to-date on test results and the day's physical examinations. He exhibited empathy for his patients and could zero in on their psychological needs as well as the needs of their families. He was trusted as the responsible doctor who would consult the "head doctor with gray hair" if there was any question.
>
> In contrast to David, Joe used to call children "wimps" if they cried during a painful spinal tap or when the nurse came in to administer medication. A parent once asked him for help in getting a bone marrow procedure

performed early in the day, instead of waiting and letting the anxiety build up. "Look," he shouted, "I've got four more (bone) marrows to do, and I'll get to yours when I can." Obviously, this family was not having their warm and fuzzy needs met by being told they were part of the "assembly line" for procedures that day. It is not an ideal world. There were another 23 patients, all seriously ill; it was not always possible to follow-up those indiscretions and allay the hurt feelings. Joe was medically competent but resistant to our suggestions to modify his style or seek psychological counseling for himself.

HOUSE STAFF: ROLES OF RESIDENTS, INTERNS AND MEDICAL STUDENTS

House staff includes physicians in training who are supervised by professors and are responsible for actual care of patients; these can include residents, interns, and sometimes medical students. Residents are responsible for the following:
- Gathering medical histories
- Performing physical examinations
- Developing and arriving at diagnoses
- Formulating treatment plans in coordination with other physicians
- Examining patients at least daily
- Monitoring responses to treatment or recovery from complications
- Placing all your orders for tests and treatment

An intern, sometimes called "Postgraduate level 1" or PL-1, is one year out of medical school and is having his first hospital care experience. This physician performs the initial evaluation and history taking, plus he usually writes orders for diet, medications, tests, and vital sign measurements (pulse, respiration, blood pressure, temperature). On the surgery rotation, this individual is the last to perform parts of the surgery and often plays a supporting role such as holding retractors or sewing up skin incisions. The PL-1 depends heavily on those with more experience – the PL-2 and PL-3s, fellows, and attendings.

> Interns and Residents are responsible for your day-to-day care.

The PL-2 and PL-3 are second- and third-year residents who supervise the interns. They take a more active role, under a professor's supervision, when additional experience is needed for procedures like spinal taps, insertion of special catheters, chemotherapy administration or surgery.

Medical students are not part of the house staff, as they are still in school and not hired by the hospital. Some may take an "externship" and will be given responsibilities like an intern but with more supervision.

Most patients and relatives are rarely negative toward a young physician who cannot answer a question quickly. Rather, they are more worried about physicians who fail to examine them, rush through exams, dismiss their concerns, or fail to provide answers in a timely manner.

Like chefs, architects, and car salespersons, there are many residents and interns who are excellent, some who are average, and an occasional few who function poorly. Their first priority is to master the basic skills of medicine: conducting procedures, ordering appropriate tests, and making accurate diagnoses. Some are naturally better than others when it comes to people skills. A few have focussed so much on medical training by the books that they are not used to dealing with people yet (especially emotional people). Attention to families' psychological needs becomes optional to them. The assumption is that they will acquire those skills, but priority is given to focusing on critical medical details, which, if done poorly, can physically harm the patient. This is understandable.

NURSE SPECIALIST AND PRACTITIONER

Over the last 15 years, a cadre of well-trained nurses has been working side-by-side with physicians. These "clinical nurse specialists" have expertise in subspecialty areas such as Neurosurgery or Neurooncology. They can assist physicians and help you by:
- Discussing the purpose of treatment and changes to be expected
- Reviewing information about a patient's condition and test results
- Explaining side effects of a medication or procedure
- Delivering instructions for postoperative care of dressings, wounds, and catheters at home
- Offering expertise that the house staff may not have
- Collecting important data for special research studies or a clinical trial

A nurse can take additional training and be designated a *clinical nurse practitioner* (CNP). They are certified and licensed to examine, diagnose, and make independent treatment decisions in the absence of a physician.

Your Nurse Specialist or PA is a great resource person for details of your care.

Physician Assistant (PA)

There is yet another professional individual that has emerged over the past 10 years called the *physician's assistant*. The PA may have been a medic in the Armed Forces, an emergency medical technician (EMT) who has received two to three years of training and is licensed by the state. Physician's assistants work under the supervision and direction of a physician and have similar roles to CNPs. In addition, they can perform procedures such as minor surgery and spinal taps, and they can prescribe medications.

CONSULTANTS HERE, CONSULTANTS THERE, BUT WHO IS MY DOCTOR?

The Process of Consultation

The process of consultation at a major brain tumor treatment center can be complex. There are usually residents and fellows on the main ward where you are admitted. The addition of consulting doctors, each with their own staff, multiplies with possible input from Neurology, Infectious Disease, Endocrinology, Neuroradiology, and so forth, depending upon the complexity of the case.

The following steps will put you more in control, prevent you from feeling overwhelmed, and assure you that the consultation is in your best interest. When someone new shows up to examine you, it's important that you ask the following questions (Table 7-2). You can refer to Chapter 5 for questions about each specialty team member.

Bottom line: You need to know who your primary, responsible doctor is. Ask that he/ she be team leader and not let you become lost among specialists.

Table 7-2 Key Questions That You Can Ask to Ensure A Successful Consultation

Question	Outcome
"Which hospital department are you from?"	You establish the pattern of interest and search for knowledge.
"Why has Doctor X asked you to consult on my case?"	You understand the purpose of the consultation if you have not been advised. You are assured that the consult is for you.
"Will you be discussing the results of your findings with me or my doctor?"	You have received clarification on objectives of the consultation and how results will be communicated to you.
"The questions I would like answered are ...." May I please have a copy of your consultation for my organization notebook?	You get answers to your specific questions. (See Chapter 5: The Team for questions to ask.) You will have in your possession: A summary of the consultant's opinion. His or her business card. Alternative recommendations, besides the final one given to you. You will have arranged to have a copy of the final written report sent to you.

EXPLAINING THE RESULTS OF A CONSULTATION

A few professionals may talk directly about their observations with you. Others will say, "Ask your physician for the results of our findings." Be patient, as the student or resident usually will want to discuss the case with his

> Always ask a consultant what question he is there to answer.

attending physician or supervisor before rendering an opinion and answering your questions. Throughout this consultation phase, you may not know if you are talking to a fellow, medical student, or nurse specialist. To tactfully determine who your consultant is, ask or look for telltale signs:

- Medical students and interns wear a different color or shorter coat.
- Their nametags should indicate their status.

Many times consultants will want to discuss the case with your primary doctor or the one who requested the consultation and have him or her explain the results. This makes sense since different consultants may disagree and your primary doctor (your team leader) can help evaluate differing opinions with you. All consultants have their own biases about treatment choices, especially when there is no clear-cut answer.

The following scenarios illustrate the importance of working with someone who understands the implications of your various options:

Scenario #1: Sam, a 66-year-old drug store manager, had not been able to eat enough to maintain good nutrition during six weeks of radiation therapy for his glioblastoma brain tumor. He and his family knew that he needed temporary nutritional support to keep him healthy. Which of the following two choices should he accept?
a) Placement of a feeding tube to the stomach performed through a small skin incision under local anesthesia and sedation by a gastroenterologist ($2,000).
b) A full operation performed by a surgeon in a hospital operating room under general anesthesia ($4,000-8,000). The outcome is the same for both.

I would vote for choice a) but choice b) could be the better one, depending upon the confidence of the patient in the doctor responsible for the procedure and whether there is anyone skilled at carrying out choice a).

Scenario #2: Selma, a 58-year-old widow, has a large meningioma on her right frontal lobe that can either be treated in three ways:
a) be removed directly or
b) be reduced in size by embolization or clotting of the tumor before major surgery. This procedure can add $3,000-$10,000 to the operation. Some neurosurgeons swear by it, and others feel it is unnecessary or complicates the tumor removal.
c) A few centers are proposing embolization as definitive therapy for small meningiomas, so that surgery will not be needed!

These are situations where even the experts are divided. Here, your primary doctor, the team leader, can help you in decision-making. I suggest that you hear all opinions before making a decision. Differing recommendations do not mean that one center is right and the others are wrong. Rather, some centers may have better results using a particular technique, while others may not. It can be difficult to accept the fact that there is not always one right answer.

> Your primary doctor should help you sort out differences in opinion among your consultants.

This is when being aggressive and proactive, when it comes to your own healthcare, is a challenge. You have to use all that you have learned and follow your gut instinct. Hopefully you have trust in one or more of your doctors to allow them to help you arrive at a decision, given all the available options. Don't be intimidated to seek even more information when making a critical decision.

BEING PROACTIVE WITH COMMUNICATION ISSUES

Not all people want to seek information or take on the establishment, and that's okay. However, to get the best care, it is in your interest to have a family member or friend serve as an advocate and request that that person speak on your behalf. If you do this:

> Have an advocate ask questions on your behalf, if you are not feeling up to it.

- You will feel better, more effective, and satisfied in knowing that specific information has been requested clearly and deliberately.
- You will spend less energy in wondering and have more psychological and physical energy for healing.
- Your physician will know that:
  - He is dealing with an informed, assertive family.
  - He must take more care to meet your needs because your needs have been clarified.
  - He may not be so sure what is going on and may need to recommend a consultation.

After a while, you learn to be straightforward and, when necessary, lead the conversations when speaking to doctors, so that all your questions get answered.

Shari, Amador, CA.
Oligodendroglioma 2/01, Dendritic vaccine trial 5/04.

Do not fear that your questions are too inquisitive, intimidating, ignorant, insulting, or time consuming, or that your doctor will respond negatively. If you have these thoughts or worry that your feelings will prevent you from speaking up, then you need support.

A recent scientific study from Boston found that physicians who are assistant professors in their first two years on the staff actually undergo great changes in their values and attitudes toward ill patients with serious diseases. They may be naive in some respects which could be an important factor in their communication style and lack of understanding the therapy choices important to you. Being proactive will allow you to get your specific information needs met in a style that is acceptable to you.

> Do not fear asking too many questions or taking up the consultant's time.

Below is one of the best examples of a family's proactive effort to obtain a medical consensus:

Ari was a five-year-old who had had successful surgery for a posterior fossa brain tumor, and he was not improving with rehabilitation. Two months after surgery, he could not stand up or speak. Neurology felt that his weakness and delayed progress were due to the chemotherapy. The neurologist interpreted the X-ray scans differently from the neuroradiologist. Rehabilitation specialists felt that the problems had something to do with the surgical procedure. As the oncologist, I did not understand how any of these diagnoses fit the current problems. The consultants argued in their chart notes for weeks. They covered themselves legally and made their different positions known to the family during their rounds. None of these activities led to any resolution.

Both parents, Daryl and Rhoda, were assertive and wanted answers. The bickering between the doctors, with no one doctor or group taking the responsibility for the future directions, caused them great anxiety. They made the only reasonable decision that they could: they requested a conference with all the specialists present. They prepared a list of questions and asked each to give his or her opinion in front of the other.

> A conference of all your consultants can be helpful in complicated cases, especially if communication has been unclear.

The parents asked the specialists to state categorically what was known about Ari's condition, and what was conjecture. The neuroradiologist stated categorically this was not recurrent tumor. The physiatrist had just returned from a national meeting and said Ari's delayed speech could be due to a newly described syndrome called "cerebellar mutism, which could last up to one year. All the specialists seemed to agree that this was the most likely explanation.

The remaining month on the Rehabilitation ward was without conflict. Ari gradually improved with his occupational and physical therapy before going home. His parents provided the setting for ongoing enhanced communication and improved their child's day-to-day care. Their anxiety about the tumor growing back was allayed. Everyone was a winner.

So that not to infer that all HTUs have communication barriers, DeeDee in Oregon thinks that her center is "user friendly:"

My son has had JPA of the brainstem for over three years. I like the team approach that our doctors use and find it convenient and less stressful. We have the perfect doctor and MRI appointment schedules via Doernbecher Childrens & Oregon Health Sciences University Hospital in Portland. Perhaps how they do things here could be a model for others? It requires the clinic nurses to spend some time coordinating. Having everything done on the same day has been a blessing.

1. *We first go to OHSU for the MRI.*
2. *Then we walk to the oncology clinic.*
3. *We meet with the pediatric oncologist and our pediatric neurosurgeon at the same time (team approach). There can be four doctors in the room, which is great. Each has his unique perspective and "bright" areas.*
4. *They have already looked at the scans via shared server, and they can eye it and tell me how the MRIs look compared with past scans. We can go to another room and look at the scans together.*
5. *If what they have told me differs greatly from the radiologist's report, they notify me. The nurse faxes me the final report later that afternoon."*

DeeDee, Portland, OR

DeeDee also has positive advice for how to be an effective patient:

You have to be an advocate. You must clearly state what your expectations are and let everyone know how you feel. Be that squeaky wheel because eventually that squeaky wheel gets the oil needed to make the ride a little smoother. If you don't get what you want, try somewhere else. Don't feel embarrassed, intimidated, or presumptuous. When it comes to our family, we must fight for their lives as much as they do!

SATISFYING MY INFORMATION NEEDS

In the past, you didn't need to know a CBC (complete blood count) from an ICU (intensive care unit) or a lymphocyte (a blood cell that fights infection) from a ventricle (a hollow, fluid-filled cavity inside your brain). But now, this language is important. You need to be familiar with it so that you can communicate with your doctors and make decisions about your care. Your life may depend on it. A medical dictionary in book or online form is a good start. (See Chapter 3: Getting Organized.)

Bottom line: Ask questions. Getting clarification will empower you because you are actively helping the physicians present the best choices for you.

THE FIVE MANTRA RULE

Most of us want to believe that the medical system will take care of us. Many times it does. To ensure your satisfaction and best possible outcome, you must take some responsibility. Families who follow the "Five Mantra Rule" are usually more satisfied

> The Five Mantra Rule allows you to satisfy your information expectations.

with their care because they get what they expect. (See Table 7-3.) This Rule allows you to manage your expectations in your treatment journey.

Table 7-3 How to Find Out About Your Actual Condition - "Five Mantra Rule" -

1. Ask your nurse and house staff once a day, "How am I doing compared with yesterday?"
2. Ask your doctor for your "problem list."
3. Ask for results the day that the test or procedure is performed.
4. Do not accept "You are doing fine."
5. Do not rely solely on the nurse to "filter" or infer information from the doctor.

**1) Ask each and every day,
"How am I doing compared with yesterday?"**

Your question will not only enhance your care, but it also will help the fellows and residents become more than just technically competent doctors. One patient advocate solved her information and communication needs by having copies of her daughter's older scans to give to the doctors for comparison with newer ones:

CHAPTER 7
Academic
Centers

> *I am not sure that doctors in training know how to talk to patients. Nor do they truly know what we go through on a day-to-day basis. A week's wait for results is nothing to them; to us it is an eternity. My daughter has had 53 MRI scans through her illness, and I have copies of the ones that show any changes (23 and counting…in my closet). Also it is handy to have copies of her medical records, hospital notes, treatments, pathology reports.*

> Shirley, Evanston, IL

It sometimes astonishes me that a family can spend weeks in the hospital and not know from one day to the next how their loved one is doing. It's easy to be lulled into just being there and watching hospital staff come in and out. Ask and then write down the answers that you hear in the consultant section of your notebook.

2) Ask your doctor for your "problem list."

You are in the hospital to find solutions for one or more *problems*, which are part of your diagnosis. Ask about progress on *each* problem for that day. Problems are what your doctor writes about in his notes. This is how your doctor knows if you are better or worse. For example:

> You are in the hospital to find solutions for one or more problems on your "problem list."

- If there is increased pressure in the head or fever: What are the causes? How has this changed since yesterday? What have been the effects of medication?
- If a patient is not waking up after surgery, paralyzed, unable to speak, gaining or losing weight, vomiting, why? What is being done to help?
- If a patient's white cell count is low, what are his or her counts? Is the bone marrow (the factory where the blood is made) responding to build up the blood naturally?
- If there is an infection, do the signs point to it getting better or worse? Why did the doctor choose that particular antibiotic? Is it working?
- Is the patient's condition improving or getting worse? If getting worse, why? What are the plans for treatment?
- It would also help to ask your doctors and nurses for written information about your condition.

Pain: Often Missing From the Problem List

Make sure to ask about pain assessment, which is often missing on the problem list. In spite of being included in almost every oncology symposium, pain continues to be under-diagnosed in most hospitals. Inattention to it leads to useless testing, prolonged hospitalization, and unhappy patients.

> Pain is often under-recognized and under-treated. This can delay healing.

I was the attending physician for another doctor's patient, Veronica. She was a sad, four-year-old girl with leukemia in her brain. Her disease was stable on our therapies after three years of treatment, yet she was losing weight. She had no fever and did not complain to the nurses. Veronica underwent two weeks of unnecessary MRI scans, daily blood tests, and bone x-rays. The parents never mentioned that she was not playing with her brothers and sisters and hardly ever watched TV; she only poked at her meals. Knowing that these are signs of early depression from chronic pain, we prescribed a morphine liquid for her. Within two hours, she was playing with her family and sharing her Barbie dolls with a roommate.

If only the doctors had been aware of the pain problem. Had the parents advised the doctors of changes in their daughter's behavior, weeks of suffering and needless testing could have been avoided. The lesson is that patients, families, and advocates should report changes in patient behavior to the doctors, as it may alert them to a specific problem. (See Chapter 9: Medications for more information about pain.)

3) Ask for test results on the day that the test or procedure is being performed.

Do not wait for the next day out of consideration for the physician, at the expense of your own increasing worry. If he or she does not know the results that day, ask tactfully if someone could call for the results because you are anxious about them.

> Ask about the progress on each problem every day. Problems are what your doctor writes about in his notes.

Ten years ago in a famous hospital where I worked, the final x-ray report took days or weeks to get back in the chart. It was common that patients could stay a few extra days because of the delay. In most hospitals today, the x-ray can be seen on the computer screen within minutes after it is taken. The dictated report should be ready a few hours later.

> Do not accept "the report is not ready" or "not back in the chart yet."

Most blood tests are completed the same day. When your doctor makes rounds, ask for the results and an interpretation of what they mean. Do not accept "the report is not ready" or "not back in the chart yet." I can assure you that families who ask for x-ray or laboratory results are discharged earlier than those who don't.

Ask for copies of all reports before you leave the hospital. These are your results and you deserve to have copies of them. The mother in the e-mail below expresses her dissatisfaction with care and how she plans to get her needs met by speaking up and making her needs known:

> *Tuesday was clinic and chemotherapy for Stacy. We had to ask the doctor for the results, and she did not have them! And her MRI was seven days ago! No preparation at all...Hours later, while Stacy was getting her Irinotecan drip, the doctor comes back and says, "We got the results... there is a little bit of shrinkage... this is good news... any questions?" I had no questions... I was dumbfounded.*

How can you respond to that? I knew more than that by looking at the printed copy. Do most parents not care to know? I am really confused! I have been on these (e-mail) groups long enough to see percentages, statistics, and dimensions. Do other doctors not pass information along, or is this just a Missouri practice? I expect more than that and am disappointed. I assumed that they would set up the MRIs side by side so we can see the difference?

Next Tuesday, I will tell her oncologist what this mommy expects and needs from her. I have her MRI from last week. I can figure out size, percentage of shrinkage, and necrosis. Just a little bit of algebra and geometry...

Lisa, mother of Stacy, Kansas City, MO.
10-29-01 bsg, IMRT 11-02/12-01,

4) Do not accept "You are doing fine."
Ask about changes in vital signs and your specific problems. They are called vital because they are part of the information that your doctor uses to determine whether or not your condition is improving. Vital signs include temperature, pulse, breathing rate, blood pressure, and weight. They are yours. You have a right to know what is going on.

5) Do not rely solely on the nurse to "filter" or infer information from the doctor. The nurse is a very important team member, but her information can be secondhand and incorrect, especially if she is "floating" and not your regular nurse. Make sure to talk with the doctors, too. If there are any discrepancies between what two professionals say, do not accept this. Go further. Discrepancies may represent the effects of a change in medication dosage, the results of a new medication about which you were not informed, or the outcome of a new test or procedure. Ask immediately to speak with the decision maker (head nurse, attending physician) and get the contradictions cleared up.

My Doctors Disagree With Each Other

Doctors do not always agree on the right approach. Ask for explanations with pros and cons of each choice.

There are rare incidents of conflicts or miscommunications that have the potential to compromise your care. One class of differences that typically occurs among specialists at university hospitals is what I call "intellectual" differences within a particular specialty area, such as cardiology, surgery, or oncology. It is problematic when the family or patient interprets these arguments to mean that the doctors do not know the correct diagnosis or treatment. This heated discussion and "can you top this?" rarely occurs in smaller private hospitals.

You can spot these discussions on formal rounds when interns, residents, and fellows are all present. A telltale sign of this dynamic is when house staff members appear to tune out or close their eyes while standing, or the nurses leave to busy themselves elsewhere. Routine arguments occur over details of treatment such as:

- Prescription of an older, tested drug or a newer one
- Cause of rash due to drug or infection
- Dietary change
- Staying put or getting out of bed
- Staying in the intensive care unit or transferring to a regular ward

For these types of the problems, the answers remain elusive and the argument serves as an intellectual catharsis for the staff, despite the stress it places on the families who observe it. During these doctor's rounds, family members may be asked to leave or the doors may be closed while discussions take place in the hall. This is done to prevent unnecessary anxiety rather than hide anything.

Personality Differences or "Turf" Wars

Miscommunications or disagreements between doctors can also be due to personality differences or "turf" wars. Specialists in surgery may abide by certain rules of thumb that conflict with conventions held by experts in Internal Medicine. Or one of your physicians may be the "black sheep" of the department. This does not mean that he or she isn't competent. It just means that other members of the department do not know how to, or choose not to, communicate with him or her. All of this can translate into less than optimal care for you.

Doctor-to-doctor communication about your case may occur via written, documented notes in your chart, rather than face-to-face encounters in your presence. Unfortunately, many points cannot be effectively communicated in the chart, either at all or in a timely fashion. Use Table 7-4 to help determine whether or not your care may be compromised by conflicting opinions or poor flow of information. If so, take steps to resolve these problems quickly using the guidelines below under "How to resolve Communication Problems with Medical Personnel, Table 7-5.

Table 7-4 Assessing Communication Among Your Specialist Consultants

1. Do they initiate a plan to meet with you and discuss the problems and plans for action?
2. Do they arrange to present your findings to one of the hospital teaching conferences or to the Tumor Board if yours is a complicated case?
3. Are you informed of the results or opinions that emerge from these conferences?
4. Do your physicians make strong efforts to accommodate and be present when your nurse tries to arrange a time for a meeting of consultants?
5. Are your physicians at ease in each other's presence?

MY ROLE AND RESPONSIBILITY TO RESOLVE COMMUNICATION PROBLEMS

You now know that it's important to assert your needs. But can persistent requests for more information label you as a "troublemaker," "pushy spouse," or "difficult patient?" Could it result in less communication from your healthcare providers? Yes... and no. There can be a downside to being proactive if you alienate the staff. The key is to find the right balance. There are a few pointers on communicating with healthcare personnel that may make an enormous difference in the outcome:

- Manner and tone of asking for information: A direct, reasonable request is better than an accusatorial, whiny, or insulting one.
- Content of question: The content of your question must be related to a particular doctor's area of expertise. If it is outside his or her specialty area, then you need to ask the right physician for this information.

SIX STEPS TO OVERCOME COMMUNICATION GAPS

What if you have asked your questions, but they have not been clarified? Here are six steps to resolve the information problem, ending with an escape clause! (See Table 7-5.)

Bottom line: Use the Six Step process to resolve communication or care issues.

Table 7-5 Resolving Communication Problems With Medical Personnel

STEP 1	Identify one physician and one family member or friend to receive information.
STEP 2	Write down your questions. Make a direct, reasonable request with the content of the question relevant to the medical provider's area of expertise.
STEP 3	Request a discussion of your concerns with the attending physician in charge of your case.
STEP 4	Ask tactfully for another consultant.
STEP 5	Demand to talk to the Chief of Service at the hospital.
STEP 6	Get transferred to another medical center.

1. Identify One Physician and One Family Member or Friend to Receive Information.

Richard, a 30-year-old surfer with a recurrent glioblastoma, was enrolled in an experimental chemotherapy trial. There was both a divorce and remarriage within this family. Four people, all having the same last name and calling themselves the mother or father, were telephoning me for up-to-the- moment information on their adult child's condition. In addition, there were phone calls from five "grandparents."

In a case like this, to whom should the doctor give progress updates? Imagine the confusion when surgery, neurology, and intensive care unit specialist consultants were also being paged. This situation got quite out of hand when one family member heard that Richard was near death, while others heard that he was doing well!

Appointing one family member to receive information and having one physician who receives all the consultations and interprets them can solve most communication problems. If this is not working, go to Step 2.

2. Write Down Your Questions.

Within the next 24 hours, talk with family, friends, clergy, nurses whom you know, or a social worker to help clarify specific questions about your medical condition.

Make a direct, reasonable request with the content of the question relevant to the medical provider's area of expertise. For example, Melodie, wife of Steve, made the following list of "points" to discuss when they met with the doctor.

Melodie's List: To Speak With the Doctors on Rounds

1. Decadron	10. Physical therapy	19. Equilibrium/Ataxia
2. Temodar	11. Facial Numbness Droop	20. Fatigue
3. Last MRI	12. Right leg numbness	21. Mental Sharpness
4. Exercise	13. Left Side Weakness	22. Self-sufficiency
5. Work	14. Eyes/Vision	23. Voice/Speech
6. Health Issues	15. Nausea	24. Weight
7. Hearing	16. Appetite/Taste	25. Swallowing
8. Testosterone	17. Bowels	
9. Blood pressure/blood counts/thyroid	18. Headache	

Talk with the doctors when they make their rounds, using the written questions in hand. Not working? Go to Step 3.

3. Request a Discussion of Your Concerns With the Attending Physician in Charge of Your Case.

Do not accept anything less. If he or she is called upon to bring you up to date on your case, you can rest assured that the message will filter down rapidly to those who *should* have been responsible for communicating more effectively with you. Not directly addressing your concerns with the powers that be for fear of retribution allows shoddy medical communication to prevail, and this helps no one. Most of the time, Steps 1-3 will solve the problem.

Does your questioning receive a negative reaction from your consultant after repeated attempts to communicate? Go to Step 4.

4. Ask Tactfully for Another Consultant (or Attending Physician).

You can say, "We need a doctor with whom we can communicate better." This is not an insult to his or her medical knowledge; it's just an expression of need for a different *style* of communication. You don't need to apologize. There are good reasons to change consultants:
- Not being given treatment choices or a discussion of their risks and benefits.
- Dissatisfaction with the type of advice that you are receiving.
- Discomfort with the communication style.

Does the new attending physician delay communication or meetings with you beyond what is reasonable (hours to a few days depending upon the problem)? Go to Step 5.

5. Demand to Talk to the Chief of Service at the Hospital.

You are taking this step to resolve your information needs. If, at this point, you still cannot talk with anyone in charge to remedy the situation, you are in great danger! Go to Step 6.

6. Get Transferred to Another Medical Center.

Do not wait one minute longer! Talk with physicians at another hospital and arrange for a transfer. The institution is not meeting your needs. They will say that you are "leaving against medical advice." Ensure that you are well enough to travel.

Despite the best of intentions, miscommunications between physicians and patients can occur. Most can be cleared up with good intentions and communication on both sides. What is important for you is to find a solution that meets your information needs, while getting the best possible care.

Now we move on to the next chapters with more information about how a diagnosis is made, how medications are often given during this time, and lastly diagnostic and treatment information about your specific type of tumor.

Table 7-6 Internet Resources – Academic Centers, University Hospitals & Institutes Where You Go for a Second Opinion

Subject	Website or Contact
Brain Tumor Centers	http://virtualtrials.com/btcenters.cfm http://www.braintumor.org
Medical Dictionaries	http://www.nlm.nih.gov/medlineplus/ http://www.medterms.com/script/main/hp.asp
Accommodations and transportation services	
Transportation	http://www.braintumor.org/pservices/ lltransportation.asp
Financial Help of Hospital Hospitality Houses	http://www.braintumor.org/pservices/llfinancial.asp
National Association	The NAHHH provides housing and associated support services for seriously ill patients and their families in order to enable patients to receive necessary outpatient care. www.nahhh.org
Road to Recovery	Road to Recovery is an American Cancer Society service that finds volunteers to provide ground transportation to and from treatments for cancer patients in need. 1-800-ACS-2345 or www.cancer.org

Table 7-7 Major Pediatric Brain Tumor Centers

• AVAILABLE EXPERTISE   ¤ Not available

STATE	CONTACT INFORMATION	Row NEW PTS SEEN YEARLY	1 MULTIDISC	2 NEUROSURG	3 RADIATION	4 NEURO-ONC	5 REHAB	6 NEUROPSYCH	7 ENDOCRINE	8 TUMORBOARD	9 CLINICAL TRIALS
AR	**Arkansas Children's Hospital** 800 Marshall St, Little Rock, AR 72202-3591. WebLink: http://www.archildrens.org E-mail: lisenbykl@archildrens.org Tel: 501-320-1448	100	•	•	•	•	•	•	•	•	•
CA	**Childrens Hospital Los Angeles,** Neural Tumors Program, Childrens Center for Cancer & Blood Diseases, 4650 Sunset Blvd., MailStop #56, Los Angeles, CA 90027. WebLink: http://www.chla.usc.org E-mail: . jfinlay@chla.usc.edu Tel: 323-906-8147	100	•	•	•	•	•	•	•	•	•
CA	**Children's Hospital, San Diego** 3020 Children's Way, San Diego, CA 92123. WebLink: www.chsd.org Tel: 858-576-5811	30	•	•	•	•	•	•	•	•	•
DE	**duPont Hospital for Children** 1600 Rockland Road Wilmington, DE 19899. WebLink: http://www.nemours.org/no/aidhc/ E-mail: awwalter@nemours.org Tel: 302-651-5500	25	•	•	¤	•	•	•	•	•	•
GA	**Children's Healthcare of Atlanta at Scottish Rite.** 5455 Meridian Mark Road, Suite 400 / Atlanta, GA 30342. WebLink: www.choa.org E-mail: michele.drummond@choa.org Tel: 404-785-3515	86	•	•	•	•	•	•	•	•	•
GA	**Children's Healthcare of Atlanta at Egleston** AFLAC Cancer Center and Blood Disorders Service 1405 Clifton Road N.E. ,Atlanta, GA 30322. Weblink: www.choa.org E-mail: joy.johnson@choa.org Tel: 404-325-6252		•		•	•					•

STATE	CONTACT INFORMATION	NEW PTS SEEN YEARLY	1 MULTIDISC	2 NEUROSURG	3 RADIATION	4 NEURO-ONC	5 REHAB	6 NEUROPSYCH	7 ENDOCRINE	8 TUMORBOARD	9 CLINICAL TRIALS
IL	**Falk Brain Tumor Center at Children's Memorial Hospital** 2300 Children's Plaza, Chicago, Illinois 60614. WebLink: www.childrensmemorial.org Tel: 773-880-4373 E-mail: WAstellp@childrensmemorial.org	110	•	•	•	•	•	•	•	•	•
MI	**DeVos Children's Hospital** 100 Michigan Ave, NE, Mail Code 85, Grand Rapids, MI 49503. WebLink: www.devoschildrens.org Tel: 616-391-2036 E-mail: Albert.Cornelius@spectrum-health.org	30	•	•	•	•	•	•	•	•	•
MN	**Children's Hospitals and Clinics** St. Paul Campus 345 N Smith Avenue, St. Paul, MN 55102. WebLink: www.childrenshc.org Tel: 651-220-6732 E-mail: chris.moertel@childrenshc.org	45	•	•	•	•	•	•	•	•	•
MN	**Children's Hospitals and Clinics/Minneapolis Campus** 2525 Chicago Avenue South, Mpls, MN 55404. WebLink: www.childrenshc.org Tel: 612-813-5940 E-mail: chris.moertel@childrenshc.org	45	•	•	•	•	•	•	•	•	•
MO	**St Louis Univ, Cardinal Glennon Children's Hosp** 3600 Vista Ave, St Louis MO. WebLink:www.slu.edu Tel: 314-577-8026 E-mail: gellertj@slu.edu	60	•	•	•	•	•	•	•	•	•
OH	**Cincinnati Children's Hospital Medical Center** Department of Hem/Oncology/Neuro-Oncology, 3333 Burnet Ave, Cincinnati, OH 45229-3039. Tel: 513-636-7197 E-mail: Judy.Dothage@cchmc.org	60	•	•	•	•	•	•	•	•	•
TN	**St. Jude Children's Research Hospital** 570 St. Jude Place, Room C-2002, Memphis, TN 38105. WebLink: www.stjude.org/brain-tumors Tel: 901-495-3604 E-mail: braintumors@stjude.org	127	•	•	•	•	•	•	•	•	•

• AVAILABLE EXPERTISE ¤ Not available

174

Location	Institution	Capacity
TX	**Texas Children's Cancer Center/Baylor College of Medicine** 6621 Fannin, CC 1410.00, Houston, TX 77024. WebLink: http://www.bcm.tmc.edu/tccc/ Tel: 1-800-CANCER9 E-mail: helpdesk@txccc.org	75
TX	**UT Southwestern Medical Center at Dallas/ Children's Medical Center of Dallas** 1935 Motor Street Dallas, Texas 75235. WebLink: http://www.ccbd-dallas.com E-mail: Daniel.Bowers@utsouthwestern.edu Tel: 214-456-6139	85
WA	**Childrens Hospital and Regional Medical Center** 4800 Sand Point Way NE, Seattle Wa 98105. E-mail: russ.geyer@seattlechildrens.org Tel: 206-9872106	80
WASH. DC	**Children's National Medical Center** 111 Michigan Ave., NW Washington, DC 20010. WebLink: www.dcchildrens.com E-mail: tmacdona@cnmc.org Tel: 202-884-2800	150
CANADA	**The Hospital for Sick Children** 555 University Avenue, Toronto, Ontario. E-mail: james.rutka@sickkids.ca Tel: 416-813-6425	150
GERMANY	**University Clinics of Muenster, Germany;** Dept. of Pediatric Hematology and Oncology Albert-Schweitzer-Str. 33; 48149 Muenster, Germany. WebLink: http://www.klinikum.uni-muenster.de/institute/paedonc/ E-mail: paedonc@uni-muenster.de Tel: +49-251-83 47742	30
GERMANY	**University Hospital, Department of Pediatrics** (Hematology/ Oncology) Robert-Koch-Str. 40, D-37075 Goettingen, Germany. WebLink: www.humanmedizin-goettingen.de E-mail: lakomek@med.uni-goettingen.de Tel: +49-551-39 6239	100
SWITZERLAND	**Neuro-Oncology Program, University Children's Hospital of Zurich** Steinwiesstrasse 75 CH-8032 Zurich, Switzerland. WebLink: www.kispi.unizh.ch E-mail: Michael.Grotzer@kispi.unizh.ch Tel: + 41- 1 2667111	25

Table 7-8 Major Adult Brain Tumor Centers

Legend: • AVAILABLE EXPERTISE   ¤ Not available

STATE	CONTACT INFORMATION	Row NEW PTS SEEN YEARLY	1 MULTIDISC	2 NEUROSURG	3 RADIATION	4 NEURO-ONC	5 REHAB	6 NEUROPSYCH	7 ENDOCRINE	8 TUMORBOARD	9 CLINICAL TRIALS
AR	**Neuro-Oncology Program, University of Arkansas for Medical Sciences** Clinical Coordinator, Mail Slot 507, UAMS 4301 West Markham St., Little Rock, AR 72205-7199 WebLink. http://www.acrc.uams.edu E-Mail: davisstephena@uams.edu Tel: 501-686-6979	205	•	•	•	•	•	•	•	•	•
CA	**Doctors Medical Center** 2000 Vale Road, San Pablo CA 94806 WebLink: www.dmcweb.com E-Mail: brenda.shank@tenethealth.com Tel: 510-970-5239	44	*•	•	¤	•	¤	¤		•	•
CA	**University of California, San Francisco (UCSF)** 505 Parnassus Ave, Box 0112, San Francisco, CA 94143 WebLink: http://neurosurgery.medschool.ucsf.edu E-Mail: kunwars@neurosurg.ucsf.edu Tel: 415-353-7500	400+	•	•	¤	•	¤	¤		•	•
CA	**University of Southern Califonia / Norris Cancer Center** 1441 Eastlake Avenue; Los Angeles, CA 90033 WebLink : http://uscneurosurgery.com/speciality%20 centers/ neurooncology/neurooncology.htm E-Mail: chamberl@usc.edu Tel: 323-865-3945	100+	•	•	•	•	¤	•	•	•	•
FL	**H. Lee Moffitt Cancer Center** Dr. Steven Brem, Neuro-Oncology Program Leader, Suite # 3136, 12902 Magnolia Drive, Tampa Fl. 33612-9497. Web Link: http://www.moffitt.usf.edu/prevention_and _ Treatment/clinical_programs/nonc/ E-mail: brem@moffitt.usf.edu Tel: 1-800-456-3434, ext. 3929	1000	•	•	•	•	¤			•	•

State	Organization	Count										
CO	**University of Colorado Cancer Center** 4200 East Ninth Avenue, Denver, CO 80262 WebLink: www.uccc.info/neuro-oncology E-Mail: CancerCenter.Webmaster@uchsc.edu Tel: 1-800-621-7621	150+	•	•	•	•	•	•	•	•	•	•
GA	**Winship Cancer Institute, Emory University School of Medicine** 1365-C Clifton Road NE, Atlanta, GA 30322 WebLink: www.winshipcancerinstitute.org E-Mail: jeffrey_olson@emory.org Tel: 1-800-WINSHIP	250	•	•	•	•	•	•	•	•	•	•
IL	**Central Illinois Neuroscience Foundation** 1015 South Mercer Ave. Bloomington, IL 61704 WebLink: www.cinf.org E-Mail: rodas56@aol.com Tel: 309-662-7500	130	•	•	•	•	•	•	•	•	•	•
MA	**Lahey Clinic** 41 Mall Rd Burlington, MA 01805 WebLink: www.lahey.org E-Mail: peter.k.dempsey@lahey.org Tel: 781-744-8698	75	•	•	•	•	•	•	•	•	•	•
NC	**Duke University Medical Center** Box 3807, 4505 Busse Building, 4th Floor, Blue Zone, Trent Drive, Durham, NC 27710 WebLink: http://www.duke.edu/~sampson E-Mail: neurosurgeon@mc.duke.edu Tel: 919-684-9041	800	•	•	•	•	•	•	•	•	•	•
NJ	**The Brain Tumor Center Of New Jersey** Overlook Hospital, 99 Beauvoir Avenue, Summit, NJ 07902 WebLink: www.atlantichealth.org E-Mail: pat.eagan@ahsys.org Tel: 908-522-5914	60	•	•	•	•	•	•	•	•	•	•
NY	**The Brain Tumor Center at NYUMC, NYU School of Medicine** 530 First Avnue, NY, NY 10016. WebLink: www.nyuhospital.org E-mail: michael.gruber@med.nyu.edu Tel: 212-263- 6267	150	•	•	•	•	•	•	•	•	•	•
OH	**Dardinger Neuro-Oncology Center** OSU Medical Center and James Cancer Hospital 465 Means Hall, 1654 Upham Dr., Columbus, OH 43210 WebLink: http://www-neuro.med.ohio-state.edu E-mail: burkart-1@medctr.osu.edu ; or newton.12@osu.edu Tel: 614-293-8930	250+	•	•	•	•	•	•	•	•	•	•

STATE	CONTACT INFORMATION	NEW PTS SEEN YEARLY	1 MULTIDISC	2 NEUROSURG	3 RADIATION	4 NEURO-ONC	5 REHAB	6 NEUROPSYCH	7 ENDOCRINE	8 TUMORBOARD	9 CLINICAL TRIALS
	• AVAILABLE EXPERTISE ¤ Not available										
PA	**Allegheny General Hospital, Allegheny Neurological Associates,** 420 East North Avenue, suite 206, Pittsburgh, PA 15212 WebLink: www.WPAHS.org E-Mail: dcantafi@wpahs.org Tel: 412-359-8850	125	•	•	•	•	•	•	•	•	•
PA	**West Penn Center for Neurooncology** 4700Friendship Ave Pittsburgh, PA 15224 WebLink: http://www.westpennhospital.com/patient/services/ index.cfm?sid=65 E-Mail: rselker@msn.com Tel: 412-578 4340	53	•	•	•	•	•	•	•	2	•
PA	**University of Pennsylvania Medical Center** 3 West Gates Building, 3400 Spruce Street, Philadelphia, PA 19104 WebLink: http://www.pennhealth.com/neuro/services/neuro_onc/ E-Mail: Felderam@nursing.upenn.edu Tel: 215-746-4707	450	•	•	•	•	•	•	•	•	•
TX	**University of Texas Southwestern Medical Center at Dallas** 5323 Harry Hines Blvd, Dallas TX 75390 WebLink: http://swnt240.swmed.edu/neuro_oncology E-Mail: laura.danly@utsouthwestern.edu Tel: 214 648 4730	400	•	•	•	•	•	•	•	•	•
AUSTRALIA	**Sydney Neuro-Oncology Group** / Royal North Shore Hospital and North Shore Private Hospital Westbourne St, St Leonards, Sydney, 2065, NSW, Australia WebLink: www.snog.org.au E-Mail: snog@snog.org.au Tel:+ 61-2-8425 3369	222	•	•	•	•	•	•	•	•	•
CANADA	**Montreal Neurological Institute and Hospital** 2801 University St Montreal Quebec H3A2B4 Canada WebLink: www.mni.mcgill.ca/btrc/delmaestro E-Mail: rolando.delmaestro@mcgill.ca Tel: 514-398 5791	600	•	•	•	•	¤	•	•	•	•

	CONTACT INFORMATION	NEW PTS SEEN YEARLY	1 MULTIDISC	2 NEUROSURG	3 RADIATION	4 NEURO-ONC	5 REHAB	6 NEUROPSYCH	7 ENDOCRINE	8 TUMORBOARD	9 CLINICAL TRIALS
CANADA	**The Gerry & Nancy Pencer Brain Tumor Centre,** Princess Margaret Hospital 610 University Ave. Toronto, Ontario, Canada, M5G 2M9 WebLink: www.uhn.on.ca Tel: 416-946-2240 E-Mail: Maureen.Daniels@uhn.on.ca	300	•	•	•	•	¤	•	•	•	•
FRANCE	**CHU Timone, Université de la Méditerranée** 264 rue Saint Pierre 13005 Marseille FRANCE WebLink: www.ap-hm.fr www.cancerologie.ap-hm.fr E-Mail: olivier.chinot@ap-hm.fr Tel: + 33 4 9138 6569	500	•	•	•	•	•	•	•	•	•

Table 7-9 Adult & Child Brain Tumor Centers

STATE	• AVAILABLE EXPERTISE ¤ Not available CONTACT INFORMATION	Row NEW PTS SEEN YEARLY	1 MULTIDISC	2 NEUROSURG	3 RADIATION	4 NEURO-ONC	5 REHAB	6 NEUROPSYCH	7 ENDOCRINE	8 TUMORBOARD	9 CLINICAL TRIALS
AL	**University of Alabama at Birmingham,** Brain Tumor Program 510 20th Street South, FOT 1020, Birmingham, AL 35294 WebLink: E-mail: www.braintumor.uab.edu Tel: 205-934-1432	300+	•	•	•	•	•	•	•	•	•
AZ	**Foundation for Cancer Research and Education** 300 W. Clarendon Ave., suite 350 Phoenix, AZ 85013 WebLink: www.azoncology.com Tel: 602-274-4484 E-mail: theresa@azoncology.com (Terry Thomas)	400	•	•	•	•			•		•
CA	**Cedars-Sinai Medical Center** 8631 West Third Street #800E, Los Angeles, CA 90048 WebLink: http://www.web.csmc.edu/mdnsi Email: csnsi@csmc.edu Tel: 310-423-7900	400+	•	•	•	•				•	•
CA	**City of Hope Cancer Center** 1500 E. Duarte Road, Duarte, CA 91010 WebLink: www.cityofhope.org E-mail: amamelak@coh.org Tel: 626-359-8111	100	•	•	•	•				•	•

STATE	CONTACT INFORMATION	NEW PTS SEEN YEARLY	MULTIDISC	NEUROSURG	RADIATION	NEURO-ONC	REHAB	NEUROPSYCH	ENDOCRINE	TUMORBOARD	CLINICAL TRIALS
		Row	1	2	3	4	5	6	7	8	9
CA	**Stanford University, Neuro-Oncology,** 300 Pasteur Drive, Stanford, Ca 94305-5235 WebLink: http://www.stanfordhospital.com/clinicsmedServices/COE neuro/neurooncology.html E-mail: referral@stanfordmed.org Tel: 650-725-8630	140	•	•	•	•	•	•	•	•	•
CA	**University of California, San Francisco (UCSF)** 505 Parnassus Avenue, M-786, San Francisco, CA 94143-0112 WebLink: http://neurosurgery.medschool.ucsf.edu E-mail: bergerm@neurosurg.ucsf.edu Tel: 415-353-7500	300+	•	•	•	•	•	•	•	•	•
FL	**CyberKnife Center of Miami** 7687 North Kendall Drive, Suite 105 Miami, FL 33156 WebLink: www.cyberknifemiami.com Tel: 305-279-2900 E-mail: info@cyberknifemiami.com		•	•	•	•	¤	¤	¤	•	•
FL	**Memorial Healthcare System Comprehensive Cancer Centers** 3501 Johnson St, Hollywood, FL 33021 WebLink: www.mhs.net E-mail: ssundararaman@mhs.net Tel: 954-985-5879	250	•	•	•	¤	•	•	•	•	•
FL	**Florida Hospital, Neuro-Oncology Center # 249,** 2501 North Orange Avenue, Orlando, FL 32804 WebLink: www.neuro-onc.net E-mail: dr-nick@neuro-oncology.net Tel: 407-303-2770	300	•	•	•	•	•	•	•	•	•
GA	**The Emory Clinic** 1365B Clifton Rd, Atlanta, GA. 30322 WebLink: www.emoryhealthcare.org or www.emory.edu E-mail: timothy_mapstone@emory.org Tel: 404-778-5770	40 peds	•	•	•	•	•	•	•	•	•

• Available expertise   ¤ Not available

State	Institution															
IA	**Holden Comprehensive Cancer Center,** University of Iowa Hospitals and Clinics, Neuro-Oncology Coordinator, Dept.Radiation Oncology, University of Iowa Hospitals 200 Hawkins Drive, Iowa City, Iowa 52242 WebLink: www.uihealthcare.com/cancercenter E-mail: elly-hochstetler@uiowa.edu Tel: 319-356-7606	121	•	•	•	•	•	•	•	•	•	•	•	•	•	•
IL	**RUSH University Medical Center** 1725 W.Harrison St #821 Chicago IL.60612 WebLink: www.rush.edu E-mail: pkhosla@rush.edu Tel: 312-942-5685	70	•	•	•	•	•	•	•	•	•	•	•	•	•	•
MA	**Dana Farber Cancer Institute, Center For Neuro-Oncology,** SW430D, Dana Farber Cancer Institute, 44 Binney Street, Boston, MA 02115 WebLink: www.DFCI.org E-mail: pwen@partners.org Tel: 617-632-2166	400+	•	•	•	•	¤	•	•	•	•	•	•	•	•	•
MA	**Brigham and Women's Hospital** 75 Francis Street, Boston, MA 02115 WebLink: www.bwh.com E-mail: pblack@partners.org Tel: 617-732-6810	200+	•	•	•	•	•	•	•	•	•	•	•	•	•	•
MD	**Neuro-Oncology Branch, National Cancer Institute** Bloch Building #82, 9030 Old Georgetown Rd, Bethesda, MD 20892 WebLink: www.home.ccr.cancer.gov/nob/ E-mail: hfine@mail.nih.gov Tel: 301-402-6298	500	•	•	•	•	•	•	•	•	•	•	•	•	•	•
MI	**University of Michigan** 1914 Taubman Center/0316, Ann Arbor, MI 48109 WebLink: www.cancer.med.umich.edu/clinic/neuroabout.htm E-mail: pagem@umich.edu or ljunck@umich.edu Tel: 734-936-9071	350	•	•	•	•	•	•	•	•	•	•	•	•	•	•
MI	**Henry Ford Health System, Hermelin Brain Tumor Center** Department of Neurosurgery 2799 West Grand Boulevard, Detroit, MI 48202 WebLink: www.hermelinbraintumorcenter.org Tel: 313-916-1796	350	•	•	•	•	•	•	•	•	•	•	•	•	•	•
MI	**Karmanos Cancer Institute and Hospital, Wayne State University** 3990 John R. Rd. Detroit, Michigan, 48201 WebLink: http://www.karmanos.org/ E-mail: mlodej@neurosurgery.wayne.edu Tel: 800-527-6266; asloan@neurosurgery.wayne.edu 313-966-5007	492	•	•	•	•	•	•	•	•	•	•	•	•	•	•

AVAILABLE EXPERTISE • Available   ¤ Not available

STATE	CONTACT INFORMATION	NEW PTS SEEN YEARLY	MULTIDISC (1)	NEUROSURG (2)	RADIATION (3)	NEURO-ONC (4)	REHAB (5)	NEUROPSYCH (6)	ENDOCRINE (7)	TUMORBOARD (8)	CLINICAL TRIALS (9)
MN	**The Cancer Center, University Of Minnesota** 420 Delaware St. Se Minneapolis Mn 55455 WebLink: www.cancer.umn.edu Tel: 612-624-2620	80	•	•	•	•	•	•	•	•	•
MN	**Mayo Clinic** 200 First Street SW, Rochester, Minnesota 55905 WebLink: www.mayoclinic.org E-mail: boneill@mayo.edu Tel: 507-284-2511	993	•	•	•	•	•	•	•	•	•
MO	**Saint Louis University School of Medicine** 3635 Vista @ Grand Blvd., St. Louis, MO 63110 WebLink: www.slu.edu E-mail: bucholz@musu2.slu.edu Tel: 314-577-8797	150	•	•	•	•	•	¤	¤	•	•
NC	**Carolina Neurosurgery and Spine Associates** 1010 Edgehill Rd. N., Charlotte, NC 28207 WebLink: www.cnsa.com E-mail: michaelheafner@cnsa.com Anthony L. Asher, MD, FACS E-mail: asher@cnsa.com Tel: 704-376-1605 Tel: 704-371-5130	250+	•	•	•	•					•
NC	**Duke University Medical Center** Duke Hospital South, DUMC Box 3624, Durham, NC 27710 WebLink: www.cancer.duke.edu/btc E-mail: btc@mc.duke.edu Tel: 919-684-5301	800+	•	•	•	•	•	•	•	•	•
NC	**Wake Forest University School of Medicine** Medical Center Boulevard Winston-Salem, NC 27157 WebLink: www.wfubmc.edu/surg-sci/ns/btc.html E-mail: eshaw@wfubmc.edu (Dr. Ed Shaw) Tel: 336-716-4047	400+	•	•	•	•	•	•	•	•	•
NH	**Norris Cotton Cancer Center** Dartmouth Medical Center One Medical Center Drive, Lebanon, NH 03756 WebLink: www.cancer.dartmouth.edu E-mail: cancerhelp@dartmouth.edu Tel: 603-650-8939	90	•								•

State	Institution	#											
NJ	**NJ Neuroscience Institute** JFK Medical Center, 65 James Street, Edison, NJ 08820 WebLink: www.njneuro.org E-mail: njneuro@solarishs.org Tel: 732-321-7950	150	•	•	•	•	•	•	•	•	•	•	•	•
NY	**Beth Israel Medical Center** 170 East End Ave, NY NY 10128 E-mail: jallen@bethisraelny.org Tel: 212-870-9407	250	•	•	•	•	•	•	•	•	•	•	•	•
NY	**Columbia Presbyterian Medical Center** Room 434, Neurological Institute, 710 W 168th St., New York, N.Y. 10032 WebLink: http://cpmcnet.columbia.edu/ E-mail: jnb2@columbia.edu Tel: 212-305-7346	400+	•	•	•	•	•	•	•	•	•	•	•	•
NY	**Weill Cornell Medical College, New York Presbyterian Hospital** 525 East 68th St, Box #99 New York, N.Y. 10021 WebLink: http://www.med.cornell.edu/ E-mail: schwarh@med.cornell.edu Tel: 212-746-5620	500	•	•	•	•	•	•	•	•	•	•	•	•
NY	**University of Rochester School of Medicine** 601 Elmwood Avenue, Box 777 Rochester, NY 14642 WebLink: www.urmc.rochester.edu Tel: 585-275-5863 E-mail: david_korones@urmc.rochester.ed 585-275-2981peds	120	•	•	•	•	•	•	•	•	•	•	•	•
NY	**Roswell Park Cancer Institute** Elm and Carlton Streets, Buffalo, NY 14263 WebLink: www.roswellpark.org E-mail: askrpci@roswellpark.org Tel: 1-877-ASk-RPCI	200+	•	•	•	•	•	•	•	•	•	•	•	•
NY	**Upstate Medical University, Department of Neurosurgery** 750 East Adams Street, Syracuse, NY 13210 WebLink: www.upstate.edu/neurosurgery E-mail: paddenl@upstate.edu Tel: 315-464-5513	300	•	•	•	•	•	•	•	•	•	•	•	•
OH	**Cleveland Clinic Foundation** Brain Tumor Institute R20, 9500 Euclid Ave, Cleveland, Ohio 44195 WebLink: http://www.clevelandclinic.org/ E-mail: eClevelandClinic@ccf.org Tel: 216-444-3223	200+	•	•	•	•	•	•	•	•	•	•	•	•

183

STATE	CONTACT INFORMATION	NEW PTS SEEN YEARLY	MULTIDISC	NEUROSURG	RADIATION	NEURO-ONC	REHAB	NEUROPSYCH	ENDOCRINE	TUMORBOARD	CLINICAL TRIALS
		Row	1	2	3	4	5	6	7	8	9
PA	**Penn State Milton S. Hershey Medical Center** 500 University Drive, Hershey PA 17033 WebLink: http://www.hmc.psu.edu/neurosurgery E-mail: rharbaugh@psu.edu or jsheehan@psu.edu Tel: 1-800-243-1455	150	•	•	•	•	•	•	•	•	•
TN	**Vanderbilt-Ingram Cancer Center, Vanderbilt University** Medical Center, 21st Avenue South and Garland Avenue WebLink: www.vanderbilt.edu E-mail: reid.thompson@vanderbilt.edu Tel: 615-343-7558	275	•	•	•	•	•	•	•	•	•
TX	**The University of Texas M. D. Anderson Cancer Center** 1515 Holcombe Blvd, Houston, Texas 77030 WebLink: www.mdanderson.org/departement/braintumor/ E-mail: dbower@mdanderson.org Tel: 1-800-392-1611 ext: 27728	500+	•	•	•	•	•	•	•	•	•
UT	**University of Utah, Huntsman Cancer Center** 2000 Circle of Hope, Salt Lake City, Utah 84132 WebLink: www.HCI.utah.edu E-mail: randy.jensen@hsc.utah.edu Tel: 801-581-6550	125	•	•	•	•	•	•	•	•	•
VA	**University of Virginia** Box 800432, Division of Neuro-Oncology, University of Virginia, Charlottesville VA 22908-0432 WebLink: www.uvabraintumor.org E-mail: ds4jd@virginia.edu Tel: 434-982-4415	400	•	•	•	•	•	•	•	•	•
VT	**Fletcher Allen Health Care, University of Vermont** 111 Colchester Avenue, Burlington, VT 05401 WebLink: www.fahc.org		•	•	•	•	•	•	•	•	•

• AVAILABLE EXPERTISE   ¤ Not available

Location	Institution		Markers
WI	**University of Wisconsin Comprehensive Cancer Center** 600 Highland Ave Madison, WI 53792 WebLink: www.cancer.wisc.edu or www.uwhealth.org E-mail: uwccc@uwccc.wisc.edu Tel: 1-800-622-8922	100+	• • • • • • • • • • • •
CANADA	**Nova Scotia Cancer Centre** 5820 University Avenue, Halifax, Nova Scotia B3H 1V7 WebLink: www.cancercare.ns.ca Tel: 1-902-473-6000	200	• • • • • • • • • • • •
GERMANY	Department of Neurosurgery, University Hospital Eppendorf Martinistrasse 52, 20246 Hamburg, Germany WebLink: www.uke.uni-hamburg.de/kliniken/neurochirurgie E-mail: westphal@uke.uni-hamburg.de Tel: 49-40-42803-3750	450	• • • □ • • • • • • • •
HUNGARY	**University of Debrecen,** Medical & Health Sciences Center + County Hospital Miskolc Department of Neurosurgery and Neuropathology, County Hospital in Miskolc, Szenpeeri kapu 72-76., Miskolc, H-3501, Hungary WebLink: http://www.unideb.hu Tel: 36-52-411-717	15	• □ • • • • • • • • • •
ISRAEL	**University of Tel Aviv, Sackler Faculty of Medicine** 6 Weizman, Tel Aviv 64239, Israel WebLink: http://www.tasmc.org.il/main/index.ie.php3?lang=e E-maill: zviram@inter.net.il (Adults) Tel: x-972-3-697 4273 sconsts@netvision.net.il (Peds) Tel: x-972-3-6974686	450	• • • • • • • • • • • •
JAPAN	**Hokkaido University Hospital** North 15 West 7, Kita-ku, Sapporo, 060-8648, Japan WebLink: http://www.med.hokudai.ac.jp/~neusur-w/ E-mail: nob_ishi@med.hokudai.ac.jp Tel: 81-11-706-5987	150	• • • □ • • • • • • • •
NETHERLANDS	**Daniel den Hoed Cancer Institute** University Medical Center Rotterdam PO Box 5201, 3008AE Rotterdam, Groene Hilijdijk 301 3075EA Rotterdam, the Netherlands WebLink: http://www.erasmusmc.nl/ E-mail: m.vandenbent@erasmusmc.nl Tel: 31-10-4391415		•
UK	**Beatson Oncology Centre** Dumbarton Road, Glasgow G11 6NT WebLink: http://www.beatson.org.uk/ E-mail: r.rampling@udcf.gla.ac.uk		•

CHAPTER 8

Traditional Approaches to Diagnosis

One of the things I learned when my daughter got sick is that all cancers are different, all brain tumors are different and all patients are different. What is true for one person is often not true for another. Our daughter's prognosis was not good… I'll admit I was envious when we heard of others getting a more hopeful prognosis. It's been over 4 1/2 years and, thank God, my daughter is still here.

Allen, father of Rachel, in a chat group e-mail

TRADITIONAL APPROACHES TO DIAGNOSIS

Ensuring an Accurate Diagnosis

Imaging and Scans
CAT (CT) and MRI scans
MR-Spect and Thallium-Spect
PET scans
Myelograms and other studies

The Problem of Recurrent Tumor or Dead Tissue (necrosis)

Biopsy of a Brain Tumor
Role of the neurosurgeon
Role of the pathologist

Key search words

- diagnosis
- imaging
- MRI scans
- myelogram

- staging
- neuroradiology
- CT scans
- Neurosurgery

- physician responsibilities
- biopsy
- MRI

By now, you know that there is a "brain tumor problem." In this chapter, I present the big picture about how diagnoses are made. The main diagnosis, treatment approaches, and options for your specific tumor follow in Chapters 10-15. The actual professionals and their roles are described in Chapter 5. I highlight here the different elements of an evaluation (examination, scans, staging and biopsy) that allow your doctors to make an accurate diagnosis. You might want to read this and Chapter 9: Medications, before you go on to read about your specific tumor.

ENSURING AN ACCURATE DIAGNOSIS

Most people assume that if you have a tumor in your brain, then you have brain cancer. While true most of the time, this is not true all of the time. In order to achieve the most accurate, final diagnosis, collaboration among your primary physician, the neurosurgeon, and pathologist must occur. This chapter and Chapter 5 highlight the roles of each professional.

> Diagnosis is collaboration among your primary physician, the Neurosurgeon, and Pathologist.

The most frequent cause of an inaccurate or mistaken diagnosis is "diagnosis without biopsy." My motto is that a biopsy always should be obtained, unless it risks the life or function of a patient, which is rarely the case. In a way, doctors are victims of their own success. The MRIs give such detailed views of the brain that it is tempting to assume that cancer is the culprit. MRIs, however, can only give us black, white and gray images and suggest possible diagnoses. The e-mail below illustrates a common dilemma when no biopsy is performed:

> *My aunt was diagnosed with a terminal brain tumor (1cm. in size) in the left pons by MRI. She was told she had 3-6 months to live and was placed on hospice. She was given morphine, chemo pills, Dilantin, and many other medications. It was said that surgery could not be performed due to location of the tumor. Six months from the day she was told she was going to die, she was taken off hospice and almost all her medications. She is in better health than ever except she is still having seizures. Now she is being told by other doctors that what she has is clinically insignificant. She is questioning that she even has a tumor. My question is this: does she have a tumor or not?*

> Kevin, nephew of Raney. Fairbanks, AK

Kevin raises the same question that any consultant would ask in reviewing this history. There are many times in the professional life of any experienced oncologist when the impossible becomes possible. Without a biopsy, there is no way to know if the "tumor" is a bleed (stroke), slow growing astrocytoma (common form of brain tumor), metastasis, infection, or loss of insulation material called myelin (white matter) from unknown causes. There is almost no excuse for not obtaining a biopsy.

> The most frequent cause of inaccurate or misdiagnosis is "diagnosis without biopsy."

There are two situations for which a scan without a biopsy is usually accepted in making an accurate diagnosis:

1. A *diffuse* brain stem tumor in the pons (lower part of brainstem near the cord).
2. A brain tumor metastasis, when the primary site is known.

IMAGING AND SCANS

It's sometimes difficult to diagnose a brain tumor because its symptoms, like head pain, can mimic other conditions such as a sinus infection, migraine or tension headache. Vomiting can be due to not only pressure from a tumor, but also to intestinal upset, nervousness, ulcers, or Vitamin A overdose. Seizures can be triggered by recreational drugs, medication or alcohol. Weakness of a hand or arm, or speech difficulty, can be caused by a stroke, medication, or the after effects of a seizure, and so on. The persistence of any or all of these symptoms, however, points to a *possible* brain tumor.

To visualize a possible brain tumor in 1968, a person with symptoms such as Harold's (below) had a procedure called a pneumoencephalogram, which required general anesthesia and recovery in the intensive care unit. This involved placing air in the spine and fluid channels of the brain, turning the patient upside down and sideways, and exposing him or her to large amounts of x-rays to obtain a picture. About 1-2 percent of patients died from the procedure. Now, we order an MRI or CT scan and in 45 minutes, we have an almost perfect anatomical picture of all layers within the head. (See Figs 8-1, 8-2, and 8-3.) For a primer on interpreting scans, see http://www.med.harvard.edu/AANLIB/hms1.html.

> Scans only suggest a diagnosis. Biopsy is the gold standard.

The following e-mail captures the complexity of the problem:

> *My husband, Harold, has had a headache for three weeks now. His memory has declined. His visual acuity has declined and is worse at night than in the day. His neck hurts and he can no longer do more than one thing at the time. He has*

had an MRI, lumbar puncture and CAT scan. All are normal and the doctors think this is all due to side effects of his heart and cholesterol medication.

Harriet in Des Moines, IA,
sent to the Frequently Asked Questions at faq@virtualtrials.com.

Harold underwent the appropriate battery of tests that completely ruled out the possibility of a tumor as a cause for his symptoms. Fortunately, we now have powerful tools like MRIs from which possible diagnoses can narrowed down, eliminating the need for a brain biopsy and with no trauma to the patient.

CAT (or CT) Scan

A Computerized Axial Tomograph (CAT) is a scan that comes from an x-ray machine linked to a computer that produces a series of cuts or levels (cross-sections) in the brain. A special dye material called "contrast" may be injected into a vein prior to the CT scan to help make any abnormal tissue more visible. The CT scan visualizes the brain and its relationship to the bony skull (Figure 8-2).

MRI Scan

MRI stands for Magnetic Resonance Imaging. MRIs produce images without the use of radiation, unlike CT scans (see Glossary.). The MRI unit consists of a large cylinder-shaped magnet that excites water molecules, measures their motion, and transmits the information about their energy release as radio waves to a computer. The water molecules in each human cell respond to the magnetic force in much the same way as metal shavings are attracted to a toy magnet. Once the magnetism is released, the water molecules relax. The computer interprets these relaxing energy waves and produces clear cross-sectional images that can be layered on top of one another to create a three-dimensional picture. (Figure 8-1). See the following site for an MRI tour of normal brain and several tumors: http://www.med.harvard.edu/AANLIB/home.html.

MRI scans show the structure of organs, which translates basically to "size." Gadolinium dye, used for "contrast" or "enhanced" MRIs, is injected into an arm vein while the scan is being run. The normal brain has a highly selective "gate" called the blood brain barrier (BBB). It keeps out all but a few types of molecules. However, tumors break down the BBB so that larger molecules, like gadolinium, can penetrate. When gadolinium

> An MRI uses magnetic energy; A CT scan uses X-rays.

shows up in the scan, it means that the BBB gate is open and a tumor may be present, appearing as white in the general location of the tumor (Figure 4-3). Many tumors, especially low grade (less malignant) ones, do *not* break down the BBB or "enhance" (take up the dye). Infections do open the gate and enhance. Gadolinium can outline the tiniest blood vessels in the brain.

SPECIAL SCANS

What Is an MR-Spect?

An MR-Spect (short for spectroscopy) is an MRI scan that measures electromagnetic signals generated by chemicals inside nerve cells, acids from metabolism, and components of all cell membranes. This is in contrast to measurement of the magnetic relaxation of water molecules as in a standard MRI. Signals from dead cells reflect acidic constitution, while live tumor cells emit "call signals" more akin to brain cells. In this way, the types of signals are a marker for distinguishing between dead and live cells. Newer machines divide the tumor into small "boxes" called "voxels" and measure the differing content in various portions of the tumor. The scans, especially multi-voxel MRI-Spect are now used to locate the ideal location for the stereotactic needle biopsy. (See section later in this chapter.)

> Dead tissue (necrosis) and growing tumor can be indistinguishable on scans.

Chemicals Detected in MR-Spect

- N-acetylaspartate (NAA) is only present in neurons. Consequently, reduced levels indicate absence of neurons, or neuronal dysfunction.
- Choline (Cho) signal arises from the cell membrane (phospholipid metabolism). Increased Cho levels may result from membrane damage, or increased membrane production due to tumor cell growth.
- Lactate production is associated with acids that indicate necrosis, which is an important prognostic factor in glioblastoma multiforme (GBM). Telling the difference between tumor and necrosis can be difficult using conventional MRI alone, as both can show increased contrast enhancement.

> MR-Spect (roscopy) is an MRI that measures chemicals inside the tumor, not just size and shape of the tumor.

- A reduction in the NAA levels, associated with an increase in Cho and lactate, is indicative of a high-grade glioma.
- High lactate and little Cho suggest necrosis.
- All three signals will be reduced or absent in the case of an abscess, or infection, providing a useful guide to tell these apart.

Often, patients can be confused, because their physician has not explained what the results of an MRI mean to them. The following question that appeared on a website is an example of a patient who is not receiving enough information from her physician:

Can a diagnosis be made from an MR Spectroscopy? Impression is of a low-grade glioma in the medial posterior temporal lobe. There is increased choline and decreased NAA and an abnormal elevation of Myo-inositol. Please advise. Dr. requests a second opinion. Still don't know what is wrong.

Arthur, husband of Ruth, New York NY.

What Is a Thallium-Spect?

A Thallium-Spect is a nuclear medicine (radioactivity) test used to tell dead from live tissue. The principle upon which it operates is that radioactive thallium (which is similar to potassium) enters live cells, while dead cells do not take it up. It is nearly identical to a thallium-stress test of heart function. Instead, however, the camera is aimed at the head and the patient lies horizontally for 30-45 minutes while radioactivity is counted in different portions of the brain. A computer then makes an image of the brain with "hot" and "cold" spots based on radioactive counts. The result is used to clarify whether or not tumors seen on scans are active tumor or necrosis.[1] The test is about 85 percent accurate to tell dead from live tumor.

What Is a PET Scan?

PET means Positron Emission Tomography. In contrast to an MRI, which shows structure, the PET scan shows cell function or "metabolic activity" in different colors. In a PET scan, the dye is a radioactive sugar or amino acid (building block of protein), that tumors use for energy or growth. The PET machine follows the uptake of the dye and makes a color-coded map of the brain that shows which areas are taking up more nutrients (i.e. which areas are metabolically active or "hot"). In contrast to the MRI-Spect and Thallium-Spect, PET picks up a high background activity by normal brain, so it may be difficult for the tumor to stand out. Metastases usually light up well on PET.

What Is a Myelogram?

This is a picture of the inside of the spine from the neck down to the sacrum and coccyx. ("tail bone"). The myelogram today is usually an MRI or CT scan of the spinal cord. It is used to determine exact location and stage or extent of tumor

Bottom line: The MRI alone is about 80% accurate. Biopsy is the only way to know for sure.

spread to the spine (from the brain or anywhere else in the body). It is often requested before or after surgery for cancers such as primitive neuroectodermal tumors (PNETs), lymphomas, melanomas, germinomas, or metastases which tend to spread to the spinal cord. (See Chapters 10-15.) Choice of therapy depends on whether the tumor is localized (in one spot) or spread through the spine. Although previously thought to be rare, spread down the spine by gliomas can also be included since up to 15 percent of glioma long-term survivors may develop spinal metastases. This is true even for patients with low-grade gliomas and ependymomas.

In past decades, an oily or heavy dye was injected into the lower spine and patients were tilted in various positions to distribute the dye throughout the spine; then x-rays were taken (myelogram). Now, the same test can be performed painlessly using CT or MRI scan techniques with and without contrast (dye) enhancement.

Myelograms are interpreted by radiologists; but, again, experience counts here. My colleagues and I have seen many cases read as "tumor in the spine," but in reality, the "tumors" were blood spots caused by surgery or scar tissue and not cancer. Such misreading or "false positive," is unlikely to happen with experts who are familiar with this dilemma. Misdiagnosis could mean unnecessary spinal radiation and corresponding bone marrow compromise, at the expense of the patient's overall health.

> Myelography is used to tell whether tumor has spread to the spine.

Other Studies for Staging

Sometimes a spinal tap may be necessary if the myelogram is negative or inconclusive. A bone marrow aspiration also can be performed, if the specific tumor is known to spread there.

THE PROBLEM OF RECURRENT TUMOR OR DEAD TISSUE (NECROSIS)

A challenge for (neuro) oncologists is to determine whether an alleged tumor on an MRI is alive and growing or composed of dead tissue. This is problematic because intuition would suggest that a live tumor grows while dead tissue does not. Often this is not the case. The careful use of scan techniques provides accurate information 80-90 percent of the time. Scans have saved many patients from having unnecessary biopsies. Experts in Neuroradiology and Neurooncology are in the best position to help you. However, as Helen states below, no test is perfect:

With any technology, there are limitations and one must not conclude that any diagnostic procedure is the "be all-end all" solution. Even the most advanced technology, in the hands of the best and most experienced technicians, with the most modern and best maintained equipment, and interpreted by the most knowledgeable medical professionals, simply is not "perfect." They all have resolution limits; they are all subject to various sources of error. As the imaging techniques are observing a living being, and not an inanimate machine, each imaged subject is unique.

Helen, monitor of the temozolomide chat group; Dearborn, MI.

Radiation treatment can cause necrosis of tumor and normal brain by premature aging of small blood vessels. This reduces or cuts off blood supply, months to years after treatment. This is particularly common after higher dosage "boosts" from Radiosurgery to the edges of the tumor cavity, or after receiving high-energy proton beam radiation (See Chapter 17, Treatments.[2]) Necrosis can relax the blood brain barrier around it, which then shows more dye uptake and it appears similar to a live tumor. Furthermore, necrosis can "grow" because new small blood vessels try to reach the dead tissue, and, when enhanced by dye, this creates the appearance of a growing tumor. Short of a biopsy, other types of scans discussed previously in this chapter can provide helpful information. Often the combination of Thallium Spect and MRI-Spect examinations can lead to the correct diagnosis. Keep the following in mind:

> Necrosis (dead tissue) can "grow" and on MRI create the appearance of an expanding tumor.

- A high-grade glioma often has a reduction in the NAA levels, associated with an increase in Cho and lactate.
- Necrosis is often characterized by high lactate and little Cho, with little or no uptake on Thallium scan.

The e-mail below describes the value of the scans in producing a definitive diagnosis:

My father has a glioblastoma multiforme tumor...had three surgeries ... six weeks of radiation and five rounds of Temodar [chemotherapy]. He had an MRI after the radiation and the doctor told us that the tumor had grown significantly in size. It was a real bummer to hear that $32,000 of radiation treatment had no effect (my dad jokes that he wants a refund). Then, after two rounds of Temodar, another MRI showed that the tumor was stable.

After many efforts, discussions with insurance, and three different oncologists, we finally were able to get a MRI/MR-Spect combo for my dad. We had two

Oncs turn us down before we were finally able to get the third Onc to give us a MR-Spect. The first "hot shot" Neur-onc insisted that he had seen so many MRIs that he could just tell the difference. The recent results of my dad's MR-Spect showed that the enhancement seen earlier was in fact necrosis and not new tumor growth. They could not detect any cancerous cells in the original tumor location. I'm not sure if anyone has had as difficult of a time getting an MR-Spect, but it has taken us seven months.

Jill, Birmingham, MI

Another e-mail highlights the worry and concern by the patient experiencing unclear answers from his physicians:

Has anyone been told that black spots in the tumor are necrosis or dead tumor and actually have it be the case? My last MRI six weeks ago showed what the docs referred to as dead tumor. It sounded good at the time. I have had an increase in symptoms. My left eye is always tearing - dry eye - I can't shut it tightly - the left side of my mouth does not shut tightly, cannot blow up a balloon, and water skirts out the side of my mouth if I gargle. Hearing in the left ear is not that good. This functionality is all controlled in the area that is showing enhancement and dead tumor near the seventh nerve on the MRI.

I sent the MRIs back to the docs to review again to determine if it is dead tumor or new growth. This does not seem good and I am scared ... about new growth.

Peter Dx 08/00 BSG. Des Moines IA

BIOPSY OF A BRAIN TUMOR

The scans are precursors to biopsies. If a scan's results call for a biopsy, then a sample of tissue taken by an experienced neurosurgeon will be given to a pathologist.

ROLE OF THE NEUROSURGEON

The neurosurgeon must decide if a biopsy is necessary and safe. He then must decide from where to extract a sample of the suspected tumor. There are two approaches for the biopsy: stereotactic or open.

Stereotactic (Closed) Biopsy

A thin, pencil-sized hole is made in the skull and the biopsy is performed and removed through a special needle. Computer-assisted MRI scans and a special frame are usually necessary to pinpoint the area of the brain in question. MRI-Spect also may be used. Advantages of this technique include:

> A biopsy can be performed using a closed (needle) or open procedure.

1. Shorter anesthesia time (many are performed while the patient is awake)
2. Twenty-four-hour hospital stay
3. No incision to heal

Rare but possible downsides include:

1. Risk of too small a sample (not representative of the tumor) to make an accurate diagnosis
2. Bleeding during or after the procedure, requiring surgery to remove the hemorrhage
3. Additional MRIs and special frame needed to set up the computer-assisted navigation for accurate targeting

Click on the links to see how neurosurgeons use MRI scans to prepare for stereotactic biopsies (Table 8-2). No personal endorsements are made. (For illustration purposes only)

Open Biopsy

Experienced neurosurgeons remove a portion of the skull bone over the suspicious area of the brain; the biopsy is taken under direct vision or through an operating microscope. The intent is to remove as much tumor as deemed safe. Your neurosurgeon has many new tools to help: electrical mapping to avoid important areas; operating microscopes to make tiny areas visible; ultrasound to remove tumor and leave brain intact; scopes to peer through small incisions in the brain; and MRI scans in the operating room. The careful application of anesthesia, constant monitoring and use of appropriate medications to prevent brain swelling has contributed to making biopsies both painless and safe. In experienced hands, this procedure has less than a one in 100 risk of death, even in the sickest of patients.

Medicine and its related technologies have come a long way, particularly in the past 50 years. Procedures that once carried an enormous risk – like Neurosurgery – are now safer than most people think. Table 8-1 shows that deaths from surgery have

Bottom line: A biopsy that proves to be only necrosis is usually good news.

decreased dramatically, even in the past 20 years. The Table summarizes reports by several authors about frequency of death following surgery in children from 1930 to 1998. Adult studies show similar results. The best-known neurosurgeon of the 1900s, Harvey Cushing, had one-third of his child patients die within a week of surgery due to complications! I have been amazed and in awe of my neurosurgical colleagues, the majority of whose patients are up and talking within hours of major brain surgery. In fact, recovery from an open brain biopsy is usually quicker and less painful than an open lung biopsy.

ROLE OF THE PATHOLOGIST

After the suspected tumor tissue is removed, a pathologist examines it under a microscope; from this comes the final diagnosis. Like any other craft, precision and accuracy of diagnosis depends upon experience. For an accurate diagnosis, the critical factors are:

a) Skill of the neurosurgeon in identifying and removing the tissue
b) A tissue specimen that is fresh and intact
c) Sample size of the biopsy tissue to ensure that it represents the rest of the tumor
d) Skill of the pathologist who evaluates the tissue

There are more than 100 brain tumor subtypes. Distinguishing a tumor from "something else" and assessing the grade of tumor can be difficult for those with less experience. For this reason, and for all but the most clear-cut situations, I always recommend that a brain tumor be reviewed by a neuropathologist. This is a specialist within Pathology who not only completed three years of general pathology training but also an extra two to four years in the study of nervous system diseases. You may recall from Chapter 1 that even the most skilled specialists in Neuropathology disagreed on the exact diagnosis in about 25 percent of the cases in one clinical trial.[3,4] This uncertainty is not due to incompetence. It is a by-product of factors such as sample size and presence of dead tissue that results in a difficult or unclear diagnosis.

Now that you have the basic elements in understanding how your doctors arrive at a diagnosis of a brain tumor, move on to Chapter 9: Medications for Pain, Fatigue, Seizures and Brain Swelling and then Chapters 10-15 for detailed information about your tumor type. Go back to Chapter 5: Doctors and other team members for reference to the roles for each of your doctors.

Table 8-1 Studies of Deaths from Surgery for Brain Tumors 1930-1998

Author	Year	Death (%)
Cushing	1930	20/61 (32)
Spitz	1947	16/67 (24)
Newton	1968	11/35 (31)
Aron	1971	3/20 (15)
Mealy & Hall	1977	4/37 (11)
McIntosh	1979	11/85 (13)
Mazza et al	1981	4/36 (11)
Zeltzer et al	1998	-/400 (<1)

Table 8-2 Internet Resources for Diagnosis

Subject	Web Address
Basic Information	http://www.cancerindex.org/medterm/medtm13.htm
Interpreting scans	http://www.imaginis.com/mri-scan http://health.yahoo.com/health/dc/003791/0.html http://www.med.harvard.edu/AANLIB/hms1.html http://cpmcnet.columbia.edu/dept/nsg
Stereotactic biopsy	http://www.mssm.edu/neurosurgery/stereotactic/biopsy.shtml http://www.yna.org/new%20pages/sbb.html http://www.neurosurgery.com.au/pdfs/OPERATION/stereobx.pdf http://www.igneurologics.com/pages/biopsy2/tx.htm http://www.fns-inc.com/stereo.html (actual case)

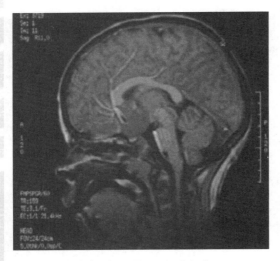

Figure 8-1 Side view. Tumor of thalamus

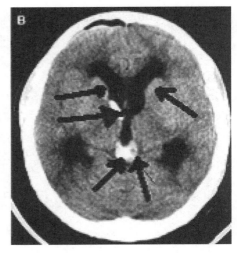

Figure 8-2 CT scan. Axial view (front to back). Arrows show tumor deposits in ventricles. White tumor takes up contrast.

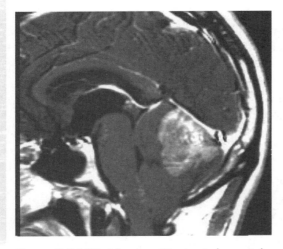

Figure 8-3 MRI side view. Contrast dye uptake (white-gray) in medulloblastoma in back of brain (posterior fossa)

CHAPTER 9

Medications for Pain, Fatigue, Seizures and Brain Swelling

Courage doesn't always roar.
Sometimes courage is the little voice
at the end of the day that says
I'LL TRY AGAIN TOMORROW.

David Bailey, Brain tumor survivor, musician

Key search words

- drug safety
- pain
- blood counts
- steroids
- dexamethasone
- medication errors
- anti-seizure drugs
- steroids
- drug interactions
- symptom relief
- side effects
- decadron
- fatigue

PROTECTING YOURSELF FROM MEDICATION ERRORS

This chapter introduces you to medications that many people take before and after surgery. Chemotherapy, anti-nausea drugs and antibiotics usually come later and those topics are presented in the companion book.[1]

The greatest danger in taking medications for your brain tumor is not the side effects of the drugs. Rather it is the possibility of an inadvertent medication error. Medical errors (the majority of which are related to mistakes in drug usage) are a public health problem: it is one of the nation's leading causes of death and injury. The Institute of Medicine estimates that 44,000 - 98,000 people die in U.S. hospitals and home each year as the result of medical errors. This means that more people die from medical errors than from motor vehicle accidents, breast cancer, or AIDS.[2]

The problem is not incompetent health care personnel; rather, good people are working in systems that need to be made safe. Your doctors are knowledgeable and responsible for timely diagnosis and recommendation of medications. However, errors occur when critical information is missing, such as additional medications you might be taking, drug allergies, other medical conditions. The theme behind this book is to help you become aware of information that is of vital importance to you, so you can team up with your physicians to get effective...and safe therapy. You must adopt a new set of skills to manage your own health. You know yourself best – your history, your hereditary health conditions, your current medications etc. – so only you can ultimately determine what's best for you.

> You are the CEO of your medical team. Your goals are to get the best care, make the wisest treatment choices, and prevent mistakes.

PREVENTING ERRORS WITH MY MEDICATION

In 2001, the Patient Safety Institute (PSI) was formed to address this issue on a nationwide basis.[3] PSI is a non-profit, consumer-oriented organization whose goal is to create a secure communications network that provides real-time access to key clinical information at the point of care and/or point of decision. PSI aims to link pharmacies, laboratory results, and physician records, so that when critical information is needed, it can be accessed. Until its goals are reached, you are principally responsible for keeping copies of your medical records and managing your health.

> Errors occur when critical information is missing.

Remember that you are the CEO (chief executive officer) of your own medical team whose goal should be to get the best care, make the wisest choices in treatment, and prevent mistakes from occurring. There are five simple questions to ask your doctor each time you receive a prescription for a medication:

> It is your responsibility to look out for your health and keep copies of your medical records.

1. Why am I on this drug?
2. What does it do?
3. What are its side effects?
4. Who is responsible for monitoring me while I am on this medication?
5. To whom do I direct inquiries, day or night, if I experience side effects?

BASIC PRECAUTIONS

When you are at home, before you take your medicine:
- Make sure that you are taking the right pills at the right dosage. Check the label.
- **Double check** each prescription to make sure that the medication has your name on the label and learn what the tablets are supposed to look like.
- **Do not** take them before talking with the pharmacist, if they are a different size, color, or shape from what you have had before.

> If your new prescription pills are a different size, color, or shape from what you have had before, <u>Do Not Take Them</u>!

Table 9-1 outlines an overall plan to prevent medication-related errors and enhance your care.

Table 9-1 How to Prevent Medication-Related Errors (adapted from[5])

Your Actions	Consequences- further action
1. Be an active member of your health care team.	Take part in every decision about your health. Those who are involved get better results.
2. Ensure that all your doctors know your weight & all your medications: over-the-counter medicines, prescription drugs, and supplements, vitamins, herbs, etc.	Once a year, bring your medicines and supplements to the doctor. "Brown bagging" your medicines can help you and your doctor discover any problems.
3. Inform your doctor of all allergies or negative reactions to medication.	This can help you avoid getting a medicine that can harm you.
4. Make sure that you can read the prescription that your doctor writes.	If you can't read the handwriting, your pharmacist might not be able to, either. Ask the doctor to print the drug's name.
5. When picking up your medicine from the pharmacy, ask "Is this the medicine prescribed by my doctor?"	88 percent of medicine errors involve the wrong drug or the wrong dose.
6. Ask for information about your medication in terms that you can understand – from your physician and pharmacist.	1. Name of the medicine. What it is for? 2. Is the dose appropriate for my weight? 3. How often do I take it? For how long? 4. Which side effects are likely? 5. What do I do if side effects occur? 6. Can I take it with other medicines or dietary supplements? 7. Which food, drink, or activities should I avoid while taking this medicine? 8. When should I see an improvement?
7. Ask about the directions on your medicine label, if you don't quite understand them.	Medicine labels can be hard to understand. Ask if "four doses daily" means every six hours around the clock, or just during waking hours.
8. Ask your pharmacist for the best device for measuring your liquid medication. Ask questions if you are not sure how to use the device.	Many people do not understand the right way to measure liquid medicines. Teaspoons vary greatly in capacity. Special devices, like marked oral syringes, help people to measure the correct dose.
9. Ask for written handout about side effects caused by the medicine.	You will be better prepared if something unexpected occurs.

DANGEROUS DRUG INTERACTIONS – FINDING INFORMATION

Knowing about resources that describe dangerous drug interactions can save your life. You can use the websites below to research your prescribed medications; see if any are incompatible with other over-the-counter or herbal agents that you may be taking or if there are any possible reactions that you might have to them. Most often, if you receive all your medications from one pharmacy, this will be done for you… but better be safe than sorry. Also, *natural, organic,* and *complementary* products can all interact with your prescription medications.

- http://www.nowfoods.com/index.php/Drug-Safety-Check/Home/cat_id/2534
- http://health.discovery.com/encyclopedias/checker/checker.jsp?&jsp Letter=B
- http://www.drugstore.com/pharmacy/drugchecker/default.asp?aid=333158& aparam=MSNFS_discountprescriptions

GETTING FINANCIAL HELP TO PAY FOR MY MEDICATION

Your insurance will pay for part, if not all, of your drug bills. You should keep receipts for submission or tax deductions. Major drug companies worldwide provide assistance in getting medications to those in need (Table 9-12). Many people are able to obtain medications free of charge by enrolling in a clinical trial.

MEDICATIONS AND SYMPTOM RELIEF

Now that safety issues are out of the way, I want to present specific information about the medications you might be taking before and after diagnosis and surgery. Symptom relief is my first topic, because it is the most immediate concern. Information about chemotherapy, prevention of its side effects, and antibiotics appears in the companion book.[5]

I want to emphasize three major areas:
- Relieving symptoms of pain and fatigue
- Counteracting inflammation and swelling
- Controlling or eliminating seizures

These "minor" discomforts can sap your energy, make you feel depressed, and not allow you to make the best use of the choices ahead. You must be proactive about getting effective symptom relief for three reasons:

1. You deserve to be with as little pain as possible;
2. Your doctor may not be aware that you have these symptoms;
3. Insurance companies and HMOs may not authorize treatments because of cost issues.

With regard to #3, health insurance organizations prefer that their doctors prescribe older drugs because of cost – $0.50-$1.00 per dose instead of $7.00-$15.00 per dose. They require physicians to fill out additional forms in order to make a "special" request. Insurance and HMO administrators do not understand that comfort is not a "minor" issue.

> Symptom relief medicines are not secondary or optional. They are critical to your success.

PAIN

Is It Normal to Suffer From Pain?

It's normal to have pain, but you don't need to suffer from it. Many physicians wrongly assume that because the brain itself does not feel pain, that pain is rare in their patients. Pain, as a complication of surgery or a by-product of disease, does not even appear in the index of two recent Neurooncology textbooks.[6,7] Yet, study after study, and regular articles in newspapers, document that pain is under-recognized and poorly treated. (See Tables 9-2 and 9-12.)

> Many studies document that pain is under-recognized and poorly treated.

Table 9-2 Possible Sources of Pain in Brain Tumor Patients

- Healing of sutures in the scalp
- Headache from inflammation, clearing of blood of meninges inside the skull
- Sutures in the skull from muscle re-attachment repair following surgery
- Headache and tension from jaw clenching
- Muscle-wasting from steroids
- Pressure on elbows, buttocks, or hips during bed rest
- Pressure on ligaments and bone due to loss of protective muscle tissue
- Hairline fractures after prolonged steroids, with or without osteoporosis
- Tumor invasion of bony skull and meninges

Myths That Allow Pain to Go Untreated or Under-Treated

Myth #1. Pain makes you tougher.
Wrong. Pain slows healing and depletes precious mental and physical resources that you need to get better.

Myth #2. Cancer patients will be addicts for life if narcotics are started.
Untrue! People do not become drug addicts from cancer pain treatment. Even if you need weeks or months of narcotics, slow tapering will stop the "addiction." If pain needs to be controlled permanently, so that living is worthwhile, then the side effects of drowsiness and constipation can be managed easily. Pain is not good for you. Appropriate and quick treatment will enhance your quality of life.

Pain Medication – The Right Type and the Right Dosage

A "pain ladder" is a guideline for increasing pain medications from the least to most toxic choices. (See Figure 9-1, Table 9-3 on drugs and dosages, and Table 9-12 on Internet resources.)

Step One – Tylenol and Advil are effective anti-inflammatory drugs for pain relief. If they do not work within one to two hours, however, then you need to march up the ladder.

Step Two – To find relief use compounds that are more powerful: Percocet, Darvoset, Percodan (contains aspirin). If these do not work, you would need to go up to the next rung of the ladder.

Step Three – codeine, oxycodone, and morphine-type medications. The highest level of Step Three analgesics come in long-acting oral forms or skin patches, so that dosing only one to three times per day is possible. Studies of chronic pain, dating back 16 years, show that adding a small dose of Ritalin (called an adjuvant) to pain medication at all Steps can enhance the (narcotic) effects and decrease any sedating characteristics.[8] (See Figure 9-1.) You can work with your physician in reporting progress of pain relief and inquire about what the next steps or choices should be.

> Pain does not make you tougher. Pain slows healing and depletes resources.

Bottom line: If you do have pain from any cause, it must be treated quickly and effectively.

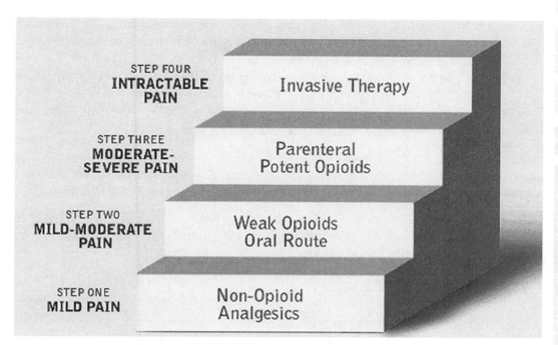

Figure 9-1 Therapeutic ladder for pain control. From World Health Organization. 1996. *Cancer Pain Relief and Palliative Care: Report of WHO Expert Committee, 3rd ed.* WHO: Geneva. Adapted with permission 2004.

The Pain Team

Most medical centers have a medical team that is dedicated to the assessment and treatment of pain. If you or your loved one has pain that is not being well managed, ask the doctor for a pain team consultation.

> Most medical centers have a Pain Team that is dedicated to the assessment and treatment of pain.

Do not wait for days to pass. If this is refused or disregarded, talk with the head nurse or chief of staff about your concerns. (See Chapter 7: Referral Hospital, effective communication sections.)

Avoiding the Side Effects of Narcotics

There are four major side effects of narcotics: sleepiness, slowed breathing, constipation and histamine release.
- Sleepiness can be relieved with an adjuvant, as above.
- Most doctors will start their patients on lower narcotic doses and work up to avoid slowed breathing. If you or your loved

> People DO NOT become "drug addicts" from cancer pain treatment.

one's breathing is dramatically slowed, there is an antidote called Narcan, which reverses the problem in less than a minute. Otherwise, skip the next dose and discuss the next step with your doctor.

- To prevent constipation, ingest four to eight tall glasses of liquid a day, prune juice, a fiber-rich diet, and/or daily Colace, a stool softener.
- Some patients will produce histamine when given morphine; this causes an itchy red rash; Benadryl can control this easily.

> Major side effects of narcotics: sleepiness, slowed breathing and constipation.

There are few conditions in which you may need to avoid narcotics: true allergies, blocked intestines, severe asthma, inadequate breathing, prostate gland obstruction, pancreatitis, and liver disease.

Table 9-3 Dose Equivalents for Pain Medications*,[9]

Drug	Usual starting dose for moderate to severe pain	
	Oral	Injection
Morphine	30 mg. q # 3-4 h	10 mg. q 3-4 h
Morphine,controlled-release (MS Contin, Oramorph)	90-120 mg. q 12 h	Not available
Hydromorphone (Dilaudid)	6 mg. q 3-4 h	1.5 mg. q 3-4 h
Oxycodone (Oxycontin) long acting	10 mg. q 12 h	Not available
Levorphanol (Levo-Dromoran)	4 mg. q 6-8 h	2 mg. q 6-8 h
Meperidine (Demerol)	Not available	100 mg. q 3 h
Methadone (Dolophine, other)	20 mg. q 6-8 h	10 mg. q 6-8 h
Oxymorphone (Numorphan)	Not available	1 mg. q 3-4 h
Combination Opioid & NSAID preparations		
Codeine (with aspirin or acetaminophen)	60 mg. q 3-4 h	60 mg. q 2 h
Hydrocodone (in Lorcet, Lortab, Vicodin, others)	10 mg. q 3-4 h	Not available
Oxycodone (Roxicodone, in Percocet Percodan, Tylox, others)	10 mg. q 3-4 h	Not available

Cautions: Recommended doses do not apply for adult patients with body weight less than 50 kg. Some combinations have added aspirin. Check with your physician for your dose.
q = every

RESPONSIBILITY FOR MONITORING MY PAIN

Any of your physicians can prescribe pain medication. At all times, whether in or out of the hospital, you must know:
- Which doctor will be responsible for monitoring your pain control?
- Who you should call for dosage adjustments.
- Who has the Federal "triplicate prescription" pads to order the narcotics?

Unfortunately, fewer physicians are choosing to carry the federal "triplicate" forms required to prescribe narcotic medications. This could be due to the fear of lawsuits, being sought out by drug addicts, or other

> Prevent constipation - 4-8 tall glasses of liquid a day, prune juice, a fiber-rich diet, and daily stool softener.

reasons. These forms are issued by the Bureau of Narcotics within the Department of Justice, and they require physician registration in order to protect against abuses. Ask your doctor if he or she has triplicate forms. And if not, who will prescribe the narcotic? Without them, there can be no prescription. In emergencies, some pharmacists will take a phone order for a one to two day supply.

> Know which doctor will be responsible for monitoring your pain.

FATIGUE

WHY DO I HAVE IT?

Tired, listless, sleepy, not wanting to move – these are all features of fatigue. It is different from muscle weakness and can have many causes. Fatigue is a signal from your body telling you that things are not right. Fighting fatigue could mean resting, avoiding fatty or fried foods, changing diet, or exercising. (See Table 9-4.)

Table 9-4 Causes of Fatigue With Brain Tumors

- Stress of anesthesia and surgery requiring time for recovery and healing.
- Brain injury or inflammation from surgery or radiation therapy.
- Poor nutritional intake and wasting away.
- Long-term use of steroids which break down muscle tissue.
- Prolonged bed stays.
- Depression that may require both talking and medication therapy.
- Low blood counts (hemoglobin).
- Response to chemotherapy drugs like Temodar.
- Recurrent tumor.

What Can I Do About Fatigue?

Many physicians are unaware of two medications that can be used to fight fatigue that's not related to other treatable causes: *Provigil* and *Ritalin*. Theoretically, your oncologist, neurologist, internist, or psychiatrist can monitor you on these anti-fatigue medications. I have included documentation of the value of these medications in case you need to convince your doctor or insurance company of their effectiveness.

> Fatigue is a signal from our body telling us that things are not right.

Provigil (modafinil) is a newer central nervous system stimulant, originally used to remedy excessive sleepiness. It can affect the metabolism of chemotherapy, anti-seizure medications, and some antibiotics. No clinical trials on this drug have been reported in people with brain tumors, but improved mood, wakefulness, and attention have been demonstrated. Adverse effects of modafinil are headache in 30 percent, nervousness, anxiety, and insomnia. Rarely does it elevate blood pressure or heart rate. With liver impairment, you should reduce dosage by 50 percent.

Ritalin (methylphenidate) is a 40-year-old central nervous system stimulant originally used to treat attention-deficit hyperactivity disorders (ADHD). It may help adult patients with malignant brain tumors by:

> Two medications to fight fatigue are Provigil and Ritalin.

- Alleviating depression and fatigue;
- Enhancing the effect of narcotics;
- Decreasing sleepiness with chronic pain;

In a study of mental functioning, 30 patients with malignant brain tumors received 10-30 mg. of Ritalin twice daily. Patients reported increased energy, improved gait, better concentration, brighter mood, improved motivation, and increased stamina. The majority of patients, who were on steroids and were able to decrease their dosage as a result of Ritalin intake, had no corresponding increase in seizures.[10]

In another study, 30 depressed patients received 10 mg. of Ritalin three times daily, increasing to 80 mg per day by week 2. Twenty-three of the 30 individuals reported benefits by Day 4 of treatment.[11]

Fatigue has also been shown to improve as a result of Ritalin. Six of 14 patients with advanced cancer who were given 5-30 mg. daily reported at least a 30 percent improvement in fatigue and significantly longer survival. Adverse effects were mild and reversible.[12]

> Patients receiving Ritalin reported increased energy, better concentration, brighter mood, and increased stamina.

212

Precautions in Taking Ritalin

Side effects are rare but can include difficulty in breathing; a fast, pounding, or irregular heartbeat; mood changes, agitation; confusion; uncontrollable muscle twitching; vomiting; sweating; fever; difficulty sleeping; or weight loss.

- Do not use Ritalin if you have had an allergic reaction, severe anxiety, tension, agitation, Tourette's syndrome, muscle tics, or glaucoma.
- You should also avoid Ritalin, if you take MAO inhibitors like Procarbazine (Matulane), Eldepryl, Marplan, Nardil, Parnate, or *possibly* Temodar.

INFLAMMATION AND SWELLING – STEROIDS

Aspirin (not to be used with chemotherapy) and ibuprofen (Advil) have anti-inflammatory effects, but steroids are much more powerful. People with brain tumors have a love-hate relationship with steroids, given the side effects that can literally drive you crazy. I answer more questions about steroids than any other medication. For this reason, here the answers to 23 of the most frequently asked questions about steroids.

WHAT IS A STEROID?

Steroids are a family of hormones (chemicals) produced by the adrenal glands (two pyramid shaped glands that

People commonly take the 4 mg dexamethasone tablets.
1.5 mg 4 mg 6 mg

sit atop your kidneys): one raises sugar levels to a stress response (cortisol); another can cause salt retention (aldosterone); and a third controls and modifies sexual development (testosterone, estrogens). Dexamethasone is the most powerful type of manufactured steroid and mimics the function of bodily-produced cortisol. Common brand names include Decadron and Hexadrol.

WHY AM I ON STEROIDS?

Your doctors think that your safety or function will be compromised without it. Steroids reduce swelling in the brain (cerebral edema) in the following situations:
- Before and after neurosurgery.
- During radiation therapy.
- If memory loss or arm-leg weakness is due to brain swelling (steroids can relieve these symptoms in hours or days).
- Anytime there is brain swelling.

What if I Miss a Dose?

- If you take two or more doses daily:
  Take the missed dose as soon as remembered, unless it is near time for the next dose. Then, take the missed and next dose together.
- If you take one dose daily:
  Take the missed dose when you remember, then resume your regular dosing schedule. If you do not remember until the next day, skip it.

Why Are Other People on Different Doses for Different Lengths of Time?

Dose ranges for dexamethasone, the most frequently prescribed steroid for brain tumor patients, are wide and responses are variable. Dosages must be individualized by severity, probable duration of need, response, and tolerance of side effects. Occasionally, patients may respond better to one steroid rather than another. Most patients take the 4 mg tablet. The available preparations in North America are listed below (Table 9-5).

Table 9-5 Dexamethasone Medications

Manufacturer	Tablet Size (mg)	Liquid
Merck	0.25, 0.5, 0.75, 1.5, 4, 6	0.5mg/5 mL
Par	0.25, 0.5, 0.75, 1.5, 4, 6	not available
Organon	4	0.5mg/5 mL
Roxane	0.5, 0.75, 1, 1.5, 2, 4, 6 Pediatric preparation	0.5 mg/5mL, 2mg/20 mL

Replacement and Treatment Doses

Each day, the normal adrenal gland makes about 20 mg of cortisol. "Replacement" dosages of steroids compensate for hormone deficiencies due to adrenal gland failure. "Treatment" or pharmacological dosages of steroids, which are higher, shut off normal secretions of cortisol and take over adrenal gland functions (Table 9-6). So your body stops producing cortisol when your taking steroids. That is why weaning off the steroids slowly (so your body can restart producing steroids itself again) is critical to treatment.

Table 9-6 Equivalent strengths for steroids (weakest to strongest)

Hydrocortisone	= 20.0 mg.
Prednisone	= 5.0 mg.
Methylprednisolone	= 4.0 mg.
Dexamethasone(Decadron)	= 0.75 mg.
Betamethasone	= 0.60 mg.

This means that ¾ or 0.75 mg Decadron is equivalent to the body's total daily production of (20 mg) hydrocortisone (a replacement dose); 12 mg of Decadron is *16 times* as much as is normally made in your body (treatment dose) (Table 9-6).

CAN I STOP THE DECADRON WHEN I FEEL ALL RIGHT?

The quick answer is no! Sudden death can occur if you have been on steroids and stop suddenly. Your body will run out of its reserve. If Decadron is stopped completely within two weeks of starting it, your adrenal glands will still make their own cortisol. The longer you are on Decadron, however, the more time it will take for your adrenal glands to begin making cortisol again. Cortisol production will not begin until dosages of Decadron are less then 0.75 mg per day.

> Sudden death can occur if you have been on steroids and stop suddenly. Your body will run out of its reserve.

It can take months to wean off high doses of Decadron. In addition, steroid supplementation may be required during periods of stress, as during an infection or surgery. With recurrence of symptoms (such as weakness, unsteadiness, memory loss), dosages should be increased and followed by a more gradual withdrawal. Obtain your doctor's recommended tapering schedule in writing… and follow it.

WHAT ARE THE SHORT-TERM SIDE EFFECTS OF DECADRON?

After three to four weeks of therapy, it's common to develop "chipmunk cheeks," a fatty hump on the back of the neck, and a larger belly, due to fat deposits. Stretch marks and muscle wasting are frequent. This is not a medication to be taken lightly (no pun intended). (See Tables 9-7, 9-8.)

The mother of John, a 29-year-old with a glioblastoma multiforme tumor, warns of the hazards of Decadron based on her son's personal experience:

"Mom... warn them about the Decadron! Weight gain is a real trauma." John had always been fit at about 170 pounds and 6 foot 3 inches. He started Decadron in September 2001 at the same time he started radiation. Initially, he lost weight so they considered Ensure supplementation. Come December, the Decadron kicked in, but we did not know that it would make his appetite increase. We were just so happy that he was eating again. Before we knew it, he had gained 60 lbs. He has lost some of the weight, but he will never be able to lose it all, especially with no more tag football, basketball, running, etc. His body image is shot with stretch marks from top to bottom. Had we known this was an effect of the Decadron, maybe we could have headed it off and not been so accommodating when he asked for food? We could have given him fruit instead of apple pie.

Table 9-7 Common Side Effects of Steroids

- Increased appetite, weight gain, indigestion, stomachache
- Difficulty sleeping, nervousness, meanness
- Fat deposits in cheeks ("chipmunk"), back of neck, belly
- Fluid retention
- Skin changes – stretch marks, acne
- Increased susceptibility to infection

Can Decadron Cause Diabetes?

Yes. When given for more than a few days, steroids may aggravate or uncover diabetes, especially in those who are "pre-diabetic," or in women who had diabetes when pregnant. Changes in dosages of insulin, oral anti-diabetic agents, or diet are often necessary.

Table 9-8 Less Frequent Side Effects of Steroids

Sugar diabetes	Stomach or intestinal ulcer (bleeding)
Osteoporosis (brittle bones)	Eye cataracts
Menstrual irregularities	Painful muscles
Slow healing of wounds	Skin rash, flushing
Behavioral changes, confusion, depression	Excitement , hallucinations, paranoia

What Are the Effects of Long-Term Steroid Therapy?

In addition to the short-term effects, sugar diabetes and protein breakdown and calcium losses in the urine are the most serious effects:

- Muscle wasting, muscle pain, or weakness.
- Delayed wound healing.
- Loss of the protein matrix and calcium in the bone – osteoporosis
- Fractures of long bones or vertebra in 25 percent of patients
- Necrosis of the femur (hip)
- Tendon rupture, particularly the Achilles tendon
- Kidney stones
- Diabetes
- Susceptibility to infections

Why Do I Get Swelling in My Feet and Hands When I Take Decadron?

The drug causes sodium retention, which pulls water into the tissues and causes edema, potassium loss, and high blood pressure. This can be counteracted with restriction of dietary salt intake. Potassium supplementation may be needed.

What Are the Effects of Steroids on the Stomach and Intestines?

Ravenous appetite is often the first side effect. Other effects can include:

- Nausea, vomiting, or anorexia, which can result in weight loss
- Development, reactivation, and delayed healing of peptic ulcers due to stomach irritation or acid in the esophagus
- Diarrhea or constipation
- Sense of fullness in the abdomen
- Pancreatitis

Can the Gastrointestinal Effects of Steroids Be Prevented or Treated?

Yes, they can.

- Antacids (such as Maalox or Tums or acid reducers (such as cimetidine (Tagamet) or ranitidine (Pepsid) can make you feel better.
- Gastric irritation may be reduced if steroids are taken immediately before, during, or after meals, or with food or milk.
- Caution: Antacids can prevent Dilantin from being absorbed. See interactions below under anticonvulsants.

What Is the Period of Risk for Bone-Related Side Effects?

- Bone wasting occurs in the initial six months of therapy.
- Decadron, 1 mg. or more, for six or more months leads to risk of bone loss and fracture.
- The risk depends upon dose and duration.
- Vitamin A can worsen and accelerate steroid-induced osteoporosis.

Which Lifestyle Modifications Will Reduce or Prevent Osteoporosis and Fractures?

- Limiting alcohol consumption
- Reducing or quitting cigarette smoking
- Engaging in weight-bearing exercise (walking, weightlifting) 30 to 60 minutes daily

Which Supplements Can Counteract Osteoporosis?

- Alendronate (Fosamax) with calcium and vitamin D supplements are used to treat steroid-induced osteoporosis. Talk to your primary doctor or endocrinologist about the pros and cons of alendronate or calcitonin therapy.
- Use the smallest effective dosage and duration of steroids.
- Calcium and vitamin D supplementation alone can be helpful.
- Sex hormone replacement therapy (HRT) is often advisable.

Why Do Steroids Make Me More Susceptible to Infection?

Steroids kill immune cells in lymph nodes (lymphocytes), so that they cannot circulate and secrete *interferons*, which stimulate other immune cells into action. This may make you more susceptible to both minor and major infections. For example, staph or strep bacteria in an infected pimple or tooth, ordinarily contained by the immune system, can spread to blood. When unchecked, shingles (Herpes-Zoster virus) can spread rapidly from the skin to the lungs and liver.

Can Steroids Affect the Nervous System?

Yes, but how they actually affect the nervous system is not understood. Common symptoms include:

- Headache, dizziness, insomnia, restlessness
- EEG abnormalities and seizures
- Elated feelings, mood swings, depression
- Anxiety and personality changes, including irrational behavior

> Steroids make one more susceptible to infection.

What Changes Occur In the Skin Due to Steroids?

- Vertical pink-brown lines of thin skin ("striae") on the abdomen or thighs.
- Incisions may take longer to heal.
- Acne on the face and shoulders.
- Increased sweating, darker and thicker hair, facial flushing, and easier bruising.

What Are Other Adverse Effects of Steroids?

- High blood cholesterol, hardening of the arteries (atherosclerosis)
- Blood clots (usually in the legs) traveling to the lungs. Steroid-induced blood clots are more frequent in patients with brain tumors.
- Patients who exhibit "allergic" reactions to injected steroids may actually be hypersensitive to the preservative paraben that is in some preparations.

When Should I Consult My Doctor While I Am on Steroids?

- At any sign of infection (fever, sore throat, pain during urination, muscle aches) or injury during therapy or up to 12 months after therapy

- When surgery is required, you should inform the physician, dentist, or anesthesiologist that you have received steroids.
- If edema develops
- If there are any other side effects that concern you

IMPORTANT MEDICATIONS AFFECTED BY STEROIDS

Before you take any additional drug, tell your doctor which prescription and nonprescription medications you are taking, especially aspirin, arthritis medication, anticoagulants ("blood thinners"), diuretics ("water pills"), female hormones (such as birth control pills), antibiotics, anti-seizure medication, and diabetes medication. Steroids can affect the blood levels of these drugs. Do not start or stop taking any medicine without a doctor's or pharmacist's approval. (See Table 9-9.)

> Steroids can affect levels of many other medications.

Table 9-9 Potentially Harmful Steroid Interactions With Other Medications

Therapy	Medication	Interactive Effects
Anti-seizure drugs	Phenobarbitol, phenytoin (Dilantin)	Reduces steroid levels
Antibiotics for infections	Ketoconazole and rifampin, amphotericin B	Increases steroid levels
Anti-diabetic therapy (grouped by drug family)	Diabinese, Orinase, Tolinase Glucotrol, DiaBeta, Micronase, Glynase PresTab, and Amaryl. Glucophage, and metformin. Glucovance. Actos and Avandia. Precose, Glyset, Prandin and Starlix.	Increase blood sugar
Anti-coagulation (blood thinner)	Coumadin or heparin	Unpredictable effects; requires careful monitoring
Diet or alertness drugs	Ephedrine, amphetamines, Ritalin, Ma Huang herbal supplement	May reduce steroid levels.
Hormone replacement (HRT)	Estrogens	Elevate steroid levels
Others	RU-486 and corticosteroids	Do not take with steroids
Anti-steroid	Aminoglutethimide (Cytadren)	Do not take with steroids

Nonsteroidal anti-inflammatory agents	Indomethacin (Advil)	Increases risk of gastrointestinal ulcers
	Aspirin	Bleeding, poor clotting paralyzes platelets. Steroids decrease aspirin blood levels. May induce symptoms of aspirin poisoning when steroids are reduced.
Potassium-depleting drugs (diuretics)	Thiazides, furosemide (Lasix), amphotericin B	Enhances the potassium-wasting effect of steroids. Serum potassium should be monitored closely.
Vaccines	Steroids may reduce the response to killed or live vaccines. Avoid contact with adults or children who have been vaccinated with live virus (measles, polio) within three weeks. Defer routine administration of vaccines or toxoids until steroid therapy is discontinued.	

WHO HAS RESPONSIBILITY FOR MY CARE WHEN I AM ON STEROIDS?

Usually, the physician who is responsible for your care is the one who originally prescribed the medication. However, if you continue taking the drug for more than a few months, it's possible that you may not still be seeing that doctor. Consult your current physician.

I have seen many patients on steroids for an extra three to six months or more because no one was in charge and automatic refills were obtained. Do not let this happen to you! Do not assume that your doctors know that you are taking steroids, let alone what dosage you are taking. Remember the 12 precautions for people on steroids (Table 9-10). Lastly, ask the following questions when steroids are first prescribed:

- "Who will be in charge of this medication?"
- "Who will be in charge of altering or tapering the dosage?"
- "To whom should I direct inquiries if I have a fever or other problems?"

Don't assume that your physicians will effectively manage either your pain or steroid medications. Get involved and be clear about their management. These are powerful drugs.

Obtain your doctor's tapering schedule in writing ... and follow it.

STORAGE CONDITIONS FOR STEROIDS

Steroids should be stored in a cool dry place. Do not store them in the bathroom. Moisture can affect their strength and shelf life.

Table 9-10 Twelve Special Precautions for People on Steroids

1. Take with food or immediately after a meal.
2. For once a day dosage, take in the morning before 9 a.m.
3. Do not suddenly stop steroids without your doctor's approval, if you have been taking them for more than two weeks. Reduce gradually.
4. Obtain your doctor's recommended tapering schedule in writing and follow it.
5. Report your entire medical history, particularly liver, kidney, intestinal, or heart disease; diabetes; high blood pressure; osteoporosis (brittle bones); herpes eye infection; tuberculosis (TB); seizures; ulcers; or blood clots.
6. Report if you are pregnant or wish to become pregnant.
7. Report if you experience vomiting, black or tarry stools, puffy face, swelling of the ankles or feet, unusual weight gain, muscle weakness, and pain in your calves.
8. Report injuries or signs of infection (fever, sore throat, pain during urination, and muscle aches) that occur within 12 months after treatment.
9. If your sputum (the mucus that you cough up) thickens or changes color to yellow, green, or gray, contact your doctor immediately.
10. Do not have a vaccination, or any other immunization, or be around any one who has recently received a live virus vaccination.
11. Limit alcoholic drinks, especially if you have a history of ulcers or arthritis medication.
12. Monitor your blood sugar level carefully if you have diabetes, as steroids may increase your blood sugar level.

> Don't assume your doctors know you are taking steroids.

SEIZURES & ANTI-CONVULSANT MEDICATIONS

About 30-40 percent of patients with brain tumors will have a seizure (involuntary movements, twitching or being "out of it" for moments to minutes) at one time or another. This has practical implications for employment, driving, and overall independence. "Anticonvulsants" reduce the chance of having another seizure.

Anti-Convulsants – How They Work

Anti-seizure medications tone down the electrical activity in the brain that sets off the seizure. Temporal and frontal lobe locations are more prone to seizures than the back part of the brain (cerebellum and brain stem). There are several classes of anticonvulsants to treat different types of seizures. Dilantin and Tegretal (carbamazepine) are best for "generalized" or Grand Mal (major motor) seizures, while Depakote (valproic acid) may be better for partial or focal motor seizures.

Reasons for Taking Anticonvulsants

> Anti-seizure medications tone down electrical activity in the brain that sets off a seizure.

You are on these medications for one of two reasons:
1. Treatment: You have had one seizure and are taking this medication to prevent another from occurring.
2. Prevention:
   - You are at risk for a seizure. Your doctors want to prevent you from having one.
   - You are about to have surgery and want to prevent one during or after.
   - Preservation of job, driving privileges, etc.

Once begun, anticonvulsant therapy is often continued for at least six months. If one drug does not control the seizure activity, then more drugs may be added. In many states, you cannot legally drive until you have been seizure-free for six months.

> You cannot legally drive until you have been seizure-free for six months in California.

There is controversy about using an anticonvulsant to prevent a seizure in a patient who has never had one. In patients with metastases who had never before had a seizure, investigators did not find anticonvulsant therapy to be useful.[13] The decision to use anticonvulsant therapy or not in this situation is a matter of risk vs. benefit. You should consider your physician's opinions on this matter. Many neurosurgeons routinely use anticonvulsants before, during, and after brain surgery to prevent seizures. They may stop the medication once they are comfortable that the period of risk for seizures has passed. The patient below is clearly in the dark about the effects and side effects issues of anticonvulsant therapy based on his interactions with his doctor:

I had a question about Dilantin. My father has a right frontal lobe glioblastoma multiforme tumor and no history of seizures. He went to a new neurologist who suggested that my father add Dilantin. The doctor said to take it… before you get a seizure, because this type of tumor often comes with seizures. So my family and I are wondering if anyone has an opinion about adding Dilantin. What kind of side effects are there? Are they worth it? My dad is currently taking 2 mg. of Decadron and 400 mg. of Temodar on the five per day for 23 days schedule, and a bunch of supplements.

Harold, London England.

AVOIDING PROBLEMS WITH ANTICONVULSANTS

Blood Levels

1. The blood (serum) level of anticonvulsant medication is too low and seizures recur. This occurs when too little medication is prescribed for a person's size, or the body is metabolizing ("digesting") the drug faster than expected. Other medicines or food can cause poor absorption. The resolution is to slowly increase the dosage and recheck blood levels. As a general principle, a drug should be administered to its maximum tolerance level before another is added. See Table 9-11 for a summary of anticonvulsant medication-related side effects.

> Medicines or food can cause poor absorption of anticonvulsants.

2. The blood (serum) level of anticonvulsant medication is too high and causing unpleasant side effects. Overdosing of anticonvulsant medication occurs in three circumstances:
   - Starting dose is too high.
   - Body metabolizes the drug more slowly than expected.
   - Other drugs are interfering with proper metabolism.

> Antacids (Maalox, Tums) can prevent Dilantin from being absorbed.

The solution is to lower the dose or spread out the doses over a longer time period (twice a day instead of three times a day).

SIDE EFFECTS

The side effects of anticonvulsant medications are unique to each one. For example:
- Dilantin can cause gum tissue to grow thicker if teeth are not brushed well. If levels are too high, then walking can become unstable.
- Carbamazapine (Tegretal) can cause low white blood cell counts, but not gum growth.

Interactions With Food, Chemotherapy, Steroids and Other Medications (Table 9-11)

Simple things like antacids (Maalox, Tums) can prevent the Dilantin from being absorbed. Many people take these for symptomatic relief of heartburn because they are also on steroids.

Dilantin also can have the unexpected effect of inactivating your chemotherapy. It has nothing to do with drug safety per se, but rather with the anticonvulsants' ability to induce the liver to degrade other important drugs, such as topotecan chemotherapy family (CPT-11, Irinotecan). The effectiveness of CPT-11 was found to be compromised in patients with brain tumors who were simultaneously on anticonvulsant medication.[14]

> Steroids and other drugs can affect anti-seizure drug levels in the blood.

It's altogether possible that in patients taking Dilantin-like drugs, serum levels of CPT-11 never reached effective concentrations. The aforementioned study is now being analyzed comparing the blood levels of CPT-11 in patients who are on or off Dilantin-like drugs. Many newer clinical trials will not allow patients to be enrolled if they are on Dilantin-like drugs.

> Some anti-seizure drugs *inactivate* chemotherapy.

RESPONSIBILITY FOR MONITORING MY BLOOD LEVELS OF ANTICONVULSANTS

The doctor who prescribes the anticonvulsant should be responsible for monitoring your condition, ordering serum level checks, and making dose adjustments. This could be your primary physician, neurologist, oncologist, or neurosurgeon. Anyone needing more than one drug to control seizures should be cared for by a neurologist who is experienced in seizure management.

Bottom line: The doctor who prescribes the anticonvulsant should be responsible for monitoring your blood levels.

Table 9-11 Side effects And Drug Interactions of Anticonvulsants

Chemical name	Trade names	Major side effects	Interactions with other drugs
Diphenyl-hydantoin	Cerebyx Dilantin Mesantoin Peganone Phenytex	• Gum thickening, Darkening hair, Drowsiness • Unsteady gait • Double vision • Constipation • Lymphoma (rare)	• Antacids (Maalox) or diarrhea medicines prevent its absorption, if taken within 2-3 h
Carbamazapine	Tegretal Atreto Epitol Tegretol Tegretol-CR	• Low blood counts Confusion • Restlessness • Pounding, slow heartbeat • Sun sensitivity	Can reduce or increase effects of these medications • Anticoagulants • Antacids • Antibiotics (Isoniazid (INH) • Corticosteroids • Estrogens, birth control pills • Pain medications (Darvon) • Heart medications (e.g., Verapamil, Diltiazem , Cardizem) • Monoamine oxidase (MAO) inhibitors (e.g., Furoxone) Marplan, Nardil, Matulane, Eldepryl, Parnate. Risperdal]— Risperidone effects may be decreased. • Tricyclic antidepressants (e.g., Elavil, Asendin, Anafranil, Desipramine-Pertofrane,Sinequan, Tofranil Aventyl

Levetiracetam	Keppra	• Tiredness, Sleepiness • Weakness • Difficulty coordinating muscles (abnormal gait) • Agitation & Anxiety • Mood changes • Worsening depression • Thoughts of suicide	
Valproate	Depakene Depakote		Can reduce or increase effects of these medications • Aspirin • Antibiotics • Herbals • Other anticonvulsants • Cholesterol-lowering meds Lamotrigine • Antiviral agents

Table 9-12 Websites for Medication Information

Patient safety institute	www.ptsafety.org
Medication error prevention	http://www.ahrq.gov/consumer/20tipkid.htm http://www.ucp.org/ucp_channeldoc.cfm/1/11/54/54-54/ 4276
Interactions between drugs	http://health.discovery.com/encyclopedias/checker/ checker.jsp?&jspLetter=B http://www.drugstore.com/pharmacy/drugchecker/default.as p?aid=333158&aparam=MSNFS_discount_prescriptions http://www.nowfoods.com/index.php/Drug-Safety-Check/ Home/cat_id/2534
Interactions between drugs, herbal, and dietary supplements	http://my.webmd.com/medical_information/drug_and_herb/ default.htm http://www.nowfoods.com/index.php/Drug-Safety-Check/ Home/cat_id/2534
Drug information	http://www.bccancer.bc.ca/pg_g_05.asp?PageID=22&Parent D=4 (Canada) http://www.bccancer.bc.ca/PPI/CancerTreatment/CancerDru gsGeneralInformationforPatients/DrugsWork.htm http://www.bccancer.bc.ca/HPI/DrugDatabase/DrugIndexPt/ default.htm www.virtualtrials.com http://brain.mgh.harvard.edu/ChemoGuide.htm
Medication access and cost-reduction information	http://www.helpingpatients.org
Discussions- pain & other symptoms	http://www.cancernetwork.com/journals/primary/ p9511e.htm http://www.cancersymptoms.org http://www.wellnessweb.com
Pain ladder	http://www.acponline.org/public/h_care/3-pain.htm
Pain treatment	http://www.acponline.org/public/h_care/3-pain.htm http://www.drugs.com/percodan.html
Morphine drug doses	http://www.stat.washington.edu/TALARIA/table10.html

Seizures	http://www.intelihealth.com/IH/ihtIH/WSIHW000/9339/10075.html
NIH drug information site	http://www.nlm.nih.gov/medlineplus/druginfo/uspdi/203051.html
Blood test interpretation	http://web2.iadfw.net/uthman/lab_test.html

CHAPTER 10

Tumors Originating In the Brain –
The Astrocytoma (Glioma) Family

In June of 2002, I entered my 13th year as a brain tumor survivor with a Brain Stem Astrocytoma (Glioma). My only explanation of this wonderful gift of time is that I have approached this disease with a "one-two punch," trying not to fold under at times from sheer exhaustion and this constant fight and always trying to beat it at its own game.

Sheryl R. Shetsky, Founder & President,
South Florida Brain Tumor Association

8— **Key search words**

- glioma
- oligoastrocytoma
- genetic analysis
- radiation
- heredity

- astrocytoma
- oligodendroglioma
- brainstem glioma
- chemotherapy
- metastasis

- glioblastoma multiforme
- anaplastic astrocytoma
- ganglioglioma
- tumor grading

GENERAL FEATURES OF ALL ASTROCYTOMAS AND GLIOMAS

WHAT'S IN A NAME?

Each year, about 34,000 people are diagnosed with gliomas in the United States. There are few things more confusing to patients and caregivers than the names that are used. They are called *astrocytomas* (astro-sy-TOE-mahz), or gliomas (glee-OH-mahz). Semantic difficulties are particularly common because one tumor can have several names. Just as a residence could be a log cabin or a brick house, mansion or a hut, a tent in the woods or an inner-city apartment, a glioma can be further named by cell makeup, pathologic grade or location. I suggest that you read Chapter 2, (The Basics), if you have not done so already, before starting this chapter.

> Astrocytoma and glioma are interchangeable terms for same type of tumor.

TYPICAL SIGNS AND SYMPTOMS OF GLIOMAS

Signs are objective indicators that doctors find during an examination, while *symptoms* are sensations or feelings that you have that do not seem normal. Signs and symptoms are always related to disruption of normal pathways in a specific location within the brain. For example:

- Tumors in the upper part of the brain (frontal, parietal, temporal lobes) often start with seizures, loss of motor (movement) control or feeling, or headache, depending upon location.

> Your symptoms always relate to location of disrupted pathways, not the type of tumor.

- Tumors in the middle of the brain may cause symptoms of hormone deficiency (thirst/frequent urination, tiredness, hair loss). Those near the optic pathway often cause impairment of eyesight, double vision, blind spots, and, rarely, bulging of the eye.
- Tumors in the brain stem (connection between the brain and spinal cord) start with arm/leg weakness, double vision, facial weakness, clumsiness or wobbliness (ataxia), but rarely headaches or vomiting.
- Tumors in the cerebellum (lower back portion of the brain) trigger headaches, nausea and vomiting (in the morning), difficulty in coordination of hand-eye movements, and unstable walking.

Facts I Need to Know About My Glioma or Astrocytoma

This section details the most frequently asked questions about gliomas that affect diagnosis and treatment. The topics below also are expanded in the individual sections for each tumor type.

Table 10-1 Basic Facts About Your Glioma Tumor

Cell types and family names

Tumor Grade: Possible areas of confusion and misdiagnosis

Location: Where is it?

Therapy choices

Cell Types and Family Names

Your brain contains about 100 billion nerve cells (neurons) that store memory, detect sensations, and tell your muscles to move. In addition, brain tissue has 10 to 50 times as many supportive and nutritional cells called "glia." There are two types of glial cells that give rise to tumors:

- astrocytes – These cells nourish and protect the neurons. (Tumors of this cell type are called astrocytomas or gliomas); and
- oligodendrocytes [o-lee-go-den-dro-sites] – These cells make fatty insulation (myelin) around nerves to prevent short circuits when electrical signals pass through (Tumors of this cell type are called oligiodendrogliomas or "oligos".

Mixed gliomas contain both astrocytes and oligodendrocytes, while a ganglioglioma (gang-glee-o-glee-o-ma) contains nerve cells and glial cells. The frequency of major astrocyte tumor types is illustrated in Figure 10-1.

Tumor Grade

Tumor (pathologic) grade refers to how abnormal (more or less cancerous) the cells looks under the microscope.

- Low-grade gliomas (grade I and II) look less malignant, closer to normal. These grow slowly and sometimes can be completely removed by surgery. Grade I tumors are sometimes called "benign" because of their appearance under the microscope. But they can still be life threatening, if located deep within vital locations such as the brainstem, or if they convert to a more malignant state. Some refer to this situation as "pathologically benign but malignant by location."

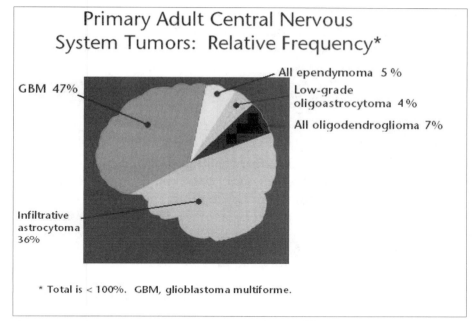

Figure 10- 1 Relative proportion of adult brain tumors[35.]

- High-grade gliomas (grade III and IV) contain cells with malignant traits, grow more rapidly and invade nearby tissue. Sometimes roman numerals may be used with a name and tumor grade. For example:
  - Juvenile Pilocytic Astrocytoma (JPA)- grade I astrocytoma
  - Anaplastic Astrocytomas- grade III astrocytoma
  - Glioblastoma Multiforme- grade IV astrocytoma

Location – Does It Make a Difference?

Yes it does.

> In children, gliomas are usually in the cerebellum. In adults, they are often in the upper brain.

- In the cerebellum the juvenile type "pilocytic" astrocytoma (grade I, low-grade), often found in younger children, usually can be completely removed with an excellent chance for cure. When the same tumor occupies valuable real estate in the hypothalamus, however, or in other parts of the brain, it's only partly resectable (removable) because it is intertwined with normal brain tissue.

- Low-grade gliomas of the brain stem in the pons are an exception to being benign. These tumors are dangerous because they are invasive, occupy valuable "real estate" and cannot be removed without severe consequences. Nonetheless, if it occurs just 2 cm (1 inch) lower in the "medulla" part of the brainstem (an *atypical* glioma), it is sometimes resectable and often is more responsive to therapy. (See section on brain stem tumors in this chapter.)

Possible Areas of Confusion in Diagnosis and Grade of Tumor

The type of tumor and its grade are critical as they determine exactly which therapies you will receive. If either is wrong, then you will not receive the correct therapy. There are many glioma "cousins," both pure and mixed, and sometimes they are difficult to distinguish from one another. Even neuropathology experts can disagree on exactly which glioma family a tumor should be assigned. (See Chapter 8, Diagnosis.)

Confusion or misdiagnosis often occurs for the following reasons:
- Grade 1 astrocytomas are slow growing and are wrongly called benign.
- Grade 3 oligodendroglioma also known as an anaplastic oligo (more malignant) can look like a highly malignant grade 4 astrocytoma, that is also called a glioblastoma multiforme or GBM for short. Treatment programs and prognoses for these two tumors are very different.
- Mixed glioma contains astrocyte and oligodendrocyte cells. It can be confused with an anaplastic astrocytoma (grade 3) and has a tendency to bleed into itself more often. The diagnosis is a reason by itself to get a second neuropathology opinion.
- Ganglioglioma is another mixed astrocytoma that contains cells that look like neurons (nerve cells) and astrocytes. It can look malignant to a pathologist unfamiliar with brain tumors, but usually it acts like a benign tumor. There is more information on this tumor later in the chapter.

> A "mixed glioma" diagnosis is a reason by itself to get a second neuropathology opinion.

INITIAL EVALUATION OF A PERSON WITH AN ASTROCYTOMA

Most physicians will use the following procedures to evaluate a patient with a suspected tumor:

1. A thorough history (medical and family) followed by a neurological exam.
2. Scans
   - Brain MRI (magnetic resonance imaging) with and without contrast is the most informative way to visualize the brain and tumor.

- MRI- Spect (spectroscopy) measures chemical components of the tumor. It can sometimes help distinguish the difference between low- and high-grade, or to tell whether the tumor is composed of live or dead cells-, after treatment. (See also Chapter 8: Diagnosis.)
- PET scan (positron emission tomography) is not commonly used at diagnosis, though it can measure the activity or the metabolic rate of the tumor and detect metastases.

3. An eye examination by an ophthalmologist (eye doctor), who evaluates "visual fields". This is important for children and adults with parietal lobe, midbrain and optic pathway tumors.
4. *Neuropsychological testing* identifies problems in different areas of higher brain function. Once specific problems are found, appropriate rehabilitation or counseling can begin. (See Chapter 5: Doctors and other Team members; and Chapter 17: Side and After Effects of Brain Tumors.[1])
5. An EEG (electroencephalogram, or brain wave test), if the patient has had actual or suspected seizures (convulsions). The electrical activity of different parts of the brain is recorded through small wires that adhere to the outside of the scalp.
6. Evaluation by a multidisciplinary team. (See Chapter 5: Team.)
7. An "open" or "closed" biopsy. (See Chapter 8: Diagnosis.)

The Outlook for Survival

The most important elements in predicting a successful result are the following:
- Tumor type, grade, and location
- Your age
- Amount of tumor that remains after surgery (i.e., skill of neurosurgeon)
- Choice of therapy and your response to it

People with lower-grade tumors typically live longer than those people with higher-grade tumors. But I have patients who are alive five and 10 years later with highly malignant tumors. Yes, having any brain tumor is a serious diagnosis, but being in expert hands can increase your chances for survival. That is why you have invested time in obtaining more knowledge. (See Chapter 6: Experts and second opinions.)

Remember, no matter how severe the situation, no physician or other person can predict the outcome of your treatment. We know how to make predictions for populations, but never for individual patients.

The Decision to Operate

Options to Try Before Deciding on Surgery

The option to have surgery, or not, depends upon the severity of your symptoms. Emergency neurosurgery to remove pressure on the brain can be lifesaving. After any emergency is resolved, there is usually time to get different opinions.

I recommend that you ask your doctors to present your case to the Tumor Board of the hospital with which your neurosurgeon is associated. Then, a team of different specialists can offer suggestions for the next series of treatments. When an aggressive tumor, such as a *glioblastoma multiforme*, has spread to the opposite side, additional surgery may not improve chances of longer life. In the case of a lower-grade tumor, however, the Tumor Board may recommend additional surgery and other treatment. Presentation to the Tumor Board usually occurs after the surgery, but it may also take place beforehand. Additionally, you can obtain consultation at any major medical center that specializes in treatment of brain tumors. (See Chapter 6: Experts and Second Opinions.)

> Successful therapy, especially surgery to remove the low-grade tumor, is equally dependent upon location, tumor type, and skill of the neurosurgeon.

Observation Without Surgery

A biopsy should be performed to determine which kind of tumor you have, except for highly unusual and rare circumstances. On an MRI scan, for example, a nervous system *lymphoma* (tumor of lymph nodes) can easily be confused with a *glioblastoma multiforme* tumor. Furthermore, blood vessels growing around dead tissue (*necrosis*), a result of previous treatment, can have the appearance of a growing tumor. A "closed" needle biopsy or open skull surgery usually removes enough tumor to make an accurate diagnosis.

> Tumor Board presentation could result in additional recommendations or alternative treatments.

Nonetheless, people for whom observation alone *could* be considered include:
1. Those with known or probable low-grade gliomas, few symptoms, and little or no swelling in adjacent brain areas as shown by MRI scan
2. Patients with mild or minimal symptoms who have had a glioma for many years without (negative) effect on their quality of life
3. Older patients who are experiencing seizures that can be controlled with medication or who have very slowly-progressing symptoms

Bottom line: In almost every circumstance, no treatment should start before biopsy proof that cancer exists.

4. Patients for whom surgery carries a very significant risk
5. Patients with the following conditions:
   - Acoustic neuroma, tumor of the "hearing nerve" (See also Chapter12)
   - Neurofibromatosis (NF-1, a genetic condition with tumors of nerves in the arms, legs, spine or brain) (See Chapter 24: Heredity and other causes of brain tumors in the companion book.[2])
   - Solitary glioma of the optic nerve that has not significantly affected vision
6. Patients choosing not to have surgery after being presented with the options

The Role of Neurosurgery for a Glioma

Surgery is important as initial therapy for at least three reasons:
1. To preserve or improve your neurological function
2. To obtain a piece of the tumor to confirm the diagnosis (biopsy)
3. To completely or partially remove the tumor

Even though the goal of surgery is to remove the tumor, the first priority is to preserve – or to improve – your neurological function. When total removal of the tumor carries significant risk of *morbidity* (any side effect that can decrease quality of life), it's better to leave some tumor behind. For a low-grade glioma, the patient could be observed over time; in some patients, the tumor may remain stable (without growing) indefinitely. In other situations where the tumor is located in a critical area, surgery might occur at a future date after radiation therapy or chemotherapy has shrunk it.

It is important to know that removing most of the tumor (90+ percent), when possible and without causing harm, often allows people to live longer than when the glioma is incompletely removed. Removal of lesser amounts of tumor usually does not affect long-term survival. The extent of removal often rests on the differences in skill among neurosurgeons. (See Chapter 5: Doctors and Other Team Members and Chapter 17: Traditional Treatments.)

LOWER GRADE GLIOMAS – SPECIAL CONSIDERATIONS

ARE THEY DIFFERENT IN ADULTS AND CHILDREN?

- Adults frequently have low-grade astrocytomas in the upper part of the brain – in the frontal, parietal, and temporal lobes.
- Children are more likely to have tumor in the cerebellum, in the lower/ back part of the brain close to the spinal cord. (The cerebellum coordinates muscle movements).
- Location – Gliomas can also occur in the midbrain and hypothalamus (an area that controls hormone regulation), and in front of, behind, and within the optic (sight) pathway that includes the optic nerve (MRI Figure 10-2). (See Chapter 2: Basics, for understanding the functions that these areas control) and Figures 2-1 and 2-2, in Chapter 2 that show differences in brain tumor types between adults and children.

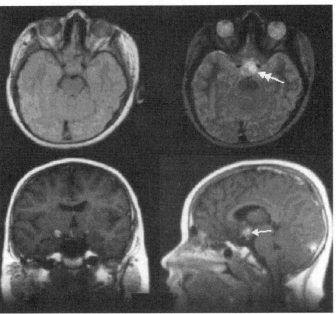

Figure 10-2 Shows an MRI of Midbrain or hypothalamic tumor.

RADIATION THERAPY FOR LOW-GRADE GLIOMAS. WHEN AND WHERE?

If further surgery is not advised, there are generally no clear-cut choices. This is when decision-making becomes complex and input from different specialists or a Tumor Board evaluation can be helpful. The recommendation of radiation therapy for low-grade gliomas is common and will cause tumors to shrink in one-third of patients; have no effect in another third; and the tumors will grow in yet another third. We are only beginning to identify who might benefit from radiation therapy.[3] Thus, many centers offer alternative experimental options such as reduced radiation or chemotherapy[4] or immunotherapy. (See Chapter 21: Clinical Trials.)

There is still major controversy whether giving radiation therapy before or after surgery or waiting for regrowth of a low-grade glioma (any kind) is the better alternative.[5,6] There is also increasing evidence that radiation can lead to significant brain damage and impairment in the very young and elderly.[7,8] The pros and cons of radiation therapy, chemotherapy, and newer experimental medications can be found in Chapter 17:Treatment and Chapter 21: Clinical Trials.

> Radiation therapy for low-grade tumors should be discussed with a brain tumor expert.

A recent analysis of radiation for some low-grade gliomas calls into question its role in improving survival.[9] There was no convincing evidence that it either improved survival or that higher vs. lower doses were more effective in children. Furthermore, 26 percent of the pathology diagnoses in this low-grade glioma group were inconsistent and varied among pathologists.[10]

CHEMOTHERAPY FOR LOW-GRADE GLIOMAS? IS THERE A ROLE?

Chemotherapy also will be discussed for each tumor subtype in separate sections. To mitigate possible collateral damage and long-term side-effects of radiation in both the young child and adult, many investigators at major brain tumor treatment centers are using chemotherapies such as Temodar (temozolomide) alone or in combination with vincristine-carboplatin, procarbazine, CCNU - lomustine, and vincristine (PCV), or high-dose Vitamin A for example.[11] In adults, my colleagues and I have observed that chemotherapy alone can shrink or stabilize low-grade gliomas in 25-50 percent of patients. Stabilizing low-grade tumors as a goal is a relatively new concept. Chemotherapy can be used to:

- Control tumor growth and shrink the tumor enough to allow for later surgical removal.
- Limit the field of radiation needed (controversial).
- Postpone radiation treatment until a later date, especially in children. (See Chapter 21: Clinical Trials.)

SPECIAL CONSIDERATIONS AND LOCATIONS

Low-Grade Gliomas and "Benign" in Appearance to the Pathologist

The *benign* diagnosis is not always predictive of how quickly an individual tumor may grow. These tumors are unpredictable, and it's imperative that you receive counsel from an experienced team regarding choices of treatment. Neurosurgery, radiation, and chemotherapy can all play a role in therapy, and the best choices are not always clear. There are trade-offs in long-term side effects on brain function, pituitary gland function, and vision. In general, survival for low-grade gliomas is good.

Low-Grade Midbrain or Optic Pathway Tumors

Problems with vision due to pressure on either of the optic nerves or the pituitary gland are possible. Tumors in front of the area where the optic nerves cross (called the optic chiasm) are usually slower growing than those situated behind the chiasm. Tumors along the optic nerves themselves (optic nerve gliomas) are often found in children and young adults with neurofibromatosis type 1 (NF-1); these tend to be slower growing. (See Chapter 24: Heredity and other causes of brain tumors.) The vignette below is typical of the treatment for a low-grade glioma and highlights both the success and long-term challenges (Figure 10-2).

Michael is six years old and has tumor on the right midbrain, optic tract, hypothalamus just over the brainstem. It was 5.5 cm. at diagnosis and the first resection got about 60 percent and 18 months of chemotherapy kept it stable. Four months later, it began to grow. The second surgery got another 70 percent of what was left. Michael went about six months before new growth. He started Temodar in September 2002, and the last MRI in May 2003 showed that the tumor actually shrank 15-20 percent. We have not had to radiate, thank God.

Michael has left-side weakness, no left peripheral vision, and some learning issues. He compensates very well for the weakness and vision (physical and occupational therapy from school and outside by a traumatic brain injury therapist/ teacher for the visually impaired.) On paper, it sounds very pitiful, but you wouldn't know all of his issues by looking at him. He is the most outgoing boy and so active. He really amazes me daily.

We take Michael to Beth Israel in New York City. They did the surgery both times, and they oversee the chemotherapy and do the MRIs. It is a long drive, but the peace of mind is well worth it. They are wonderful and the best as far as we are concerned.

Bess, mother. Clifton, NJ.

Cerebellar Astrocytomas and the Classical "Juvenile Pilocytic Astrocytoma" (JPA)

These are more common in children and affect balance, coordination, and movement because of their location near the spinal cord. A biopsy is mandatory in almost all cases. When completely removed, most children are cured with no return of tumor. The exact same tumor in an adult has a greater chance of re-growth.

Long-term side effects resulting in learning difficulties and "mutism syndrome"

This can occur despite complete tumor removal and cure. With mutism, the child or adult wakes up from surgery intact but within hours or days, speech, swallowing, balance and limb movements are affected. Rehabilitation will help most patients, but it can take months or years for recovery. (See Chapters 20: Side and Long- term effects and 22: Children: Special Considerations.)

GLIOBLASTOMA MULTIFORME (GBM)

FACTS I NEED TO KNOW

"Glioblastoma" in a child or young adult should be reviewed by a Neuropathologist.

What is a Glioblastoma Multiforme?

The *glioblastoma multiforme,* also called grade 4 astrocytoma, is the most malignant form of glioma or astrocytoma. It is the most common brain tumor in adults, but accounts for fewer than 15 percent of childhood brain tumors. The word "multiforme" refers to the many sizes and shapes of cells that can be seen under the microscope.

Table 10-2 Important Facts About Glioblastoma Multiforme

Location (Lobe)	Symptoms	Factors affecting survival	Therapy Choices
Frontal	Memory loss Executive function -Initiating tasks & priorities? Confusion, Seizures, headache	Age 40 or less Remaining tumor Function level (Karnofsky Score)	Surgery, Radiation Chemo-CCNU, Gliadel, Gliasite Immunotherapy, Gene therapy, Clinical trials
Temporal	Word-finding difficulty, Seizures		
Parietal	Weakness, Paralysis, Blind spots		
Occipital	Blind spots		
Spine	Arm, leg weakness or numbness; bowel, bladder control		

What are Typical Signs and Symptoms?

The common symptoms are confusion, seizures, weakness, paralysis, or partial loss of vision or feeling. Rarer symptoms when the tumor is located in the lower, back part of the brain include headaches, nausea and vomiting (in the morning), poor eye-hand coordination and difficulty in walking. Some people may have a headache for a few days, while others may exhibit confusion and forgetfulness for weeks or months. Still others may experience "stroke" symptoms or seizures, only to discover that these are caused by a tumor that is found on a scan. Symptoms are always related to disruption of normal pathways in specific areas of the brain that are affected by the tumor (Table 10-2).

Are all Glioblastoma Multiforme's Alike?

No, they are not. People who have tumors a) near the surface, b) in the occipital lobe (back of the brain), c) or are aged 40 years or younger, and d) have a high level of functioning before and after surgery, generally have better survival. Glioblastoma multiforme inside the brain near the thalamus (top of the brain stem) usually cannot be removed completely.

There are many glioma "cousins" that can be difficult for pathologists to distinguish from glioblastoma multiforme. Even neuropathology experts can disagree on the exact glioma family to which a tumor should be assigned. For example, a malignant *oligodendroglioma* can look like a glioblastoma multiforme to some pathologists; however, their treatment programs and prognoses are quite different (Chapter 17, Treatments). The reasons why one GBM will respond, and another will not, have recently been discovered.[12] Just looking at the tumor under the microscope is not the whole story.

Glioblastoma Multiforme in Adults and Children? Are They Different?

- Adults: frequently in upper part of the brain: frontal, parietal, and temporal lobes
- Children: infrequent; more likely in lower rear part of brain, close to spinal cord or cerebellum
- Tumors look alike under the microscope, but they differ in their active genes
- Children generally have a better response to combination therapies than do adults

What Are the Tests Needed for Initial Evaluation?

Refer to previous section under astrocytomas in this Chapter.

What Is the Outlook for Survival?

The most important elements in predicting successful results are the following[13]:
- Functional capabilities, expressed in the *Karnofsky* Score (See Glossary.)
- Location of the tumor
- Amount of tumor that remains after surgery (skill of the neurosurgeon)
- (Younger) age

I have patients who are alive five and 10 years later with highly malignant tumors and have seen people with low-grade tumors that continued to grow. Yes, having any brain tumor is serious, but being in expert hands can increase your chances for survival.

> Patients with GBM might benefit from being on a clinical trial.

THE ROLE OF NEUROSURGERY

Surgery as Initial Therapy for Glioblastoma is Important

- To preserve or improve your neurological function
- To obtain a piece of the tumor to confirm the diagnosis (biopsy)
- To completely or partially remove the tumor, as this can influence your survival.

Additional Surgery is Not Indicated – What Are the Other Choices?

If further surgery is not advised, then there are generally no absolute choices; but there are options to consider with your physician. Even if the tumor is completely removed, additional therapies including radiation are still needed for maximum benefit. Why? Because before the tumor was diagnosed, it released cells that spread beyond the boundaries seen on the MRI scan. Choices include:

1. Standard radiation and a stereotactic boost and/or simultaneous Temodar[14]
2. Radiosurgery for smaller tumors
3. GliaSite radioactive implant.[15] (See Chapter 17: Traditional Treatment)
4. Radioactive seeds[16] implanted into the tumor
5. Gliadel wafer[17]
6. Chemotherapy, including CCNU (lomustine, CeeNU) alone or in combination chemotherapy in a clinical trial
7. Clinical trials using newer individual or combination chemotherapy agents,[18] gene therapy, or immunotherapy (See Chapter 21: Clinical Trials)
8. Alternative and complementary medicine. There are clinical trials for these therapies, too. (See Chapter 18: Complementary and Alternative Therapy)

The decision making can be complex and the choices depend upon your functional state (how well the activities of daily living are performed, as measured by your *Karnofsky* score), age, rehabilitation potential, other medical conditions, etc. You should obtain input from different specialists involved in your care. This is another reason for Tumor Board discussion or referral to a medical center that specializes in brain tumor treatments. Research shows that patients

> **Karnofsky score**- A measure of your ability to perform activities of daily living like getting dressed, feeding your self. It is used to determine your eligibility to enroll on a clinical trial.

who enter into experimental clinical trials generally live as long as or longer than those who get their doctor's best guess or recommendation. This is probably due to the closer monitoring of patients on clinical trials.

RADIATION THERAPY

A booster dose of radiation to tumor cavity borders after standard radiation treatment has been reported to give increased survival time for newly diagnosed patients with glioblastoma multiforme.[19] Unlike Radiosurgery, stereotactic radiation therapy (SRT) is delivered during frequent treatment sessions, rather than all in one dose. There are no size limitations on the tumors to be treated. Both Radiosurgery and SRT require the head to be in a special frame or device to allow precise and accurate delivery of radiation beams.

> Stereotactic Radiation (SRT) for glioblastoma can be delivered during frequent treatment sessions, rather than all in one dose. There are no tumor size limitations.

Your radiotherapist should discuss with you the pros and cons specific to your particular tumor. (See Chapter 5: The Team, "Questions to ask your radiation Oncologist", and Chapter 20: Side Effects and After Effects of Treatment.)

CHEMOTHERAPY

At Initial Diagnosis

BCNU (or CCNU in oral, pill form) is the only chemotherapy medication approved by the U.S. Federal Drug Administration (FDA). It was approved in 1979 after a controlled clinical trial showed a survival advantage of about 10 weeks for glioblastoma patients who received it along with radiation therapy, compared with radiation therapy alone. Some people may think that taking chemotherapy for an extra eight to 10 extra weeks of life may not be worth it. But this is a misunderstanding of statistics. In fact, about 15-20 percent of the patients

> 15-20% of GBM patients were benefited from chemotherapy, experiencing a longer time without tumor progression. Similar results have been shown for the Gliadel wafer.

benefited, and they experienced a much longer time without tumor progression.[20] Similar results have been shown for the Gliadel wafer in its clinical trials.[17] As yet, there is no accurate test that can predict which patients might benefit most from chemotherapy. New research, however, is testing sensitivity to BCNU and Temodar in a new way that may be predictive.[18] This test detects and measures a gene that reverses the damage caused by the drug.

Temozolomide (Temodar in North America) is used by many oncologists to treat glioblastoma multiforme, based on preliminary findings of clinical trials.[14,21,22] It's officially approved only for use in recurrent grade 3 astrocytoma and is awaiting FDA approval for treatment of glioblastoma multiforme. Many physicians are using it "off label" for glioblastoma.

Chemotherapy has been used in various combinations and concurrently with radiation therapy in some studies (www.virtualtrials.com). A recent clinical trial reported that the use of cisplatin with BCNU yielded no particular advantage in survival and its benefits were offset by more severe side effects.[23] Temodar and concurrent irradiation have yielded some hopeful results.[14]

RECURRENT GLIOBLASTOMA MULTIFORME AND ANAPLASTIC ASTROCYTOMAS

There is no standard treatment for recurrent tumors, if you have had both radiation and complete or partial chemotherapy with lomustine (CCNU), or procarbazine, vincristine (PCV). Temodar is approved for recurrent anaplastic astrocytomas but not glioblastoma multiforme. Radiosurgery boosts to previously radiated areas in the form of SRT (fractionated or divided stereotactic radiation), have been studied with generally life extending results. The doses are given daily or less frequently for one to three weeks.

There are now more studies (clinical trials) for recurrent brain tumors than there have been in any other time in history. For these reasons, many patients enroll in clinical trials of experimental yet promising chemotherapy and/ or radiation therapy. Patients who enroll in clinical trials usually live longer than those who are treated by the best available therapy. Descriptions of the various approaches to therapy are listed in Chapter 17: Traditional Treatments and Chapter 21: Clinical Trials; and Table 10-4.

THE OLDER ADULT – IT'S ULTIMATELY UP TO THE PATIENT AND FAMILY TO INQUIRE ABOUT CHEMOTHERAPY OPTIONS

Older people may not be offered chemotherapy, because some oncologists believe that they do not tolerate side effects as well as younger patients. Many reports have shown that patients whose function in daily living (Karnofsky score) is less than 60 percent and who are more than 60 years of age do not show a benefit from additional chemotherapy. Recent reports, however, refute this and suggest aggressive treatment.[4,11]

Bottom line: Do your research, talk with knowledgeable doctors and fellow patients, and then decide on your options.

My colleagues and I conducted a clinical trial using five-day continuous infusion of vincristine at Cedars-Sinai Medical Center in Los Angeles from 1999-2001 and found that even persons aged 70 to 85 years exhibited no more toxicity than younger patients, and some patients showed significant life extension. One intriguing study[11], yet unconfirmed, has shown that patients aged 70 years and older, who took Temodar for five days per month, had survivals equal to those who received radiation therapy. Given the older population's poor tolerance for radiation to the brain, this study provides an unconfirmed chemotherapy alternative for older patients.

ANAPLASTIC ASTROCYTOMA, OLIGODENDRO-GLIOMA AND "MIXED" TUMORS

COMMON QUESTIONS

At the beginning of this chapter, I stated that the glioma family includes many members, including anaplastic (fairly aggressive) astrocytomas and oligodendrogliomas (oligos). Technically speaking, "mixed" tumors are those with features of *both* astrocytoma and oligos. These three are so closely related that most features of diagnosis and treatment apply equally. Moreover, they can be confused with one another in diagnosis.

The most important point is that anaplastic astrocytomas, mixed tumors, and oligodendrogliomas are responsive to similar current therapies and for many people the tumor does not return. The "package" of radiation therapy and at least procarbazine, CCNU-lomustine and vincristine (PCV) chemotherapy offer prolonged survival compared with radiation alone or with any one drug.[24] There are several clinical trials for this tumor group, and these can be found on websites (Table 10-4).

> "Anaplastic astrocytoma" should be reviewed by a Neuropathologist.

What Is an Oligodendroglioma?

An oligodendroglioma (oligo) is a type of glioma in which the tumor cells resemble oligodendrocytes (o-lee-go-den-dro-sites), cells that make the insulation (myelin) around nerves. Oligos can be low grade (slow growing), or higher grade (malignant, or more quickly dividing and growing). They can be large (diameters of 2.5 inches or more) and seen easily on CT scans because many contain calcium.

How Common Are Oligodendrogliomas?

Oligos represent 7-20 percent of all gliomas in the brain. In the United States alone, about 3,000 to 6,000 people each year are diagnosed with them. Some are called "mixed tumors" when they contain elements of both anaplastic astrocytoma and oligodendroglioma. Pathologists have been recognizing "mixed glioma" more frequently than in past years, because of their awareness that this is a responsive tumor. (Figure 10-1)

What Are Typical Symptoms of Anaplastic Astrocytomas and Oligodendrogliomas?

Symptoms depend upon the location of the tumor. Often, a person between the ages of 20 and 40 has a first-time seizure or severe headache. Tumors in the frontal and temporal lobes often begin with loss of motor control (movement) and/or changes in sensory function (feeling) and can mimic a stroke.

Are There Unique Features of Oligodendrogliomas or Anaplastic Astrocytomas?

These tumors can be the most survivable of all brain tumors, if treated correctly. Over the past 20 years, neuropathologists have not been consistent or precise about the way that they diagnose anaplastic astrocytomas and oligodendrogliomas. This has occurred for four major reasons.

> Anaplastic astrocytomas, mixed tumors, and oligodendrogliomas are responsive to similar current therapies with longer life and sometimes cure.

1. Astrocytoma tumors often may contain some "oligo"-looking cells. Confusion exists over how many cells need be present to call it oligodendroglioma.
2. Oligos and anaplastic astrocytomas respond well to combinations of chemotherapy and radiation therapy with many long-term survivors.
3. A specific test, called the 1p/19q tumor DNA deletion, predicts response probability to chemotherapy for some types of oligos.[25] To be absolutely sure of the diagnosis and possible therapy options, it's vital for you to have this test done and have your pathology slides reviewed as a second opinion. (See below under 1p/ 19q test.)

> If you have a malignant oligo or mixed oligo, discuss the 1p/19q deletion test with your physician.

4. About 15 percent of people who have an oligodendroglioma will have a significant bleed into or around their tumor sometime during their course. I have seen several patients in whom a stroke was first diagnosed, and only later was a tumor considered as the cause for the bleed. Tumor expansion

Bottom line: It is important for you to be absolutely sure of the diagnosis with a second opinion. Ask about a 1p/19q test if you have an oligo tumor.

from bleeding, rather than cancer cell growth, can be mistaken later for progressive or unresponsive tumor.

Mike, a 39-year-old software company entrepreneur, noted tingling and weakness in his left arm and leg and was diagnosed with a malignant oligodendroglioma. Six months later, while receiving his third cycle of 'PCV' chemotherapy, he noted more headache and arm weakness. His doctor in Seattle ordered a follow-up MRI scan; it showed enlarging tumor. Mike was despondent. Our group reviewed his scans, comparing them to scans of two months earlier. It was clear that the 2-cm. Enlargement was due to new blood and *not* cancer growth. His symptoms were worse in spite of being on high doses of steroids. Dr. Keith Black made the decision to operate and surgically remove the clot. Both the blood clot and dead tumor were removed, and Mike's strength returned dramatically over the next two weeks. He continued to be tumor-free.

What Is the Outlook for Survival?

Fifteen years ago only about 20-30 percent of patients with malignant or mixed oligodendroglioma or anaplastic astrocytomas lived more than five years. Now about 60 percent are alive and well five years later.[24,26] That is progress! There are a host of new and tested therapies that are powerful and effective. However, one must be both knowledgeable about the choices and treated by a team that keeps abreast of the latest developments. The following are important factors in predicting outcome:
- Exact type of oligo (low or high grade)
- Location of the tumor
- Amount of the tumor that remains after surgery
- Skill of the neurosurgeon
- Results of the 1p/ 19q genetic test
- Sensitivity to chemotherapy
- After-surgical therapies like radiation and choice of chemotherapy

Oligodendrogliomas – Differences Between Adults and Children

Oligodendrogliomas in children are rare. They are more likely to involve the back part of the brain (cerebellum), which is closer to the spinal cord and in the midbrain, an area that controls hormone regulation. Due to its significant effects on the developing brain, radiation should be delayed for children less than three years of age, if possible. Chemotherapy delays or could preclude the need for radiation in younger children. Radiation in very young children is considered experimental.

Bottom line: Chemotherapy is part of a possibly curative therapy but is not recommended as the only therapy for an oligodendroglioma tumor.

DIAGNOSIS

For most people, like Michael in the vignette above, their symptoms bring them to the doctor. Thereafter, the only radiographic study needed is a MRI scan. Computed tomography (CT) is often obtained initially, because it is a less expensive screening study to rule out a stroke. On the other hand, the CT scan allows us to see whether the tumor contains calcium or blood or has invaded the bones of the skull better than the MRI. This is informative for how the surgeon will approach the tumor.

What Tests Are Needed to Evaluate an Oligo or Anaplastic Astrocytoma (AA)

1. For items 1-7, see this Chapter, in previous section under astrocytoma
8. The 1p/19q deletion test on the tumor specimen
9. Angiography (a study of the major blood vessels in the brain) is indicated sometimes, depending upon tumor location. This gives information about the blood supply to the tumor and will help the neurosurgeon design the best angle of approach and avoid complications like cutting important blood vessels
10. Biopsy and removal
11. Pre-surgical and surgical studies: functional MRI, Brain Mapping etc.

The 1p/19q Tumor Deletion Study – Why Is It Important?

In 1998, Dr. Geoffrey Cairncross reported on a genetic test for malignant oligos, called the *1p/19q deletion* test. It detects the presence or absence of a DNA sequence, which in turn predicts whether or not the tumor will respond to PCV chemotherapy and radiation therapy. It is now widely available. The missing DNA (deletion) that this test measures is found only in the tumor, not in other cells the body. Be forewarned that this is different from a tumor *chemo-sensitivity* test that many doctors will order. For the 1p/19q, cells are tested for their DNA, while a chemo-sensitivity test incubates tumor cells with a drug to see if it stops their growth or kills them.

Tumor Grade – How Does This Affect My Treatment Options?

Tumor grading by the neuropathologist is very important. It is reason enough to get a second opinion. Pathologists use at least three different systems for grading gliomas, based on their microscopic appearance. For the most malignant and most benign, there is no controversy. But, for everything in between, there can be confusion. The World Health Organization (WHO) tried to solve this problem with one (four)-category system for glioma family tumors that neuropathologists are starting to use:

1. Grade 1 - benign (very slow growing tumors)
2. Grade 2 - atypical (usually slow growing but can recur)
3. Grade 3 - anaplastic (more malignant, faster growing)
4. Grade 4 - highly malignant (essentially a glioblastoma multiforme)
5. Mixed oligodendroglioma-astrocytoma can be graded as above, but usually as grades 2-4

Lower grade (1 or 2) oligos and gliomas usually grow slowly, may be completely removed and have a better prognosis than higher-grade tumors.[27] Survivals of 10 to 30 years or more are common. Management of low-grade tumors is controversial. The usual approach is surgery for both diagnosis and removal of as much tumor as is safe. Some doctors then recommend a "wait and see" approach, while others recommend therapy[28] (radiation and/ or chemotherapy). The tumors are unpredictable, although most remain unchanged for months or years. Follow up with MRI scans two to three times per year is typical. There are no blood tests currently available to monitor gliomas.

Grade 3 means it is anaplastic or malignant, and will grow if untreated. Up until 10 years ago, treatment involved radiation therapy alone. With recent progress in treating mixed tumors, most patients now receive chemotherapy as well as radiation.[26] Most doctors will order a 1p/19q genetic deletion test on the oligo tumors to determine the likelihood of it responding to chemotherapy and radiation. The best combination therapy is not yet known, but PCV and radiation currently is the standard.

Grade 4 is a glioblastoma multiforme (see glioblastoma multiforme sections earlier in this chapter). However, neuropathologists may not always agree on the exact grade of any given specimen.

Mixed gliomas (called mixed oligodendrogliomas, mixed astrocytomas, or oligoastrocytomas) are at the center of the "oligodendroglioma controversy," because there is imprecision and subjectivity in naming them. Many "mixed" tumors have areas of anaplastic astrocytoma and a few areas of oligodendroglioma, or vice versa. Is it an astrocytoma with some oligodendroglioma, or an oligodendroglioma with some anaplastic astrocytoma? Small sample biopsies also complicate matters, because there is not enough tissue to know if it is representative of the whole tumor. Do you see the problem? For this reason, I recommend that everyone with an astrocytoma or oligodendroglioma have his tumor reviewed by neuropathology experts and his/her case presented to a Tumor Board.

Differences Between Oligo and AAs Are Important for Four Reasons

1. Clinical trials are specific for different grade tumors.
2. Many oncologists suggest giving chemotherapy first for oligo tumors followed by radiation later.
3. If the tumor does not have the 1p deletion, then the decision to switch chemotherapies, if there is no or questionable response, could be made sooner.
4. Some major centers are using the 1p/19q test to determine initial therapy choices.

Two e-mail messages to the www.virtualtrials.com website highlight this confusion:

Question #1: *A friend recently had an oligodendroglioma tumor, grade 3, removed from the right frontal lobe. I have tried to look up oligodendroglioma and category 3. I couldn't really understand what I was reading. Could you provide a better explanation?*

Robert Q. New York

Question #2: *My husband has a recurrence of a grade 3 oligodendroglioma. He had partial surgery and the path report now calls it a mixed glioma (oligo and astro) grade using the WHO grading system. My question: What is the difference between a grade 3-mixed glioma and a glioblastoma multiforme? My confusion is that I thought grade 4 with any glioma was called a glioblastoma multiforme?*

Ethel in San Diego, CA.

Answers: Both people have a right to be confused! We physicians have been imprecise in our use of terms. The "mixed" category crosses boundaries between tumor types. Usually brain tumors are graded by their worst component. However, we know that some tumors, like a grade 4 mixed glioma, can respond better than the usual glioblastoma multiforme.

If you followed the steps outlined in Chapter 3 (Getting Organized), then you and your physician can look at the pathology report in your notebook and see what the pathologist said. This is another reason why you should collect the reports.

Surgery – To operate... or Not to Operate?

Importance of Location for an Oligodendroglioma

As in real estate, the property value is always spoken in terms of "location, location, location." The same holds true when it comes to brain tumors. If the tumor is near the surface and has not invaded deep structures or major blood vessels, then *resection* (tumor removal by surgery) can be carried out more easily and safely. Oligodendrogliomas tend to invade both the brain and its covering, called the *meninges*. If the oligodendroglioma is invading any large draining veins, major arteries, *ventricles* (hollow, fluid-filled cavities inside the brain) or the undersurface of the brain, then the success of complete resection is less likely, and chances of complications can increase.

Options Before Deciding On Surgery

- Not every patient needs a complete resection, but in my opinion, all individuals need a biopsy and tissue diagnosis.
- A "closed" stereotactic (needle) biopsy can be performed safely, with the patient returning home in 24 hours or less.
- In patients with low-grade tumors, periodic evaluation with regular MRI scans might be best, while for malignant tumors, aggressive combination therapies are recommended.

After the diagnosis, you will need to choose between the options of more surgery, radiation therapy, chemotherapy, or a combination.

I recommend that your case be presented to a Tumor Board and that you receive guidance from a brain tumor team.

Unique Roles For Neurosurgery

Surgery is important initial therapy for six reasons:
1. To preserve – or improve – your neurological function
2. To completely or partially remove the tumor
3. To obtain a piece of the tumor to confirm the diagnosis (biopsy)
4. To provide tissue for genetic 1p/19q deletion studies
5. To help control the seizures
6. To remove blood at any time during treatment (to prevent further damage to the brain)

Bottom line: For oligo tumors, chemotherapy is part of a possibly curative therapy but is not recommended as the only therapy for an oligodendroglioma tumor.

With technical developments in neurosurgery, such as computer-assisted navigational devices and monitoring of brainwaves during surgery, and mapping, the neurosurgeon can aggressively remove greater amounts of tumor, while sparing permanent functional loss in most cases. Although the goal of surgery is to remove all or most of the tumor, the first priority is safety and preservation or improvement of your neurological function. When total tumor removal carries significant risk of morbidity (any side effect that can cause decreased quality of life), it's better to leave some tumor. New York University's Dr. Patrick Kelly lists principles of surgery on his website. Though written in 1995, they are still valid. (See Table 10-4.)

Observation Alone?

Those patients for whom observation alone might be considered include:
1. Older patients who are experiencing seizures that can be controlled with medication
2. Any patient with a stable or very slow growing, low-grade tumor
3. Patients for whom treatment carries a more significant risk than the tumor itself
4. Those with a completely removed low-grade oligodendroglioma
5. Patients who choose not to have surgery after hearing all the options

What Medications Will I Receive Before or During Surgery?

See the surgery section in Chapter 17: Traditional Treatments.

RADIATION THERAPY

Do I still need Radiation?

One question that frequently comes up from both physicians and patients alike:

If the tumor responded to chemotherapy (Temodar or PCV combination) and I have no evidence of tumor on the follow-up MRI scans, do I need to have the radiation therapy?

The only cures (10+ year survivals) have resulted from combined chemotherapy *and* radiation. Thus, for me it is difficult to withdraw chemotherapy or radiation from the effective combination and expect the same results. My general advice usually has been to accept the combination package even with the chance of radiation-induced neuro-cognitive deficits that can occur over time.

Different Types of Radiation Therapy

Several different techniques are used to irradiate brain tumors. They all have advantages and disadvantages. Your radiotherapist should discuss with you the pros and cons specific to your particular tumor. One common treatment dilemma is illustrated below. It highlights one potential problem with Radiosurgery.

Question: I was diagnosed with a brain tumor of my right temporal lobe in May 2001. The surgeon could not take out the entire tumor as it extended into the ventricle. He recommended Cyberknife to treat 5-cm. residual tumor. The pathology report indicated a Grade II oligodendroglioma. Do you have any information on Cyberknife radiation?

James, Athens, GA.

Answer: This is a difficult management problem. I do not have your complete history. From what you write, most centers are unlikely to recommend Cyberknife alone at this point. All radiosurgery procedures work best when the tumor is less than 3 cm. In addition, you have a lower grade tumor, which means you do have time to get second or third opinions on the choices of therapy. Many centers might suggest a combined chemotherapy and radiation approach. At this time, the chemotherapy-radiation therapy combination offers the best chance for long life and possible cure.

Another letter illustrates the process, the problem and a possible solution:

Question: I've recently had an oligodendroglioma (4.5 x 4.5x 4.7cm, grade III) and the surgeon removed 70 to 90 percent of the tumor. I assume the remaining tumor is a shell, carved out like a potato skin. The surgeon said that the demarcation point between tumor and brain is indistinguishable. He used a special image-guided microscope to clean the wall of the tumor, being very careful to stay within the tumor. He told me that the tumor has fingers that invade brain matter.

I know that "shaped-beam" surgery (Radiosurgery) could remove more, if not almost all of what remains. I've also heard that the GammaKnife can be pointed at brain tissue without causing any harm. My hypothesis is that I would need the Gamma Knife as opposed to the more advanced shaped-beam technology, because the GammaKnife would be able to get those fingers that invade my brain. Help, thanks in advance.

Ron M, Des Moines, Iowa.

Comment: Ron had obviously done a lot of research on his tumor type and is knowledgeable, but he missed an important point. The most effective therapy that has led to long-term survival (cure) of oligodendrogliomas includes *both* radiation and chemotherapy. It was not the shape of the radiation beam that made the difference. He should go to a major medical center that specializes in brain tumors to obtain expert opinions on pathology and total treatment recommendations. The different radiotherapy techniques are a minor issue at this point.

The Changing Role for Radiation Therapy – Best Advice

Radiation therapy will slow or stop the growth of higher-grade oligodendroglioma and anaplastic astrocytoma tumors. For malignant oligos, the chemotherapy-radiation therapy combination has produced longer survivals.[29] Currently, oligodendrogliomas are one of the few tumors for which most treating physicians use chemotherapy *before* radiation. Radiation is often used to treat:

> Unlike most other brain tumors: for oligo tumors, radiation follows chemotherapy.

- Fragments of tumor left behind by the surgeon
- Tumor that has recurred
- Low-grade tumors that start to grow, before or after chemotherapy
- Mixed or anaplastic tumors, after chemotherapy

CHEMOTHERAPY

Chemotherapy for oligodendroglioma and anaplastic astrocytoma has a proven role. The survival results using it over the past 10 years have been dramatic. There are at least five different roles for chemotherapy:

> The "Gold Standard" for initial therapy of anaplastic astrocytomas and oligodendrogliomas remains chemotherapy first (PCV). This could change with new information.

- Treat the tumor prior to radiation therapy.
- Treat tumor that recurred after radiation therapy.
- Delay radiation treatment.
- Control and shrink the tumor enough to allow for later surgical removal.
- Limit the field of radiation needed, sometimes.

Best Chemotherapy Combination – Newly Diagnosed Oligodendrogliomas

We do not yet know the best combination since oligodendrogliomas do not represent one tumor type. In addition, I have seen many patients who were initially diagnosed with glioblastoma multiforme or anaplastic astrocytoma, who on later review of their pathology analysis were diagnosed with a high-grade oligo, "mixed glioma" or oligoastrocytoma. True oligodendroglioma tumors can be chemotherapy-sensitive and there is great enthusiasm to treat them.

Dr. Geoff Cairncross in 1992 reported the effectiveness of the PCV (Procarbazine, CCNU, Vincristine) chemotherapeutic combination, which is still considered the gold standard of treatment.[30] Temozolomide (Temodar in the USA) has been used in Europe since 1993, and it is very effective and approved for use in the relapsed setting.[31] While the 1p/19q deletion study predicts with 80 percent accuracy which tumors will respond to *PCV* and radiation, we do not yet know if the same prediction holds true for Temodar, although it is likely.

PCV or Temodar?

PCV combination has the best-proven record of accomplishment for long-term survival. However, many clinicians and patients have agreed to use Temodar off label as the first-line drug, because it causes fewer toxic problems to blood than PCV. About 20 percent of oligodendroglioma tumors do not have the 1p/19q deletion and are more resistant to chemotherapy by other tests as well. For these tumors, there is no known best initial therapy. I have led a clinical trial that used both Temodar and PCV for oligodendroglioma tumors.[32] Major brain tumor centers will be aware of the treatment subtleties and can offer either a clinical trial or choice of the latest known effective therapies.

Best Chemotherapy Combination – Recurrent Oligodendrogliomas and Anaplastic Astrocytomas

Oligodendroglial Tumors- Treatment Options. Many reports suggest that temozolomide is effective for recurrent oligodendroglioma tumors, and it has been approved by the FDA for recurrent oligodendrogliomas.[33] The best information suggests that if you have not received "complete" PCV (all three drugs) as the chemotherapy part of combination therapy, then treatment with complete PCV is the next best option. For tumors that have recurred within a year off PCV, then Temodar or Phase 1, 2 drug or combination on a clinical trial could be considered. Cisplatin (possibly carboplatin) and VP-16 have produced responses in 40 percent of patients with recurrent tumors.[34] If radiation has not been given, then your team should determine whether there is time to give chemotherapy first or whether it would be best to go directly to radiation.

Recurrent Lower-Grade Oligodendrogliomas – Treatment Options. You should be followed closely with an MRI scan taken three to four times a year in the first year after surgery, with gradual lengthening of the period between scans. Repeat surgery, radiation and/or chemotherapy can be considered, if the tumor grows. Radiation has not shown an overall proven benefit, and each case should be considered on its own merits. A Phase 1 or 2 clinical trial will offer the latest in chemotherapies, radiation sensitizers (like Xcytrin), or immune molecules (like Avastin) that block a type of vascular endothelial growth factor (VEGF). Secreted by the tumor, VEGF allows an oligodendroglioma to travel by dissolving cell connections as it invades normal tissue and create its own blood supply.

Recurrent Anaplastic Astrocytomas –Treatment Options. If you have had both radiation and PCV chemotherapy, then Temodar is usually the next option. On the hopeful side, there are more studies (clinical trials) for recurrent brain tumors than ever before. As I stated before, patients enrolled in clinical trials live longer than those who are not, owing in part to the fact that they are monitored more closely. For these reasons, many patients participate in clinical trials of experimental, yet promising chemotherapy or radiation therapy. (See Table 10-4, and Chapter 21: Clinical Trials.)

BRAIN STEM TUMORS

DIAGNOSIS

Brain MRI Scan Is the "Gold Standard"

Brain stem *tumor* is a location, while brain stem *glioma* is a real or presumed tissue diagnosis.

Throughout North America and Europe, MRI is used for diagnosis and treatment decisions. Biopsy is *almost* never obligatory for "typical" brain stem tumors, unless the diagnosis is in doubt, because biopsy bears risk. Most neurooncologists (brain tumor specialists) and other physicians will use the initial battery of tests cited in the astrocytoma section of this chapter for evaluation.

> For your brain stem tumor: you must know location and if it is "typical" or "atypical."

Symptoms of a Brain Stem Glioma

Typical symptoms in older children and adults include double vision, clumsiness or wobbliness (ataxia), weakness of a leg or arm, and sometimes headaches, vomiting, or facial weakness. For people with "atypical" brain stem gliomas, symptoms like double vision and unstable walking occur gradually and more than 6 to 12 months may pass before the tumor is diagnosed. This contrasts with the typical brain stem glioma in which diagnosis is usually made within three months of first symptoms. (See Table 10-3.)

All Brain Stem Tumors Are Not Alike

Over the last 15 years, we have learned that not all brain stem tumors are created equal. They are usually described by their location. It's critical to know your type *and* location of brain stem tumor, because the atypical form of glioma responds to many types of therapy. Even though they are "low grade," unfortunately, typical brain stem gliomas (BSGs) still cause damage. If you are misdiagnosed, then you will not receive the correct therapy.

- "*Typical*" brain stem gliomas (80 percent)
  These originate in and invade the pons (the middle portion of the brain stem). Sometimes, they spread upward to the midbrain (the upper part of the brain stem) or downward to the medulla (the bottom portion of the brain stem). When this happens, they are called diffuse pontine gliomas. Their crucial location is central to important brain functions such as breathing, heart rate and movement. Typical brain stem gliomas are usually not biopsied unless you are enrolled in a clinical trial or there are unusual features that make the diagnosis questionable.
- *Atypical* brain stem gliomas (20 percent)
  These include more localized tumors (with less invasion of normal brain) that begin in the medulla or grow onto the outside surface of the brainstem. Careful assessment of the MRI is needed to make these distinctions. These tumors can appear with cysts that originate from the brain stem.
- Ependymoma brain stem tumors
  These are not gliomas, are less common, and grow around the brain stem and can resemble a glioma on an MRI scan.

The Need for a Team of Doctors to Treat My Brain Stem Tumor

Brain stem tumors are uncommon and require complex management only available in a comprehensive cancer center where a team of doctors with different areas of expertise work together. Such teams might include neurooncologists, neurosurgeons, neurologists, oncologists, radiation oncologists, neuropathologists, neuroradiologists, and rehabilitation specialists. Because of its rarity, patients and families should be encouraged to participate in clinical trials to improve and optimize therapy.

What Is the Outlook for Survival?

The most important elements in predicting a successful result are the following:
- Type of brain stem glioma (defined by location) and either typical, atypical, or other
- Amount of tumor that can be removed at surgery (skill of the neurosurgeon)
- Response to therapies
- As yet unknown factors

This is a good time to revisit the first quote in Chapter 10:

In June of 2002, I entered my 13th year as a brain tumor survivor with a Brain Stem Glioma. Many professionals can safely say that I have significantly beat the "statistics." My only explanation of this wonderful gift of time is that I have approached this disease with a "one-two punch," trying not to fold under at times from sheer exhaustion from this constant fight and always trying to beat it at its own game.

Sheryl R. Shetsky, Founder & President.
South Florida Brain Tumor Association

As Sheryl attests, people with atypical brain stem gliomas will usually have long, productive lives. I treated my first patient with an atypical brain stem glioma in 1978. She is still alive after three surgeries, chemotherapy, and radiation. This is not unusual. Yes, having any brain tumor is serious, but placing yourself in expert hands can increase your chances of survival. Remember, no matter how serious the situation, no physician or anyone else can predict for the individual what will happen with treatment. Predictions apply to populations as a whole, but never to any one person.

TREATMENTS

Location of a Brain Stem Tumor and Therapy Choices

Brain stem tumors occur anywhere in the brain stem, regardless of pathology grade. The *atypical* brain stem glioma often can be partially removed by a skilled neurosurgeon, and the remaining tumor can remain dormant for years. Frequently, the atypical types arise above the pons in the midbrain or below in the *medulla*. The grades 1 and 2 and juvenile "pilocytic" astrocytomas (JPA) are often the atypical types, which mean that they can be treated effectively with surgery, chemotherapy, and radiation. Conversely, the diffuse pontine type is treated by radiation and may progress to a higher grade.

Table 10-3 Important Facts About Brain Stem Gliomas

Types	Location in brainstem?	Symptoms	Survival Factors	Therapy Choices
Typical	Pons, thalamus, Diffuse growth	Weakness of cranial nerves, double vision Swallowing and speech problems Arm/leg weakness, wobbly walking Headache, vomiting	Age 40 or less High function (Karnofsky score) Slower development of symptoms	Classic forms not biopsied (except in clinical trials); Radiation Phase1,2 studies
Atypical	Medulla; one sided or outer parts of brain stem	Arm/ leg weakness or speech problems	Response to therapy	Biopsy/ removal Radiation Chemotherapy Phase 1,2 studies

The e-mail below describes a 10-year perspective on chemotherapy, submitted by a mother whose son was diagnosed at age two with an atypical brain stem glioma at a leading institution:

Hello everyone, my name is Cindy. My 12-year-old son, Eric, has a cervico-medullary glioma (brainstem tumor). He is currently in a study at the NIH using temozolomide and O-6-Benzleguanine. Eric is doing fine, and the tumor is stable. He just completed his 10th cycle of chemo on Sat Nov 2.

Cindy, mother of Eric age 12 dx
cervico-medullary Glioma at age 2 Dec 1992

THE ROLE OF NEUROSURGERY

Can Surgery Help?

Yes. It can confirm the diagnosis when the tumor may actually be an ependymoma or atypical glioma. Surgery with less than total removal can preserve or restore function, especially for tumors growing out from the brain stem. This often results in quality long-term survival. The extent of removal and freedom from complications depends upon the skill and experience of your neurosurgeon.

The biopsy is also to justify experimental treatment and to prove that it is cancer and not something else. These tumors invade the brain stem, growing and spreading between normal nerve cells. Aggressive surgery could cause fatal damage to normal nerve cells that are vital for swallowing, breathing, and movement of the limbs and eyes.

> Successful therapy, and specifically surgery to remove the tumor, is dependent upon location and whether atypical or typical.

A Shunt Operation – What Is It and Why Is It Necessary?

About half of adults and children with brain stem tumors will develop a pressure build-up from blockage. This is called "obstructive hydrocephalus." It occurs when cerebrospinal fluid is trapped in the brain's ventricles, behind the blockage. Shunts are simple mechanical tubing devices that the neurosurgeon uses to divert this fluid to another location in the body, typically into the abdomen where the fluid is absorbed. (For a diagram, see Chapter 17:Treatment.)

If Surgery Is Not Possible, What Are Other Options?

1. Observation of your atypical brain stem glioma, if its stable and you have no symptoms.
2. Radiation or chemotherapy.
3. Radiation therapy often has been the next step.

However, investigators at major brain tumor treatment centers are using different combinations of radiation and chemotherapies and newer approaches. The following e-mail from Angelique illustrates how atypical brain stem gliomas can continue to shrink even after the completion of therapy:

Hillary was diagnosed May 16 at age four with a brain stem glioma. Finally, after two years of treatment her MRI shows 30 percent shrinkage. This is the first time we have had any change on her MRIs. We were so excited, crying and yelling and hugging. She had chemo from May 2001-March 2002, which was stopped early because her bone marrow was slow to recover. She was supposed to be on chemo for three years and then start radiation at age seven. Since chemo was stopped, she began radiation five days after turning five years old.

We were in the Emergency Room last Friday night because she "passed out" upon waking and said she couldn't see. I panicked and was sick to my stomach. Hillary had CT and MRI scans. Long story short, they found that she was dehydrated and had not enough sodium. She was hydrated and improved. The best news is – the tumor is smaller! We are loving life right now! Thank you.

Angelique, mother. Paris, France.

RADIATION THERAPY

"Typical" Brain Stem Tumors

Radiotherapy, limited to the involved area of tumor, is the most common and effective treatment for "typical" brain stem gliomas. It is usually administered daily over a period of six weeks. Twice-daily radiotherapy (hyper-fractionation) had been used to deliver higher dosages of radiation, but it did not improve survival and may have longer-term toxicities.

Generally, there are few radiation side effects to other parts of the brain. Most patients will return to near normal function, although the tumor may recur in 6 to 18 months. As I have stressed many times in this book, there should be input from the different specialists involved in your care, using the team approach as well as a Tumor Board evaluation.

Different Radiation Therapy Options for Brain Stem Gliomas

There are several different techniques that all have pro's and con's. Your Radiation Oncologist should discuss with you the specifics for your tumor. Remember, clinical trials offer additional options. For example, a recent clinical trial used Xcytrin (gadolinium-texaphyrin), a radiation sensitizer, in a Phase 1 study for brain stem gliomas and glioblastoma multiforme with positive safety results (Table 10-3).

CHEMOTHERAPY

The role of chemotherapy for typical brain stem gliomas is unclear. Although used to control tumor growth, chemotherapy alone has rarely cured these gliomas, and it's still considered experimental. High-dose chemotherapy using the patient's own bone marrow or stem cells has so far shown little effect. Finally, one type of immunotherapy, using white blood cell "hormones" called interferons, was tried but had disappointing results in one study in 1990.

> Clinical trials might benefit people with recurrent brain stem gliomas.

- "Atypical" brain stem gliomas in children and adults. Chemotherapy has led to tumor shrinkage in about 30 percent of patients. In children younger than three years old, chemotherapy is preferable as initial therapy because of the side effects that radiation can produce in the developing brain.
- Recurrent or progressive brainstem gliomas. Several adult and pediatric clinical trials of new chemotherapies and immunotherapies are underway and can be accessed on the Internet. The trials are available through national research consortiums like the New Approach to Brain Tumor Treatment (NABTT), the Children's Oncology Group, National Cancer Institute, and others. (Table 10-3).
- *Atypical* brain stem gliomas are a chronic condition with ups and downs. The e-mail below is from the mother of a child with a brain stem glioma. It points to the need for multidisciplinary teams:

My nine-year-old daughter, Blossom, was diagnosed with a 4 cm brain stem glioma when she was six years old. We were referred to Duke. Her tumor is at the top of the brain stem next to her optic nerves. She also has a genetic condition, Neurofibromatosis type 1 (NF-1). A biopsy was done in 1999; her tumor was classified as glioblastoma multiforme. Her only options were chemo and radiation. She received 18 months of CPT-11 (March 99- Sept. 2000), followed by six weeks of radiation. By this time, there had been over 50 percent "shrinkage" and there was "very little activity" in the tumor by PET scan. She progressed in Oct. 2001 and began 12 months of alternating CPT-11 and Temodar. She came off treatment Nov. 2002 and is going to school full time. Tumor is stable.

Radiation stimulated her body into starting puberty at eight years old. She will be returning to Duke, May 30 for an MRI and meeting with an endocrinologist. She still has some weakness on the right side, her handwriting is poor, and she is not at the top of her class. As for me, I'm still taking things one day at a time, and today looks like it will be a good one.

Tonya mother of Blossom. Charlotte, NC

Here is another example of the uncertainties involved in determining the progression of a brain stem glioma and the need for knowledgeable specialist care:

Question: *I am a 30 year old construction worker and have a JPA [Juvenile-type "pilocytic" astrocytoma] in the medulla, biopsied in May 2002 when the cyst was drained out. Radiation was in June-July, and control MRI in October said shrinkage was due to disappearance of the cyst. Yesterday's MRI states slight progression when compared to the MRI in October.*

a) Can an MRI differentiate growth of tumor from edema caused by radiation?
b) Can a PET test help in answering this?
c) Can it be that the growth is due to the cyst, which is now visible again?
d) Can edema be present six months after the radiation when it was not there two months after treatment?

Fred, New York City, NY

Answers:
a) Can an MRI differentiate the growth of tumor vs. edema caused by radiation? Sometimes, yes. But it can be difficult and many times we are wrong in our interpretation. For "atypical" tumors, in which growth is the outer side of the brain stem (exophytic), enhancement means dye has crossed the blood-brain barrier. Dye uptake does not always indicate tumor, but rather the state of "leakiness" of the blood vessels; tumor or irradiated blood vessels are leakier than blood vessels of the normal brain. Enhancement can also indicate necrosis (dead tissue) or inflammation from surgery or radiation. In many instances, the necrosis acts like a "tumor" and must be surgically removed.

b) Can a PET help in answering this? If the area is all tumor then PET scans can be useful; some institutions swear by them, while others believe that the MR-Spect or Thallium-Spect is more accurate. The most important consideration is accuracy. Together all these tests are more than 90 percent accurate, but not 100 percent. If an MRI shows possible tumor, we use the Thallium-Spect to confirm the presence of live cells and the Magnetic Resonance Spectroscopy tests to indicate the chemical signal of dead or live brain tissue. Repeat testing is often performed to see if the answer is clearer four to eight weeks later (Chapter 8: Diagnosis).

c) Can it be that the growth is due to the cyst, which is now visible again? Cysts can occur alone or along with a tumor. They also are called "syrinxes" when they occur in the cord. A cyst is usually distinguishable from a solid tumor by MRI.

d) Can edema be present six months after the radiation when it was not there two months after treatment? Yes. The amount of edema can be affected by the dosage of radiation and the length of time over which it is administered. With a radiosurgical boost, edema can last longer. Necrosis is often associated with edema. The generally accepted approach for necrosis, however, is treatment with steroids, usually for many months. The steroid dose can affect the appearance of edema too.

Steroids – When Are They Used for Brain Stem Tumors?

Dexamethasone (trade name Decadron®) is a steroid drug frequently administered to patients with brain stem tumors. It is used to reduce the swelling and "tightness" caused by the tumor, particularly before and after surgery or radiotherapy. Dexamethasone has side effects that include mood changes, increased appetite and weight gain, fluid retention, blood sugar instability, high blood pressure, and increased susceptibility to infection. (See Chapter 9: Medications.) A few patients and families have voiced that there is a dramatic negative trade off in quality of life when on long-term steroids.

GANGLIOGLIOMAS

DIAGNOSIS

Symptoms

Gangliogliomas are more frequent in persons under 30 years of age and occur commonly in the upper and frontal part of the brain. Seizures are often an initial symptom. In older children and adults, complaints may include weakness of a leg or arm, or face, double vision, and sometimes headaches or vomiting. These symptoms can be present for months or years before the diagnosis is made. Gangliogliomas can originate from the brain stem and midbrain, in addition to their more common location in the upper lobes. Gangliogliomas grow very slowly and most patients will be long-term survivors.

Evaluation and Tests

Diagnosis starts with a thorough neurological exam by your primary physician or neurologist and then a CT or MRI scan (steps 1-7 under "Initial evaluation of a person with an astrocytoma.") Thirty-five percent of tumors contain deposits of calcium that can be distinguished more easily on CT than on MRI scans. The presence of calcium or accompanying cysts is a tip-off to the neuroradiologist that the tumor is a ganglioglioma.

Confirmation by Biopsy and Resection

This is usually indicated, since the scan appearance alone is not 100 percent proof. Necrosis (dead tissue) that surrounds gangliogliomas can give a false appearance of a more malignant tumor. Even oncogenes (growth signal genes in cancers that are more malignant) have been detected in gangliogliomas. Despite these potentially misleading attributes, there is usually little confusion in making the correct diagnosis.

How Are They Graded?

More than 95 percent of all gangliogliomas are low grade and usually do not recur after removal. They are composed of a mixture of astrocytoma and neuronal (nerve) cells. A small percentage of these malignant tumors can invade brain or spread to other parts of the body. Refer to the section on astrocytomas.

TREATMENT

A Team of Doctors to Treat My Ganglioglioma

Gangliogliomas are uncommon and management may be complex, especially if they are not completely removed or are located in critical areas of the brain that govern speech, movement, breathing, etc. A child or adult requires evaluation in a comprehensive cancer center where doctors who have different areas of expertise can work together. The kinds of professionals that you will need may include neurooncologists, neurosurgeons, neurologists, oncologists, radiation oncologists, neuropathologists, and neuroradiologists. If your case is presented to a Tumor Board, you will also benefit from their combined wisdom, experience, and technical expertise.

> Most gangliogliomas are cured with complete surgical removal.

Surgery Issues

- Options before deciding on surgery for my ganglioglioma
  Whether to have surgery or not depends upon the severity of your symptoms. Emergency neurosurgery to remove pressure and/or insert a shunt can be life saving. After the emergency is resolved, there is usually time to get second opinions.
- The role of surgery
  Surgery is useful for making the correct diagnosis as well as relieving symptoms. It is the recommended therapy and is considered by most experts to be the only effective treatment. Gangliogliomas are usually distinct from normal brain and can be completely removed 75 percent of the time. For the rest, however, surgical removal is less than complete; yet, the tumor can remain stable for years. Even for tumors that grow out from the brain stem, surgery often results in quality, long-term survival. Shunt placement to treat pressure build-up may be necessary. (Refer to the brain stem glioma section under "Shunt Operation" and Chapter 17: Treatment, under section, "What is a shunt operation, and why is it necessary?)

The Ganglioglioma Cannot Be Removed By Surgery – So What Are My Other Options?

Generally, if surgical removal is incomplete and additional surgery is not advised, many centers will suggest a "watch and wait" approach. Gangliogliomas generally grow slowly, if at all. Some centers offer radiation or clinical trials using chemotherapy or immunotherapy. Since there are no clear directives beyond "watch and wait," I suggest that your physician present your case to a Tumor Board at your hospital or get a referral to a center that specializes in treatment of brain tumors.

Radiation Therapy

For the past 70 years, radiation has been used to treat most brain tumors as the first line of offense. There are no definitive studies, however, to show that radiation is effective for gangliogliomas. Most are benign and, if they are completely removed, radiation is not usually suggested. If, however, you have a more malignant type of ganglioglioma, then post-operative radiation is often recommended.

Chemotherapy

Chemotherapy has been of little help, although efforts are underway to explore newer drugs in recurrent gangliogliomas. While some dramatic responses have been reported with recurrent tumors, it is difficult to estimate what percentage of people will benefit. For young children, chemotherapy is preferable to radiation therapy (lesser of the two evils) because of the severe side effects of radiation on the developing brain. Several adult and pediatric clinical trials of new immunotherapies and chemotherapies are underway for recurrent brain tumors. As of January 2004, eight therapeutic clinical trials are open (Table 10-4).

What Are Steroids and How Are They Used?

Refer to Chapter 9 in this book and Chapter 19: Medications.

Table 10-4 Useful Websites and Chat Groups for Specific Glioma Brain Tumors

Tumor	Website and Chatgroup contact information
All brain Tumors	http://www.cancer.gov/search/clinical_trials **or** http://www.cancer.gov/templates/doc_wyntk.aspx?viewi d=b5500bd0-3da6-496a-8080-3052a630ba57
General	http://www.neurosurgery.org/health/patient http://www.virtualtrials.com/serchfrm.cfm http://www.cancer.gov/clinicaltrials
North American Brain Tumor Consort.	http://www.nabtt.org
Healing Exchange	http://www.braintrust.org/services/support/othergroups
BRAIN TRUST online email groupsLow-grade gliomas	http://www.med.nyu.edu/neurosurgery/articles

Table 10-4 continued

Childhood Brain Tumors	http://www.childrensoncologygroup.org http://clinicaltrials.gov/ct/screen/BrowseAny

Malignant Astrocytomas
  Glioblastoma Multiforme
	http://www.neurosurgery.org/health/patient/
	  detail.asp?DisorderID=79

Oligodendroglioma	http://www.med.nyu.edu/neurosurgery/articles/ braintumors_5.html mailto: oligo-captain@braintrust.org
Brain Stem Tumors	http://www.virtualtrials.com/serchfrm.cfm# http://www.virtualtrials.com www.virtualtrials.com/trialdetails.cfm?id=60900391 mail to: adultbsg-captain@braintrust.org
Gangliogliomas	http://www.emedicine.com/radio/topic291.htm http://www.virtualtrials.com/Ganglioglioma.cfm

CHAPTER 11

Tumors Originating in the Brain – Medulloblastomas, PNETs and Ependymomas

Foolishly, I waited 7 months before I joined this (or any) group. By that time, my son had radiation, chemo, and a recurrence of his medulloblastoma while on treatment. Because of advice from a person on this group, we decided to travel to St. Jude's for Maurice's second surgery. You will not find more comprehensive knowledge about childhood brain tumor care than on a listserv such as this one. Definitely not from an oncologist! I wish you and all the rest of us the best.

Mitch, Father of a son with medulloblastoma.

MEDULLOBLASTOMAS AND PRIMITIVE NEUROECTO-DERMAL TUMORS (PNET)s

⚷ Key search words

• metastases	• PNET	• MRI, MR-Spect and PET scans
• ependymoma	• staging	• myxopapillary ependymoma
• M stage	• tumor grade	• tumor markers
• therapy options	• internet resources	• obstructive hydrocephalus

The most important fact I can share with you about PNETs is that we have one good chance to treat them – the first treatment. Our success with re-treatment, after they recur, is much less effective. That is why everything that you can have going for you must be used in the beginning. This tumor is not nice and it will not wait. (See also Chapter 22: Children-Special Considerations.)

MEDULLOBLASTOMAS AND PRIMITIVE NEUROECTODERMAL TUMORS (ALSO CALLED PNETS) GENERAL QUESTIONS

WHAT IS A PNET?

PNETs are a family of brain tumors that typically occur in younger children and also are diagnosed in the 18 to 40-year-old group. Most grow in the back part of the brain (cerebellum) and are called *medulloblastomas*. About 20 percent start in the upper brain and are called *supratentorial PNETs* (SPNET)s.[1] No one used the term PNET until 1973, when a group of pathologists devised a new category for tumors they could not classify by their system at that time. It is generally accepted that despite the similar appearance under the microscope, medulloblastoma in the cerebellum and SPNET in the upper hemispheres respond differently to treatment.

> PNETs occur in the upper or lower parts of the brain.

WHAT ARE SYMPTOMS OF A PNET?

Typical symptoms of medulloblastoma in older children and adults include headaches, vomiting, double vision, clumsiness or wobbliness (ataxia), or weakness of a leg or arm. For SPNETs, a seizure can be the first symptom. In infants, the symptoms are less obvious. A baby may be fussy, vomiting off and on for weeks, or register a large head size during routine checks with the pediatrician. Average time from symptoms to diagnosis in our study of more than 400 children was 90 days, with some as long as 18 months.

HOW ARE PNETS CLASSIFIED OR STAGED? IS THE TYPE IMPORTANT?

PNETs are usually described by their location. Typical medulloblastomas (infratentorial PNETs) start out at the top-center of the cerebellum in the fourth ventricle; a minority grows within the cerebellum. (See Chapter 2 for basic anatomy.) SPNETs begin in the upper brain and can invade the ventricles. Over the last 20 years, we have learned that not all PNETs are created equal. Some grow slowly and can be completely removed. Others invade locally or spread and lodge along the spinal cord. The invasive ones wrap around the pons (the middle portion of the *brain stem*), sometimes extending up to the *midbrain* (the upper portion of the brain stem) or downward to the *medulla* (the bottom portion of the brain stem).

| All PNETs are malignant. None are benign. |

Under a microscope, PNETs appear different from astrocytomas (Chapter 10); they look more like (immature) fetal cells to the neuropathologist. By definition, all are malignant; none are low grade.

Table 11-1 Tumor (T) and Metastasis (M) Stage for PNETs[1]

T-stage	
T-I	Tumor < 3 cm in diameter and limited to the classic midline position in the vermis, the roof of the 4th ventricle, and less frequently to the cerebellar hemispheres.
T-2	Tumor > 3 cm and invading one adjacent structure or partially filling 4th ventricle.
T-3a	Tumor further invading two adjacent structures or completely filling the 4th ventricle with extension into the aqueduct of Sylvius, foramen of Magendie, or foramen of Luschka, thus producing marked internal hydrocephalus.
T3b	Tumor arising from floor of 4th ventricle and filling 4th ventricle.
T-4	Tumor spread through Aqueduct of Sylvius to involve 3rd ventricle, midbrain, or down into upper cervical cord.
M-stage	
M-0	No gross subarachnoid or blood-borne metastasis
M-I	Microscopic tumor cells found in cerebrospinal fluid
M-2	Gross nodular seeding in cerebellum, cerebral subarachnoid space or in 3rd or 4th ventricles
M-3	Gross nodular seeding in spinal subarachnoid space
M-4	Spread outside the nervous system into bone marrow, bones, liver, or lungs (Extra-neuraxis metastasis)

The most common staging system is called the M-stage. (M stands for "metastasis.").

It is absolutely critical to know the M-stage before any treatment begins, as the choice and intensity of therapy depends upon it. T-stage is a measurement of size and extension but is not as important as M stage, which measures how far the tumor has spread.[3] (See Table 11-1 and Chapter 22: Children – Special Considerations.)

ARE THERE FACTORS THAT HELP PREDICT LONGER OR SHORTER SURVIVAL?

Studies by our group and others over the last 10 years have indicated that while tumor spread at diagnosis (M-stage) is most important in tailoring therapy, it is not the only factor. I have heard some physicians say, "You have a 40 percent chance of being cured, because you have widespread tumor." You are one specific and unique case; the doctor is merely stating his understanding of PNETS for all patients. In actuality, for the individual the odds are either 100 percent or 0 percent with nothing in between. If it works for you, it is 100 percent.

> It is critical to know the M-stage before any treatment begins.

DIAGNOSIS

DOES THE LOCATION OF MY PNET MAKE A DIFFERENCE?

Yes it does.
- Tumors in the upper brain (SPNETs) may not be quite as responsive to the same therapies as the medulloblastoma (infratentorial PNET).
- SPNETs metastasize *less* frequently (10 percent) compared with medulloblastomas (35 percent).
- Most clinical trials place SPNETs in a higher risk category, requiring therapy that is more intensive.
- A tumor that has not spread will be easier to remove than one that has invaded wider areas.

WHAT TESTS ARE NEEDED FOR THE *INITIAL* EVALUATION OF A PNET?

Throughout North America and Europe, the brain MRI is the "gold standard" for diagnosis and treatment decisions with typical PNETs. A CT scan may show the tumor, but details that allow the neurosurgeon to plan a maximal resection usually are better appreciated on the MRI. For an explanation of the MRI and CT, see

Chapter 8: Diagnosis. The sites listed in Table 11-2 have good scans and general information, but chemotherapy recommendations may be outdated.

Most brain tumor specialists will evaluate a patient with a suspected PNET with the following:
1. Thorough medical and neurological examination
2. Brain MRI with and without contrast, to visualize the tumor prior to surgery
3. MRI or CT scan of the spine (myelogram) to detect "drop" (spinal) metastases
4. Spinal tap to look for malignant cells and protein concentration (if MRI is negative)
5. Biopsy to confirm the diagnosis and maximal resection of the tumor

WHAT ARE MY CHANCES OF A CURE?

It's fair to say that groups of people with localized, completely resected PNETs usually will live longer than those whose tumor has spread. However, I treated my first patient with a stage M-3 PNET in 1978, and she is still alive 26 years later. I also recently met an independent, vivacious 41-year-old woman who was treated as a two-year-old! The most important elements in predicting a more successful result are the following:
- Amount of tumor that remains after surgery (skill of the neurosurgeon) – Less is better
- Stage of tumor – tumor spread within the nervous system – M-0 stage is better than M-1+
- Response to therapies
- Age of the child – 3 years or more is better (adults follow a similar pattern to older children)

Note: Size of the tumor, big vs. small, was not important.

About 40 percent of patients who have residual disease or spinal spread will be alive for five years or more. Again, these are the general odds for the entire population, not for specific individuals.

Bottom line: Successful therapy is dependent upon location, tumor "M" stage, and skill of your neurosurgeon.

TREATMENTS

Do I Need a Team of Doctors to Treat a PNET?

PNETs are uncommon. Only 500+ cases occur annually in the U.S. and most of these are children. A child or adult with a PNET requires evaluation in a comprehensive brain tumor center where doctors with different expertise can offer you the latest approaches. Initially, this might include neuroradiologists, neuropathologists, neurooncologists, neurosurgeons, neurologists, (pediatric) oncologists, radiation oncologists, and later, neuropsychologists and endocrinologists. (Chapter 5: Doctors and other Team members.)

Everyone should be encouraged to participate in clinical trials to receive the most advanced therapy and to improve and optimize therapy. Consultation at a major brain tumor center will increase your chances of longer survival and a better quality of life. (Chapter 22: Children-Special Considerations.)

SURGERY

Do I Have Options Before Deciding on Surgery?

If the pressure inside the head is high, most neurosurgeons will prescribe steroids. In an extreme emergency, a drain will be inserted to relieve the pressure and settle the patient down for 24 to 48 hours before attempting to remove the tumor. After the emergency is resolved, there is usually time to get opinions from the local Tumor Board and to obtain consultations at a major medical center that has a pediatric neurosurgeon or one who specializes in treatment of PNETs. At the least, a biopsy is mandatory before beginning any treatment program. (See Chapter 6: Experts and a Second Opinion; Chapter 8: Traditional Diagnosis; and Chapter 22: Children-Special Considerations.)

What Is the Importance of Surgery for a PNET?

Surgery is important initial therapy for four reasons:
1. Preservation or improvement of neurological function.
2. Biopsy of the tumor to confirm the diagnosis.
3. Removal of as much tumor as possible and staging.
4. Insertion of a shunt to decrease pressure that cannot be managed by other means.

WHAT IS THE ROLE AND IMPORTANCE OF YOUR NEUROSURGEON?

The neurosurgeon's removal of the tumor is the only prognostic factor over which we have any control. That is why it is so important to be in the hands of an experienced (pediatric) neurosurgeon (more on this below). Our 1999 study showed, quite convincingly, that if a surgeon left more than 1/4 teaspoon of tumor behind (about 1.5cc), the chances of living more than five years was reduced from 75 to about 50 percent. The amount of tumor removal affects survival five years later![3]

> Tumor removal = critical to survival.

Neurosurgeon Dr. Leland Albright at the Univerity of Pittsburgh reported that resections performed by a pediatric neurosurgeon, generally resulted in 10 percent more complete resections with no more complications than outcomes of surgeries performed by non-pediatric neurosurgeons.[4] If you can, go with an expert.

Dr. Albright, I, and other investigators reviewed the MRI scans of all 200+ patients in our trial. We believe that for more than half of the children and young adults who had *incomplete* resections, it would have been possible to leave less than 1.5 cc of tumor with an additional resection, and thereby improve their chances for survival. Thus, if the first attempt or neurosurgeon did not get a complete resection, it is possible that the second opinion neurosurgeon may be able to get the job done.

> Second opinion - if incomplete resection.

A SHUNT OPERATION – WHY IS IT NECESSARY?

As mentioned, about 50 percent of children and adults with PNETs will develop a pressure build-up in the head known as "obstructive hydrocephalus." This happens

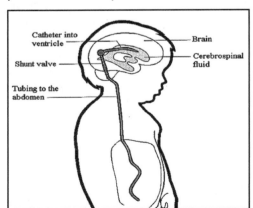

when cerebrospinal fluid is trapped in the brain's ventricles and not reabsorbed. If this condition is not responsive to steroids, then a shunt (mechanical tubing device) can be used to divert this fluid to another location in the body, typically to the abdomen where the fluid is absorbed. The neurosurgeon's skill and experience is essential to a shunt that is free of complications. (See Chapter 17, Figure 11-1 and Table 11-2.)

Figure 11-1 Diagram of a shunt and tubing.

Bottom line: 75% of people who have a complete or near complete resection and no tumor spread will be alive five years later.

WHAT MEDICATIONS WILL I RECEIVE BEFORE OR DURING SURGERY?

See Chapter 9 and Chapter 17 for information on this topic.

ADDITIONAL THERAPY OPTIONS

For incomplete resection:
- Radiation therapy is typically the next step for older children and adults, after biopsy and maximal tumor removal.
- A Tumor Board or your neurosurgeon may recommend a second surgery to remove more tumor.
- Referral to a major brain tumor center and second opinions
  - Clinical trials of radiation, chemotherapy, and/or immunotherapy
  - Testing intensive, combination chemotherapies along with lowered radiation doses for children and adults may be offered

For recurrent disease:
- Intensive chemotherapy with stem cell rescue (or temozolomide alone or in combination with other agents)
- Tumor maturing agents (e.g., high dose Vitamin A)
- Growth receptor inhibitors such as Iressa™ are being studied in Phase 1 and 2 clinical trials.
- Phase 1 and 2 studies. Sites in Table 11-2 review the results of different clinical trials and offer new ones. For more information on clinical trials, see Chapter 21.

> Clinical Trials offer advanced treatments.

RADIATION

WHY IS RADIATION THERAPY USED TO TREAT PNETS?

Radiotherapy is the most well-studied and effective therapy for PNETs. In 1930, Dr. Harvey Cushing reported that when patients received no radiation therapy, 60 of 61 with medulloblastoma died within two years.[5] This contrasts with 75 percent five-year survivals with a combination of radiation and chemotherapy in 2003. Radiation to PNETs is directed not only to the tumor area, but also to the head and spine.

The major controversy about radiation and PNETs concerns the dosage of radiation to the normal brain and spinal cord to prevent relapse. Older studies reported that

3600 cGy (cen-ti-gray, a measure of the amount of radiation) to the spine and unaffected brain was effective, while newer studies are using 2400 and 1800 cGy.

WHAT ARE THE DIFFERENT TYPES OF RADIATION THERAPY FOR PNETs?

Several different techniques have been used to irradiate PNETs; each has advantages and disadvantages. For example, twice-daily radiotherapy (hyper-fractionation) delivered higher dosages of radiation but did not improve survival. Your radiotherapist should discuss the pros and cons specific to your particular tumor with you (Chapter 17: Treatments; Chapter 22: Children-Special Considerations).

CHEMOTHERAPY

HOW IS CHEMOTHERAPY USED TO TREAT PNETs?

The role of chemotherapy for typical PNETs has been evolving over the past 15 years. Chemotherapy has been used to improve survival and reduce radiation exposure to the brain. Therapy intensity is determined by tumor stage.

For Stage M-0, Lower Risk, Completely Resected PNETs

Recent studies have attempted to give lower doses of radiation (2400 cGy) to the brain-spine of lower- risk M-0 children. The largest of these clinical trials showed more tumor recurrences in children who received the lower spine radiation dose (2400 cGy vs. 3600 cGy) and no chemotherapy.[6] The survival for these patients (70 percent at five years) was slightly *worse* than that of higher risk children treated with radiation and chemotherapy (75 percent alive at five years). The best treatment combination for Stage M-0 (best prognosis-lowest risk) individuals with a completely resected medulloblastoma/ PNET is not yet established. Current clinical trials are the best way to obtain the most advanced therapy combinations (Table 11-2).

Stage M-1+, Higher Risk, or Incompletely Resected PNETs

Radiation plus chemotherapy offers the best chance for survival among those who have residual disease after surgery or if spread has occurred into the head or spine. Dr. Roger Packer developed a protocol for lower brain and spinal radiation doses (2400 cGy) plus vincristine, cisplatin and lomustine. Early results showed that survival at five years was 79 percent; survivals at 10 years have not been reported.[7]

Bottom line: Your tumor stage determines the type of treatments you will receive.

A number of children suffered significant cisplatin-related kidney damage and hearing loss. No comparison data from clinical trials are available on quality of life improvement with 2400 cGy vs. 3600 cGy doses of radiation to the brain and spine.[8] The best dose and combinations are still being developed in current clinical trials (Table 11-2).

The lack of a known best therapy naturally makes parents and patients uncomfortable. The following exchange from a medulloblastoma e-mail chat room exemplifies the dilemma:

> My 4 year old is undergoing chemotherapy for medulloblastoma and recovering from cerebellar mutism. Damian is high risk with a second inoperable tumor in the brain and three small tumors in his spine. He received high dose radiation, but five weeks later, all these tumors were still on his MRI. He has completed two rounds of high dose chemotherapy with a stem cell transplant. Today his spinal MRI is clear and the tumor in his brain is smaller. I don't believe that we would have these results without chemotherapy.
>
> I have read studies of radiation alone that had terrible results. I think of it like the war in Iraq with the radiation being the smart bombs taking out major targets and the chemotherapy being the troops on the ground that finish the job….Having a child with cancer or mutism is a nightmare by itself. Dealing with both and the financial strain thrown in for good measure is a parent's worst nightmare.
>
> Reginald, father of Damian, Ottowa CN.

How Can the Internet Help Me Obtain Information About Medulloblastoma?

This is an actual e-mail that shows how the people in the "Internet community," who have never met personally, can support one another.

Question: *Hi: I tried to access the medulloblastoma list from Yahoo groups without my ID and couldn't find it.*

Answer: *Try sending an e-mail to moderator medulloblastoma-owner@ yahoogroups.com. The medulloblastoma list is still up and running, you should be able to find it there. Also, there is a pediatric brain tumor group for all kinds of tumors. Try sending an e-mail to pediatricbraintumors-owner@*

yahoogroups.com. They are very active sites. I just read about another child with medulloblastoma in the pons and spine. If this doesn't help, send another e-mail or a public e-mail asking to join medulloblastoma@ yahoogroups.com and pediatricbraintumors@yahoogroups.com. Let me know if this works.

Lorry, Yael's mom

Although they may be geographical strangers, fellow brain tumor survivors on the Internet will help you to gather the information that you need to find expertise, optimal care, and a selection of treatment choices.

EPENDYMOMAS – GENERAL QUESTIONS

EPENDYMOMAS – WHAT ARE THEY? WHERE ARE THEY FOUND?

Ependymal tumors arise from cells that line the ventricles (hollow fluid-filled cavities within the brain) or the central canal of the spinal cord. They can be located in the supratentorial (top-frontal) or infratentorial (lower, rear portion) parts of the brain. Ependymomas can appear anywhere in the brain, brain stem or spinal canal.

Ependymomas are rare, accounting for only 3 to 6 percent of all primary brain tumors. Yet, they are the third most common brain tumor in children. In adults 60 percent are found in the brain stem or spinal cord, while in children 85 percent are in the brain; the majority of these are in or around the cerebellum.

WHAT ARE THE COMMON SYMPTOMS OF EPENDYMOMAS?

Symptoms of an ependymoma are related to the location and size of the tumor. In older children and adults, nausea, vomiting and headache are the most common symptoms. These are signs of increased pressure, which may develop if the tumor blocks the drainage of cerebrospinal fluid (the liquid that bathes the brain). In infants, enlargement of the head is one of the first symptoms. Irritability, sleepiness and morning vomiting develop as the tumor grows. Neck pain may result from a tumor growing near the brainstem or the upper part of the spinal cord. Seizures and weakness may occur on one side or one part of the body. Spinal cord tumors cause bladder control problems, leg or back pain.

Types of Ependymomas — How Are They Graded?

Pathologists classify ependymomas into four major types:
1. Myxopapillary ependymomas
2. Subependymomas
3. Ependymomas
4. Anaplastic ependymomas

The cells of a grade 1 tumor look somewhat unusual, whereas grade 4 tumor cells look definitely abnormal. Most grade 1 tumors do not recur after complete removal. Grades 2-4 tumors need additional treatment and have a higher likelihood of recurrence. General considerations of lower- and higher-grade tumors are as follows:
- Lower-grade ependymal tumors
  - Myxopapillary ependymomas occur in the lower part of the spinal column and are more frequent in young adults.
  - Subependymomas usually occur near a ventricle in the brain. These and myxopapillary types are slow growing.
  - Ependymomas (classical) are the most common of the ependymal tumors and are considered grade 2. They are usually located along the ventricular system, in the posterior fossa or in the spinal cord.
- Higher-grade ependymal tumors
  Anaplastic ependymomas are high-grade tumors (grades 3 or 4). They are faster growing than the low-grade tumors. They usually occur in the posterior fossa.

What Tests Are Used for Diagnosis and Staging of an Ependymoma?

Magnetic Resonance Imaging (MRI) is the gold standard for surgical planning and staging. The MRI scan of the brain provides details about the location of the tumor and which parts of the brain are involved prior to surgery.

MRI or CT scans of the spine are mandatory for staging, as 10-15 percent of ependymomas spread or metastasize through the cerebrospinal fluid. Staging uses the Chang system (Table 11-1).

If the spinal MRI is negative, a lumbar puncture (spinal tap) is performed to determine whether the tumor has spread. The fluid should be tested for the presence of tumor cells and the results will guide treatment. In our clinical trial for ependymomas, we found that tumor grade did not predict whether the tumor would recur or even develop metastases.[9]

WHAT IS THE OUTLOOK FOR SURVIVAL WITH AN EPENDYMOMA?

Overall, 10-year survival rates are about 50 percent. But the site of the original tumor plays a big role: spinal cord tumors have a high cure rate near 100 percent, while infratentorial are 45 percent and supratentorial tumors 20 percent. Remember, no one knows your survival ahead of time. It is zero percent or 100 percent with nothing in between!

TREATMENT FOR EPENDYMOMA

SURGERY

The goal of surgery is to remove as much tumor as possible. Patients who can have a "gross total resection" (removing the tumor that can be seen) have the best chance of long-term survival. Our trial showed that the Neurosurgeon's ability to perform a complete removal was of prime importance. For ependymomas, no other factors, including centrally reviewed tumor pathological type, location, metastasis and tumor (M and T) stages, patient age, race, gender, or chemotherapy treatment regimen seemed to predict survival.

The amount of tumor that can be removed, however, depends on location. Removal of all visible tumor is not always possible, especially if it is attached to the brainstem or involves other important areas of the brain. In children, ependymomas often fill the fourth ventricle and extend through its floor into the brainstem, making safe removal of those sections of tumor difficult.

Some patients will require the placement of a shunt to by-pass the blockage.

An MRI of the brain should be done within three days after surgery to determine how much tumor remains.

Bottom line: For PNETs & Ependymoma, survival depends upon the skill of your neurosurgeon.

RADIATION THERAPY

The initial treatment of an ependymoma will vary depending on location, grade, and whether the tumor has spread to the spine. Radiation therapy is usually recommended for older children and adults with pathology grade 2-4 tumors, even if all visible tumor was removed. Patients treated with radiation therapy following surgery generally have a better chance of long-term survival than patients treated with surgery alone.

Focal radiation therapy is given, often just to the tumor area. For example, with a myxopapillary ependymoma of the spine, surgery (and sometimes radiation) can produce cures and long-term survival in nearly all cases. If the tumor is widespread, radiation is usually given to the entire brain and spine, with an extra amount of radiation (called a boost) given to the area of the brain where the tumor started. You should ask the radiation oncology specialist about the different techniques that would be best for you.

> Spinal cord ependymoma has a high cure rate near 100%.

CHEMOTHERAPY

Chemotherapy's role in the treatment of newly diagnosed ependymoma is not clear. Some tumors respond for a while, while others continue to grow. For infants and young children, chemotherapy may be used to delay radiation, or to treat tumors that have grown back after radiation therapy. Treatment studies using cisplatin in combination with other chemotherapy drugs have shown the best results. There are active clinical trials for ependymomas (Table 11-2).

FOLLOW-UP STUDIES AFTER TREATMENT IS CONCLUDED

MRI scans of the brain and/or spinal cord are performed every 3 to 4 months for the first two years following diagnosis. These scans are used initially to determine the effectiveness of treatment and to watch for possible recurrence. Scans are done less frequently thereafter, unless symptoms develop that indicate tumor growth.

THE EPENDYMOMA THAT RETURNS AFTER OR DURING THERAPY

The completeness of tumor removal is the strongest factor influencing recurrence and survival.[9] Almost all recurrences occur at the initial site. Thus, if it were a spinal or parietal lobe tumor, those are the places to scan and be most concerned about. Isolated spinal metastases are rare.

For patients whose tumor recurs after initial treatment, re-operation, followed by additional therapy, can be helpful. Newer investigational treatments include chemotherapy, re-irradiation (possibly with radiosurgery) or radiation implants to the site of recurrence. A search of the clinical trial databases will put you in touch with the latest clinical trials for ependymomas. There were 37 open studies as of February 2004 (Table 11-2).

> You must know the type, location, and stage of your ependymoma for best treatment options.

Table 11-2 Internet Resources for PNETs & Ependymomas

Subject	Web Address
Metastases to brain	http://www.emedicine.com/radio/topic101.htm
Pineal region tumors (general)	http://neurosun.medsch.ucla.edu/diagnoses/braintumor/ braintumordis_11.html
Clinical trials	http://www.centerwatch.com/patient/studies/cat564.html http://www.virtualtrials.com/new.cfm (newer trials) http://www.virtualtrials.com/mmenu.cfm http://www.cancer.gov/clinicaltrials/finding
Medulloblastoma general	http://www.emedicine.com/neuro/topic624.htm http://www.emedicine.com/ped/topic1396.htm http://www.nci.nih.gov/cancerinfo/pdq/treatment/ childmedulloblastoma/healthprofessional http://www.neurosurgery.org/focus/august99/7-2-1.html
Medulloblastoma scans	http://www.uchsc.edu/sm/neuroimaging/T6107/T6107.htm http://www.rad.uab.edu:591/tf then go to "Browse by category" and then "Neuro".
Surgery- Shunts/ Hydrocephalus	http://www.yoursurgery.com/proceduredetails.cfm?br=4&proc=44

Medulloblastoma clinical trials	http://clinicaltrials.gov/ct/screen/BrowseAny;jsessionid=D6025 0162CF0EC060340F73E62D2B47E?path=%2Fbrowse%2Fby-condition%2Fhier%2FBC04.b%2FD008527%2BMedulloblast oma.k&recruiting=true; www.cancer.gov www.virtualtrials.com http://www.nci.nih.gov/cancerinfo/pdq/treatment/ childmedulloblastoma/healthprofessional http://clinicaltrials.gov/ct/show/NCT00053872;jsessionid=2BB B502D754A72CF25F2ADE094D6808E?order=18
E-mail medulloblastoma list – Pediatric brain tumor group for all tumors.	medulloblastoma@yahoogroups.com medulloblastoma-owner@yahoogroups.com pediatricbraintumors-owner@yahoogroups.com pediatricbraintumors@yahoogroups.com
SPNETs	http://www.nci.nih.gov/cancerinfo/pdq/treatment/ childSPNET/patient http://www.acor.org http://www.jncicancerspectrum.oupjournals.org/cgi/pdq/ jncipdq;CDR0000062775 http://www.neurosurgery.org/focus/august99/7-2-1.html (treatment)
Ependymoma (General)	http://www.abta.org/Ependymo.pdf http://clinicaltrials.gov/ct/screen/BrowseAny;jsessionid=D6025 0162CF0EC060340F73E62D2B47E?path=%2Fbrowse%2Fby-condition%2Fhier%2FBC04.b%2FD008527%2BMedulloblast oma.k&recruiting=true E-mail to: adultependy-captain@braintrust.org http://www.braintumorkids.org/Medical_News/ ependymoma.asp

CHAPTER 12

Tumors in the Head – Meningiomas, Pituitary Tumors and Acoustic Neuromas

Fear is life's one true opponent. It is a clever, treacherous adversary. Disguised as doubt it slips into your mind as a spy…you make rash decisions. You dismiss your last allies: hope and trust. You must fight hard to express it… to shine the light of words upon it. Because if you don't… if your fear becomes a wordless darkness that you avoid, perhaps even manage to forget, you open yourself to further attacks… because you never truly fought the opponent who defeated you.

Yann Martel 2001[1]

TUMORS IN THE HEAD

Key search words

- metastases
- staging
- microadenoma
- therapy options
- pituitary adenoma

- meningioma
- tumor grade
- macroadenoma
- acoustic neuroma

- MRI, MR-Spect, and PET scans
- Internet resources
- hormones
- neurofibromatosis

MENINGIOMAS - GENERAL QUESTIONS

WHAT IS A MENINGIOMA? HOW COMMON ARE THEY?

A *meningioma* grows out from the meninges, which are coverings of the brain and spine. It occurs frequently in people with a hereditary disorder called neurofibromatosis type two, NF-2, not type 1. (See Chapter 24: Heredity and other causes.) Meningiomas represent about 20 percent of all tumors originating in the head and 10 percent of tumors of the spine. (See Chapter 2, Figure 2-1.) This means that about 6,500 people are diagnosed with meningiomas each year in the U.S. Most tumors do not invade or spread. Many can become quite large; diameters of 2 inches (5 cm) or more are common.

> **Fast Facts** • Tumors of the covering of brain and spine • Most are benign • Cures are frequent • Residual tumor may need radiation

ARE MENINGIOMAS A FORM OF CANCER?

This is a frequently asked question. I answered it on an Internet website:

Question: *There has been a lot of discussion within the meningioma community about a meningioma as being "benign." The implication is that a meningioma is not harmful, which of course is not true. What is your opinion?*

Answer: Most meningiomas are called "benign" because they are a form of low-grade, slow-growing "cancer" with a low potential to spread. Those that are incompletely removed by surgery will be treated with radiation therapy, since they respond and can be cured with this. I think the word "cancer" frightens a lot of us, and we would prefer not to use it. It is emotionally charged. Physicians and scientists use the term more liberally since they view cancer in a less personal context.

(You might want to go back to Chapter 2, where I discuss how the modern interpretations of Noah and the Ark highlight the emotional challenge of the word "cancer" and how you might become less sensitive to its use.)

What Are Typical Symptoms of Meningioma?

Symptoms that lead people to seek medical consultation depend upon location of the tumor. Common symptoms are pain (headache) for weeks to months, weakness or paralysis, visual field cuts, or speech problems (Table 12-1).

What Are My Chances of Cure With a Meningioma?

Eighty-five percent of all people with meningiomas are cured with surgery. In other words, the tumors do not return after removal. Location, the amount of the tumor that is removed by surgery, and the skill of the neurosurgeon are the important elements in predicting a successful result. The goal of the operation is to remove the meningioma completely, including fibers that attach it to the covering of the brain (dura) and bone.

> 85% of all people with meningiomas are cured with surgery.

DIAGNOSIS

How Is a Meningioma Diagnosed?

For most people, symptoms cause them to consult their doctor. Only an MRI scan can give the most definitive diagnosis of a meningioma. Sometimes a computed tomography (CT) scan is obtained initially as a screening scan in the evaluation of a headache; it's a less expensive diagnostic tool. The CT scan is better in showing whether or not the tumor has invaded the bones of the skull, but is not best for details of the brain itself.

How Are Meningiomas Classified or Graded?

Meningiomas are classified by pathologists into three types:
- Grade 1 – benign, very slow-growing tumors (75 percent of all meningiomas)
- Grade 2 – atypical, usually slow growing but can recur
- Grade 3 – anaplastic (more malignant, faster-growing)

The 15 percent of meningiomas that recur often progress to a higher grade. Grade 2 and 3 tumors recur more frequently than grade 1 growths (Table 12-2).

Does the Location of My Meningioma Make a Difference?

Yes. Again, as in the price of real estate, the answer is "location, location, location." Meningiomas are more frequent in some locations and rarer in others. The ease of removing them is dependent upon both their accessibility and the skill of the neurosurgeon. Where is your meningioma? (See Table 12-1.)

Table 12-1 Most Common Sites and Symptoms for Meningiomas in the Head

Location	% of Total	Common Symptoms
Frontal-Parietal	20	Seizures, local neurological deficits, intracranial high pressure, headache, extremity weakness, personality changes, dementia, urinary incontinence, difficulty speaking, visual field loss
Midline	25	Seizures, local neurological deficits, intracranial high pressure, lower extremity weakness, sensory seizures, headache, personality changes, dementia, increasing apathy, flattening of affect, unsteadiness, tremor
Sphenoid Ridge	18	Eye bulging, decreased visual acuity, cranial nerve (III, IV, V, VI) palsies, seizures, memory difficulty, personality change, headache
Posterior Fossa	10	Unsteadiness and incoordination, hydrocephalus (increased pressure inside the brain & large ventricles), voice and swallowing difficulties
Pituitary Gland	8	Lateral field visual deficit
Olfactory Groove	7	Loss of smell (anosmia), subtle personality changes, mild difficulty with memory, euphoria, diminished concentration, urinary incontinence, visual impairment
Optic Sheath	5	Decreased vision in one eye
Other, including head and spine	7	Variable depending on location

If the meningioma is near the surface and has not invaded deep structures or major blood vessels, resection (tumor removal by surgery) can be carried out safely. If it invades any of the large draining veins, major arteries of or on the brain surface, or if it is on the underside of the brain, chances of a complete resection decrease and risk of complications increases. The experience of the neurosurgeon is critical. (See Chapter 5: Doctors and Other Team Members.)

□ **Bottom line: Ease of removing a meningioma is dependent upon accessibility and skill of your neurosurgeon.** ➔

What Are the Options Before Deciding on Surgery? – Is There a Role for a Tumor Board?

Not every patient with a meningioma needs immediate surgery. In some patients, observation and periodic evaluation with MRI scans is the best course to follow. Beyond this, the options include surgery, embolization, radiation therapy, or a combination. I recommend that your case be presented to the Tumor Board of the hospital with which your neurosurgeon is associated. There, a team can have input into the next sequence of treatments, if necessary. Tumor Board deliberations usually occur after surgery, but they can also take place beforehand.

When Would Observation Alone Be Sufficient?

The following are situations where observation alone is sufficient:
- Those with mild or minimal symptoms, whose tumor has not interfered with their quality of life, or who have little or no swelling in the adjacent brain.
- Older patients who have very slowly progressing symptoms. If they are experiencing seizures, these can be controlled with medication.
- Patients for whom treatment carries a significant risk of reducing ones quality of life.
- Patients who choose not to have surgery after being presented with all the options.

TREATMENTS

Surgery

Surgery vs. No-Surgery – What Are the Considerations?

Question: *I have a friend who has a large meningioma that started in the ear. She had surgery four years ago and has been told that it is too big and cannot be operated on. A hospital in Sheffield England offers a laser treatment to shrink the tumor and not damage vital parts of the brain. Has anybody heard of this treatment? The original surgery left her face paralyzed on one side.*

Answer: This patient has a rarer tumor in a more hidden location. She might go to a major center that has a team of neurosurgeons, and ear surgeons, radiation therapists, and neurooncologists who specialize in the treatment of meningiomas. There are various surgical and non-surgical alternatives, including Radiosurgery, depending upon the exact size of the tumor and its location. Experience counts for a lot here.

Although the goal of surgery is to remove the tumor and all its attachments, the first priority is to preserve - or improve neurological function. When total removal of the tumor carries significant risk of morbidity (any side effect that can decrease quality of life), it's better to leave some tumor tissue in place. There are four choices:

> Surgery, radiation therapy and embolization are the major treatments for meningioma.

- Observation over time (the tumor may remain stable indefinitely);
- Surgery now or at a future date
- Radiation therapy
- Embolization (clotting of tumor blood supply)

What Are Angiography and Embolization? Are They Useful?

Angiography is the name of the x-ray test that uses injections of dye to locate and create an image of the major blood vessels in the brain and those feeding the tumor. *Embolization* is the threading of a thin tube (catheter) up the leg veins or arteries directly into the blood vessels that feed the tumor. Then, a glue-like clotting substance is injected to choke off and shrink the tumor. Some neurosurgeons prefer to shrink the meningioma before surgery, while others do not feel that it is necessary. It is rare for embolization to be used as the only form of therapy.

What Medications Will I Receive Before or During Surgery?

See Chapter 9 and Chapter 17 for the answer and more information.

RADIATION

Why is Radiation Therapy Used to Treat Meningiomas?

Radiation therapy is effective in slowing or stopping the growth of most meningiomas. It is often used to treat fragments of tumor left behind by the surgeon, a tumor that has recurred, or tumors that could not be treated surgically.

What Types of Radiation Are Used to Treat Meningioma?

Most meningiomas are cured by complete surgical resection. For those with incomplete resection, either conventional radiation or fractionated stereotactic methods are very effective. Meningiomas have sharp margins, which mean that they usually do not invade beyond what can be seen visually or by MRI scans; they also have smaller amounts of residual tumor after surgery. Thus, they are ideal tumors for focused, well-localized, shaped radiation fields using GammaKnife or Intensity modulated radiation therapy (IMRT) or fractionated stereotactic radiation therapy. (See Chapter 17: Treatments and Table 12-2.)

CHEMOTHERAPY

What Chemotherapy Options Are There for Meningiomas?

There is no standard chemotherapy for meningiomas. However, new chemotherapies are being tested for the 15 percent that recur:

- Several investigators have reported stability or responsiveness of meningiomas to the drug hydroxyurea,[2] although this chemotherapy has not been tested rigorously.
- The drug RU-486, that blocks progesterone receptors, is also being tested, since meningiomas have surface receptors for the female hormones progesterone and estrogen. Whether RU-486 affects these receptors is not yet known. One study of 12 patients suggested an anti-tumor effect, but this finding remains unconfirmed. For more information, see Table 12-2. The anecdote below illustrates how chemotherapy may not be the best first option.

At a Florida Brain Tumor Association meeting in 2003, I was consulted by Constance M., a 32-year-old mother of three young children. She was having difficulty obtaining a prescription for RU-486 to treat her recurring, right temporal lobe meningioma. Constance had the tumor for 12 years and never received radiation, even after two surgeries. She feared its side effects and wanted to try the RU-486 pill.

I explained that trying an experimental medication might not be in her best interest when she had not had curative radiation. The tumor was localized in an area of her brain where modern radiation techniques could be applied without damaging her normal brain functions. I encouraged her to see an experienced radiation oncologist at her local cancer center.

INFORMATION RESOURCES

You can access general information on meningiomas from the Internet. Many people share their experiences by going to a meningioma website (Table 12-2).

Printed below are comments from its founder, as well as remarks by the founders of other meningioma-related websites. This will give you an idea of the extensive networking that these sites can offer.

About 18,000 individuals have visited my meningioma website in the two years that it has been up. Two to six new members sign up each day. Over half return more than once to the site; http://meningioma.intranets.com.

My Yahoo site is just getting enough members to sustain a regular conversation. It now has 93 members. http://groups.yahoo.com/group/meningioma.

My Meningioma Talk bulletin board has 146 subscribers that get a list of new postings each day. There are 20 to 30 new postings each day and the site had about 45,000 hits in six months. Perform a Google search "meningioma talk bulletin" for latest URL address.

PITUITARY TUMORS

GENERAL QUESTIONS

What and Where Is the Pituitary Gland?

The *pituitary gland* is often referred to as the body's "master gland" because it controls secretion of most *hormones* from the other glands. Pituitary hormones are chemicals that circulate in the bloodstream and regulate functions like thyroid activity, sugar levels, menstrual cycles in women, sex drive, growth in children, adrenal gland activity, salt balance, urine production and concentration, initiation of labor during pregnancy, and milk-production. These functions can be affected by pituitary tumors and tumors affecting the pituitary gland (Table 12-2).

What Is a Pituitary Adenoma?

Pituitary adenomas are non-cancerous tumors that account for 7-10 percent of tumors occurring inside the head. "Adenoma" is simply another word for tumor. (Figure 12-2) Although they are called "brain tumors," adenomas really start in the pituitary gland, which is located directly behind the nose and at the base of the brain. Figure 13-1) Pituitary adenomas can enlarge and put pressure on surrounding structures. (Table 12-2).

> Pituitary is the master gland that controls secretion of hormones from other glands.

What Types of Pituitary Adenomas Are There?

- Small adenomas, less than ½-inch (10 mm), are called *microadenomas*.
- Larger tumors (often ½ to two inches) are *macroadenomas*. They can press on and damage adjoining structures.
- There are two subtypes: *hormone secreting* and *non-hormone secreting*.
  - 75 percent of adenomas do not produce any hormones and are called non-secreting or non-functional tumors. They grow and damage normal pituitary gland tissue, which ultimately leads to a drop in normal hormone production.
  - 25 percent are "secreting" or functional tumors that produce the same hormones as normal tissue, but more of them and in greater quantity.
  - Recurrences can be either secreting or non-secreting.

> **Types of Pituitary adenomas**
> • Small and large • Hormone secreting or non-secreting

How Do Pituitary Tumors Cause Problems?

Pituitary tumors can cause local and distant (hormonal) problems.

Local harm to structures: Locally, the optic nerves and chiasm (where the optic nerves cross over), which connects the eyes to the brain, are particularly vulnerable because they are so near. With tumor growth, peripheral vision is affected, and without treatment, blindness may occur (Table 12-2 chiasm). Although benign, pituitary adenomas can spread into the cavernous sinus. This area is behind and below the pituitary gland and contains the carotid artery and several cranial nerves. When this spreading occurs, the tumors may be particularly stubborn and difficult to remove (Table 12-2).

Distant harm by non-functioning adenomas: At a distance, adenomas cause hormonal imbalances by affecting the production of hormones. With non-functional adenomas, the first hormones affected are often the ones controlling sexual characteristics and milk production. Low output of sexual function hormones (follicle stimulating hormone [FSH] and luteinizing hormone [LH]) cause irregularity or cessation of menstruation (periods) in women and sterility with loss

> Hormonal supplements are needed if pituitary is damaged by tumor.

of sex drive in men and women (low hormone output). Strangely enough, pressure on the stalk of the pituitary gland *releases* prolactin hormone, which in turn can cause milk production in non-pregnant women and men.

Distant harm by functioning adenomas: Functional adenomas have the opposite effect, causing an overproduction of hormones. They secrete growth hormone, which leads to excessive growth in children (gigantism). In adults, these tumors cause a disease called *acromegaly,* characterized by abnormal growth of the facial bones, enlargement of the hands and feet, excessive sweating, and heart disease. An excerpt from faq@virtualtrials.com illustrates a common question about pituitary tumors that start out as secretors and recur as non-secretors:

> **Question:** *Six years ago, I had endoscopic, transphenoidal surgery performed for a secreting pituitary tumor followed by 28 weeks of radiation. I was just diagnosed with a non-secreting tumor and they want to do surgery again. Is there any medication that I can try first?*
>
> **Answer:** You need to ask your surgeon and endocrinologist exactly what type of tumor you have. Blood tests can be performed for about 8-10 hormones to determine if the tumor is really non-secretory. If it is a growth hormone or prolactin hormone-secreting tumor, there are blocking drugs for this. Ask your doctors for more information.

What is Cushing's Disease?

A rarer example of a functioning adenoma may cause Cushing's Disease. It is named after the most famous American neurosurgeon of the early 1900s, Dr. Harvey Cushing. It refers to symptoms of a functional pituitary adenoma that secretes a hormone called "adreno-cortico-tropic hormone" (ACTH). This, in turn, causes the adrenal glands to make and release elevated levels of the steroid hormone *cortisone.* The main function of cortisone is to regulate the body's response to stress and sugar. Patients with Cushing's Disease may suffer from several problems including sugar diabetes, high blood pressure, weight gain, and depression.

You can be "cushingoid" when taking steroids. This refers to fat under the cheeks giving the face a rounded appearance, thinning of the muscles, and a protuberant belly. More information about Cushing's Disease can be found on websites (Table 12-2) and in Chapter 9.

Bottom line: Pituitary functions affect thyroid, menstrual cycles, sex drive, sexual development, growth in children, adrenal gland, salt balance, urine concentration, initiation of labor, milk production.

DIAGNOSIS

Which Tests Need to Be Performed?

An MRI scan: Enhanced and Unenhanced MRI with "special views of the pituitary area" and gadolinium enhancement is sensitive and can detect most, but not all tumors. Sometimes CT scanning is used, but CT scans can miss smaller *micro*adenomas.

Complete hormone testing: This is important, and you may need to consult with an endocrinologist. Tests of follicle stimulating hormone, luteinizing hormone, morning cortisol, thyroid stimulating hormone, thyroxine, prolactin, growth hormone (somatomedin-C), and other hormones can determine the level of pituitary function.

A complete neuro-ophthalmologic evaluation: This includes a visual field exam which is needed to determine any visual loss.

Fast facts for Pituitary tumors: • MRI better than CT scan
• Complete hormone testing • Complete neuro-ophthalmologic evaluation • An experienced Neurosurgeon is a must!

TREATMENTS

The Medical and Surgical Goals for Treatment

- Normalization of hormone excess
- Restoration of normal pituitary function

The most important factor in pituitary surgery is your access to an experienced neurosurgeon. Radiation therapy is used primarily when surgical or medical therapy is not successful in reversing symptoms.

Options Prior to or Instead of Surgery

For the most common prolactin-secreting tumors, medical therapy with dopamine agonists (drugs which act like dopamine) is considered the first-line treatment. They are effective in decreasing adenoma size and restoring normal prolactin levels. Bromocriptine (Parlodel) and cabergoline (Dostinex) prevent prolactin secretion and shrink the tumor before surgery. They can be given after surgery, if tumor is left behind.[3]

For treatment of gigantism (acromegaly), taking octreotide (Sandostatin and long-acting Sandostatin LAR Depot) results in normalization of pituitary effects in about 70 percent of patients. The most common side effects are diarrhea, abdominal pain, and nausea. The most serious side effect of octreotide is gallstones, which occurs in up to 25 percent of patients on chronic therapy. Growth hormone receptor antagonist (B2036-PEG) has been recently developed and is expected to be released for use soon. It is more effective than octreotide.

Low thyroid stimulating hormone (TSH) production requires thyroid replacement therapy.

Occasionally, a small pituitary tumor may be discovered as an unexpected finding on a MRI scan performed for some other reason. The size of the tumor, coupled with the patient's symptoms and hormone status, all enter into the decision-making process. If vision is not threatened, the choice can be made to observe the small tumor over time with repeated MRI scans and visual field studies.

What Is the Role of Neurosurgery?

The majority of pituitary adenomas must be treated surgically. A few may be treated with medication before, after, or instead of surgery. It's important to reduce the pressure placed on the optic nerves and chiasm (vision, sight) and to restore normal hormone production. The major surgical goals are
* Reduction or complete removal of tumor
* Elimination of mass effect on surrounding structures

How Is the Tumor Removed?

The pituitary gland, located under the brain, sits in a small saddle-shaped area of the skull called the *sella* that forms the back wall of the sphenoid sinus (Figures 13-1, 13-2). This sinus is next to and behind the nose. Therefore, almost all surgery for removal of pituitary adenomas is performed via the "trans-sphenoidal" approach that is done through the nose.[4] This approach is very direct and does not leave any visible scars on the patient. An incision is usually performed under the lip or nostril.

A surgical microscope or "endoscope" with a mini-camera attached to a computer monitor guides the surgeon through the area. In some cases, the neurosurgeon that performs your surgery will be assisted by an ear, nose, and throat (ENT) surgeon.

Surgery is sometimes performed via a "trans-cranial" approach (through the skull). This larger operation is reserved for tumors not suited for a trans-sphenoidal approach due to their location or size.

What Are the Risks of Pituitary Surgery?

The major risk is diabetes insipidus, in which the kidney produces large volumes of urine due to lack of the water-saving, anti-diuretic hormone (ADH) from the posterior pituitary. This occurs in about six of every 100 operated patients and is usually temporary. The problem is in the risk of becoming severely dehydrated. It can be controlled with pills or nose spray. Recovery from surgery is usually quick, and most patients are discharged from the hospital in two to three days. Incomplete removal of tumor is another risk.

Radiation Therapy – When Is it Used for Pituitary Tumors?

Radiation therapy is sometimes recommended for people who have remaining or recurring tumor. For example, if a large tumor has invaded neighboring parts of the brain, partial surgical removal can relieve pressure-induced symptoms. Radiation therapy can further reduce the chances of tumor re-growth.

Another radiation technique, called *stereotactic radiosurgery*, delivers a high dose of radiation directly to the tumor in two to five treatments. Stereotactic radiosurgery has been used to treat both residual and recurrent pituitary tumors. In some cases, it might also be used for newly diagnosed tumors. Stereotactic radiosurgery can be performed either after surgical removal or as primary therapy.[5] See Chapter 17.[6]

ACOUSTIC NEUROMAS

WHAT IS AN ACOUSTIC NEUROMA?

An *acoustic neuroma*, also called vestibular Schwannoma, is a benign tumor that grows from Schwann cells coating the vestibular, hearing (8th) nerve. It often grows first in the auditory canal of the skull (where the 8th nerve lies) and then expands inward to compress the brain.

How Are Acoustic Neuromas Diagnosed?

Acoustic neuromas commonly cause slowly developing, progressive hearing loss, ringing in the ear (tinnitus), and balance problems. An MRI scan is diagnostic and also gives information about the *opposite* ear canal for comparison purposes. Schwannomas also can occur on other nerves, too.

What Are the Major Challenges?

MRI scan for Acoustic Neuroma: • Gold standard for diagnosis • Comparison of left and right sides is important (NF-2)

- Prevention of further tumor-related neurological disability
- Maintaining function of the surrounding nerves that control facial movement, balance, and swallowing
- Avoiding deafness or other damage from the tumor or treatment
- Minimizing post-surgery risks (e.g. spinal fluid leakage, infection)
- Avoiding hydrocephalus (obstruction of spinal fluid)
- Maintaining quality of life and employment
- Understanding possible hereditary implications (NF-2) and having other tumors in the head or spine (meningiomas)

What Are the Treatment Options?

Acoustic neuromas usually are slow growing. For some patients, observation is advised. As the patient, you have to shop around with different specialists (Radiosurgery or Surgery) as each specialist may not offer you all the options. For more details on surgical and radiation therapies, see Chapter 17. The following are possible treatment alternatives to ask about:

Treatments: • Surgical or Radiosurgical • Choices depend on tumor size • Prevention of tumor-related neurological disability.

- **Surgical resection** is indicated for patients with larger acoustic neuromas that have caused major neurological deficits from brain compression. Often a neurosurgeon and an ear, nose, and throat surgeon (ENT) will operate together, particularly if removing bone near the hearing apparatus is necessary.
- **Stereotactic radiosurgery** has become the main alternative to acoustic tumor resection for smaller tumors; the goals are to preserve neurological function and prevent tumor growth. The long-term outcomes of radiosurgery, particularly with GammaKnife techniques, have justified its role in the primary management of this disease.[7]

- **Fractionated radiation therapy** can be offered to the few patients who have larger tumors for which radiosurgery may not be feasible.
- Careful observation with no intervention
- Combinations of the above

GENETIC ASPECTS OF ACOUSTIC NEUROMAS

When tumors are present on both sides, a condition called neurofibromatosis type 2 (NF-2) almost certainly exists. Patients with NF-2 pose specific challenges, particularly with preservation of hearing and function of other cranial nerves. These patients should be treated at a major center that has seen many such cases. For more information about NF-2, see Table 12-2 and Chapter 24: Heredity and Other Causes of Brain Tumors.[6]

> NF-2 is almost conclusive if neuromas are on both sides.

SUMMARY

You have learned many details about your specific tumor in this chapter. Now it's time to arm yourself with additional information. By now, you should know about some of the medications you will receive (Chapter 9) and how to get an expert opinion (Chapter 6). In the second book, I'll give you more information about medications (Chapter 17) and you'll learn about complementary and alternative therapies in Chapter 18. It may also be helpful for you to review how to use the Internet to investigate your options (See Chapter 4), especially if you have not used this resource already.

Table 12-2 Internet Resources for Meningiomas, Acoustic & Pituitary Tumors

Subject	Web site and contact information
Metastases to brain	http://www.emedicine.com/radio/topic101.htm
Meningiomas	http://meningioma.intranets.com (Internet group) http://groups.yahoo.com/group/meningioma http://disc.server.com/Indices/148753.html
RU-486	http://www.medscape.com/viewarticle/456128 http://www.cbctrust.com/ru486.96.html

Meningioma Pathology, Classification	http://www.brighamandwomens.com/neurosurgery/
	    meningioma/WHOclassification.asp
	http://www-medlib.med.utah.edu/WebPath/CNSHTML/
	    CNS115.html

Pituitary Network Association	http://www.pituitary.org **or** E-mail: P.O. Box 1958, Thousand Oaks, CA 91358 (805) 499-9973, Fax: (805) 480-0633 http://www.pituitary.com

Pituitary- General	http://www.graphmed.com/Movies/anatomie.html (active cartoon)
	http://www.thedoctorsdoctor.com/diseases/pituitary_
	    adenoma.htm
	http://www.clevelandclinicmeded.com/diseasemanagement/
	    endocrinology/pituitary/pituitary.htm#anatomy (Extensive
	    review)
	http://www.iis.com.br/~jgcc/chiasm1.htm (optic chiasm)

Pituitary-Cushing's Disease and Effects	http://www.uic.edu/depts/mcne/homepage/neurofounders.html http://www.niddk.nih.gov/health/endo/pubs/cushings/ cushings.htm

Pituitary Cases	http://pathweb.uchc.edu/eAtlas/CNS/243.htm
	http://www.medhelp.org/forums/neuro/messages/31350a.html
	http://www.iis.com.br/~jgcc/pitaden1.htm
	    (Adenoma effects)
	http://www.ghorayeb.com/PituitaryMRI.html
	    (Diagnosis)

Pituitary Treatment	http://www.irsa.org/pituitary_tumors.html (radiation)
	http://www.cksociety.org/PatientInfo/MedicalConditions/
	    pituitary_adenoma.asp
	http://www.medscape.com/viewarticle/456137?WebLogicSessi
	    on=P1tL82p8ZnhzguZTXES1nl2naQFnliwUEa2unQ477nGu9P
	    MiTgfo|-1935058065519272500/184161393/6/7001/7001/
	    7002/7002/7001/-1 (Radiosurgery)
	http://www.c3.hu/~mavideg/jns/4.html (medication)

Table 12-2 continued

Pituitary:Trans- sphenoidal surgery Cranial surgery	http://apollo.med.unc.edu/ent/oto-hns/whatsnew.html#MIPS http://www.endotext.com/neuroendo/neuroendo13/ neuroendo13.htm_Toc61071910
Acoustic neuromas	http://www.anausa.org (Acoustic Neuroma Association)

Acoustic neuromas
(Schwannoma)
	http://www.anarchive.org (all the options)
	http://www.acousticneuroma.neurosurgery.pitt.edu (balanced)
	http://www.emedicine.com/ent/topic239.htm (general, extensive)
	http://www.uscneurosurgery.com/glossary/s/schwannoma.htm
	  (general)
	http://www.med.uc.edu/neurorad/webpage/bra.html (other
	  nerves)
	http://www.neurosurgery.org/focus/may03/14-5-2.pdf
	  (Radiosurgery)
	http://www.hopkinsmedicine.org/radiosurgery/disorders/
	  acoustic.cfm

Acoustic Neuroma Scans	http://www.mribhatia.com/braintf10 http://www.mribhatia.com/braintf10/l2-braintf10_t1- coronal.html
Acoustic Neuroma Neurofibromatosis NF-2	http://www.nf.org http://www.nf2crew.com http://www.acousticneuroma.neurosurgery.pitt.edu http://www.emedicine.com/radio/topic7.htm http://www.nf.org/schwannomatosis http://www.webcrossings.com/nf2crew/links.html http://neurosurgery.mgh.harvard.edu/NFR/nf2.htm

CHAPTER 13

Tumors Originating in the Head Outside the Brain – Germ Cell Tumors

I wish I could tell you that everything will be fine and you have nothing to worry about but you know that is not true. There are going to be good days, and not so good days. This is hard work, and many hard decisions have to be made… This is a scary journey my friend, but you are in good company.

Luanne, a brain tumor survivor. Las Vegas, NV.

Key search words

- metastases
- germinoma
- tumor grade
- staging

- MRI, MR-Spect and PET scans
- non-germinomatous germinoma
- alpha fetoprotein (AFP)
- human choriogonadotrophin (h-CG)

- germ cell tumors
- therapy options
- tumor markers
- Internet resources

GENERAL QUESTIONS

WHAT IS A GERM CELL TUMOR?

A *germ cell tumor* (GCT) is made up of cells looking like those seen in early embryos. Some GCT types even have the potential to form teeth, hair or muscle. Pathologists who study these tumors under the microscope assign family names ("germinoma") and grades (low grade or malignant) following biopsy or removal. As I mentioned in Chapter 1, neuropathology experts can disagree on which family a germ cell tumor should be assigned. (See World Health Organization Classification[1] and Table 13-2.)

Over the past 75 years, various names have been used to describe different members of the germ cell tumor family. The two main groups that are discussed in this chapter are: a) germinoma

> **Major Groups of Germ Cell Tumors:**
> • Primary brain or metastasis • Germinoma or Non-germinomatous germ cell

and b) non-germinomatous germ cell tumors. The latter include endodermal sinus tumor, extra-gonadal germ cell tumor, teratoma, malignant teratoma, and choriocarcinoma (from the placenta). (For a general review, see references[1,3] and Table 13-2).

A BRAIN TUMOR OR A METASTASIS – WHAT IS THE DIFFERENCE?

Germinomas can be either primary in the brain or metastatic tumors ("mets" or secondary tumors) that have spread from cancer originating elsewhere in the body.[1,2] A *primary brain tumor* starts in the brain. The astrocytic (Chapter 10) and neuronal tumors (some also called PNETs) start from actual brain tissue. Technically speaking, many tumors in the head do not come from brain, but rather from its coverings (meningiomas), nerve linings (neuromas, Schwannomas), glands inside the head (pituitary adenomas), and other tissues (lymphomas and pineal gland tumors). Metastases are discussed separately in Chapter 15: Brain Metastases).

IS THE GERM CELL TUMOR (GCT) A PRIMARY TUMOR OR METASTASIS?

This is a crucial first question. Germ cell tumors can start anywhere in the body, but usually they begin in the chest, ovaries or testicles, and later spread to the brain. As a metastasis they can grow anywhere inside the brain, even in the fluid cavities, called ventricles. In contrast, most primary GCTs (starting in the head) develop from above the pituitary or pineal gland (pineal region tumors) (Figures 13-1 and 13-2). If the tumor starts from outside the head, different forms of therapy are needed. Knowing the exact type and source (primary or metastasis) are critical for your treatment success.

How Common Are Germ Cell Tumors?

Germ cell tumors make up about 5 percent of all brain tumors in adults and children, are twice as frequent in males and are more common in persons aged 20 to 40 years. For some reason, they also appear to be more common in Australians and people of Asian ancestry. (See Table 13-2, General information.)

What Are Typical Signs and Symptoms?

The signs (objective findings that a doctor finds after examination) and symptoms (sensations or feelings that do not feel normal) of a brain tumor always result from interference by the tumor with normal brain pathways in specific areas and not the tumor type (Table 13-1). For example:

- The pineal gland (Figure 13-1) regulates melatonin secretion and sleep cycles. With a tumor in the pineal gland, four inches behind the nose, nearly at the center of the head (Figure 13-2), many people complain of headache, nausea and vomiting (in the morning), unsteadiness, or inability to look upward. If the tumor is nearer the pituitary gland, symptoms include headache, visual field difficulties, and frequent urination, because the pituitary gland regulates water release from the kidney by its anti-diuretic hormone, ADH. This site is also near the optic nerves.
- A tumor in the third ventricle (Figure 13-2) will block the outflow of cerebrospinal fluid, causing headache and vomiting.

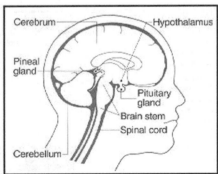

Figure 13-1 Pituitary and Pineal gland locations.

Bottom line: Knowing whether your tumor is primary or a metastasis is critical for treatment success.

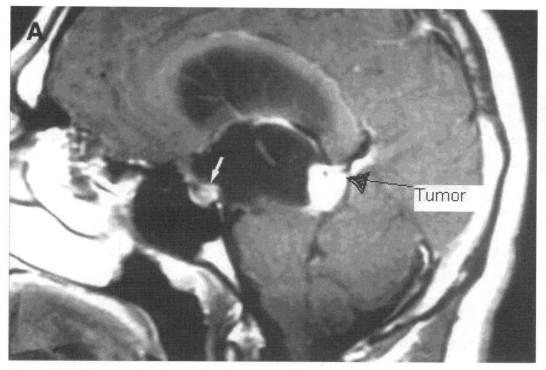

Figure 13-2 MRI scan. Pineal tumor (black arrow, right). Pituitary gland (white arrow).

HOW ARE GERM CELL TUMORS DIFFERENT IN ADULTS AND CHILDREN?

Mixed (malignant) teratomas are more frequent in children, while pure germinomas tend to be a disease of young adults. As a result of the potential side effects of radiation on a child's brain, recent studies have focused on initial, more intensive chemotherapy approaches to delay or omit radiation.[4] This approach is now being evaluated in two international studies, one being conducted by the International Pediatric Oncology Society (SIOP) in Europe[5] and the other by Dr. John Finlay's group[6] in Los Angeles.

Table 13-1 Important Facts About Your Germ Cell Tumor

Symptoms	Possible Locations	Tumor Grade	Tumor Family	Therapy Choices
Weakness Field of vision Blind spots Frequent urination Dehydration Headache Seizure Vomiting	Metastasis or Primary Pineal Pituitary Ventricle Meninges Frontal or Parietal lobe	Low grade or malignant	Germinoma (Pure) Nongerminomatous germ cell tumors • Embryonal • Mixed germ cell • Endodermal sinus • Choriocarcinoma • Teratoma with AFP, hCG secretion Pineocytoma Pineoblastoma	Surgery for diagnosis and removal Radiation alone Chemotherapy and radiation Chemotherapy alone* Radiation implants* * =Unestablished effectivenes

WHAT ARE MY CHANCES OF CURE WITH A GERM CELL TUMOR?

In 2004, more than 90 percent of people with germinomas will be cured. Even non-germinomatous tumors are having phenomenal survivals with newer approaches.[7] The most important elements in predicting a successful result are the following:

- Type and grade of tumor
- Location(s) of the tumor
- Stage or amount of spread (metastasis within the nervous system)
- Age
- Amount of the tumor that is left in after surgery (skill of the neurosurgeon)
- Response to and type of therapies you receive

I have many patients with highly malignant, and sometimes recurrent, tumors who are alive five to 20 years later. Yes, having any brain tumor is a serious diagnosis, but being in expert hands will increase your chances for survival.

Bottom line: Successful outcome is dependent equally upon location, stage, and tumor type.

DIAGNOSIS AND TREATMENTS

WHAT IS THE INITIAL EVALUATION FOR A GERM CELL TUMOR?

Foremost, you and your doctors *must* know if your brain tumor is primary (i.e., it originated in the brain), or if it was a metastasis (spread) from another part of the body. The stage and degree of spread is critical in planning your treatment options. Most brain tumor specialists and other physicians will evaluate a patient with a suspected germ cell tumor using the following series of tests:

1. A thorough history, physical examination, and neurological exam
2. Scans for complete staging (evaluation of extent or spread)
   - High-resolution brain and spinal MRI scans, with and without gadolinium contrast, to visualize the brain, spine, and tumor
   - CT scans of chest and abdomen, both unenhanced and enhanced with contrast media
   - MR Spect (spectroscopy) to measure chemical components of the tumor. This is usually reserved to estimate the difference between low- and high-grade, or to tell whether the "tumor" is composed of live or dead cells, after treatment.
   - PET scan (positron emission tomography) is not commonly used initially, though it can measure the activity or the metabolic rate of the tumor.
3. Measurement of alpha-fetoprotein and human choriogonadotrophin markers in blood and spinal fluid
4. Examination of spinal fluid for cells, if spinal MRI is negative (staging)
5. Screening tests for pituitary hormones and their function, especially water retention (ADH activity)
6. An EEG (*electroencephalogram* or brain wave test), if the patient has had actual or suspected seizures (convulsions)
7. Visual field (blind spot) examination by an ophthalmologist (eye doctor), if the tumor is near the pituitary gland or optic nerves/ pathways, or is causing visual symptoms
8. Neuropsychological testing to help recognize problems in different areas of higher brain function before and after radiation is given

The recent case history below illustrates what can happen when appropriate staging is not performed:

Erin, a wife and 26-year-old mother of two young boys, and also a Jehovah's Witness, was referred to me because her doctor noticed that she had a pineal gland cyst. Two years earlier, she had received radiation for an unbiopsied, "classic glioma" of her upper spinal cord. Her original treating doctors were confident of the "glioma" diagnosis.

I explained that in order to treat her appropriately, she needed a biopsy of the pineal gland, since it was likely that her spinal tumor two years ago was really a metastasis from the pineal tumor, and not a glioma. Spinal fluid studies looking for hormones and proteins to diagnose the tumor type were not helpful. She asked to delay decision-making.

A year later, the tumor spread to and destroyed her posterior pituitary gland, causing her to urinate frequently. She underwent a biopsy and a mixed teratoma/ germinoma was found, not a glioma. We recommended a special, intensive chemotherapy protocol to be followed by customized radiation fields so as to not damage her spine from the previous treatment. This combination is curative in over 50 percent of patients. She refused further therapy and died one year later.

The principles here are: 1) biopsy before therapy is mandatory; and 2) biopsy, not guessing, leads to the best choice of therapy. If the original tumor had been

> Biopsy before therapy is mandatory.

accurately diagnosed in Erin's case, then surgery to the spine and brain followed by radiation and a short course of chemotherapy could have been curative, and she could possibly have lived to see her sons grow up.

SURGERY

Do I Have Any Options Other Than Surgery for Diagnosis?

Except in highly unusual circumstances, a biopsy should be obtained to identify the exact type of germ cell tumor. For a probable small benign teratoma, a patient could be observed with frequent MRI scans, and the tumor could remain stable indefinitely.

If there is extensive spread and initial surgery is unwise, then the diagnosis and

> Biopsy, not guessing, leads to the best choice of therapy.

treatment decisions can be made based on the presence of alpha-fetoprotein (AFP) or human choriogonadotrophin (h-CG) in the blood and spinal fluid. The case below illustrates this point:

Muriel, a 45-year-old woman who volunteers to prepare food for the homeless, presented a complicated situation to her doctors in July 2002. She

Bottom line: You must know if you have pure germinoma or non-germinomatous type. Accuracy can be a matter of life or death!

had been having morning headaches for a month, but thought they were due to the odors from the kitchen. She was also a diabetic on insulin, had high blood pressure and an aneurysm in her abdomen. Her brain MRI showed a tumor wrapped around her pituitary gland and projecting back into the ventricle. Her blood studies showed elevated AFP and h-CG, diagnostic of a malignant mixed teratoma.

Muriel's case was fully discussed at the Tumor Board of a major University hospital. The decision was made to administer chemotherapy first, without surgery or biopsy, because of her precarious state, the aneurysm, and that we knew from the blood studies which kind of tumor she had. If there was no response by MRI, radiation would commence. Muriel's tumor shrank 75 percent with chemotherapy, and three months later, her tumor was 95 percent removed with only a six-day post-operative stay in Intensive Care. The pathology report showed only a few malignant cells and a lot of dead tumor. She received all her recommended treatments and is back as a volunteer.

The vignette above is another example of why I recommend that your case be presented to the Tumor Board of your hospital. Usually, this happens after biopsy or surgery. In this case, the Tumor Board provided management suggestions for the sequence of treatments prior to surgery.

What Medications or Precautions Should Occur Before or During Surgery?

If the pituitary gland is affected, then steroid and other hormone supplements should be given to increase your capacity to undergo stress. Lack of water retention (dehydration) from posterior pituitary gland failure also may need to be controlled through careful use of medications like vasopressin (DDVAP) and intravenous fluids. See (Chapters 9,17, and 19.[8]) Talk to your surgeon and anesthesiologist about this.

AFTER SURGERY OPTIONS

If My Germ Cell Tumor Cannot Be Removed, What Other Therapies Are There?

Generally, if further surgery is not advised, there are no standard choices. Decision-making is complex and requires input from different specialists involved in your care. This is when presentation of your case to a Tumor Board at your local hospital or at a medical center specializing in brain tumors is key.

Bottom line: Regardless of "grade," if a germ cell tumor has spread to brain or spinal fluid pathways, aggressive treatment is needed.

ARE LOW- AND HIGH-GRADE GERM CELL TUMORS TREATED DIFFERENTLY?

Treatment of a germ cell tumor depends on its family type and status as a primary or metastatic tumor.[9] Accuracy here can be a matter of life or death. This is why many people obtain two or three opinions on the pathology diagnosis and therapy options before approving a treatment plan. (See Chapter 6: Experts and Second Opinions.)

- **Low-grade (benign) germ cell tumors: teratomas**
  Often they can be removed and shelled out completely during surgery. If the pathologist determines that no malignant cells remain, then no further treatment is recommended, but regular follow-up scans are needed. About 5 percent of tumors will recur, but the timeline between 6 months and 20 years is not predictable.
- **Malignant germ cell tumors:**
  Pure germ cell tumors (germinomas are called seminomas when they occur in the testes) are malignant and used to be treated by radiation therapy only. This was curative in most patients whose disease had not spread. The debate was whether just local radiation, or whole brain plus spinal radiation, should be given. (See Table 13-2, Germ cell tumors, General, and Clinical Trials.) However, discovery of late adverse radiation effects including dementia, mild memory problems, vascular disease and stroke have resulted in the study of chemotherapy to delay or omit radiation therapy. Recent studies suggest only local radiation is needed for localized disease.[10] Several centers are involved in national and international clinical trials of chemotherapy for germinomas to reduce the brain damage effects[4] (Table 13-2).
  - Mixed teratomas are also called non-germinomatous germ cell tumors (non-ger-min-o-ma-tous germ cell tumors, a mouthful to pronounce), extra-gonadal, or mixed germ cell tumors. These contain both benign-looking and malignant cells. They used to be treated with radiation alone, but the addition of chemotherapy has resulted in many more cures, from 30 to 70 percent! These tumors secrete special proteins, alpha-fetoprotein (AFP) or human choriogonadotrophin (hCG), into the spinal fluid and blood which can be monitored regularly to determine tumor activity and even can be used for diagnosis, if biopsy is not possible. Several clinical trials for these tumors were open to patients in 2004 (Table 13-2).
  - Embryonal germ cell tumors and endodermal sinus tumors (AFP, hCG secretors) are malignant and usually need both radiation and chemotherapy.

- Choriocarcinomas secrete human choriogonadotrophin (h-CG), which can be detected in the serum or spinal fluid. These respond to different chemotherapy combinations. Metastases from the testicles to brain respond to combined therapies, and many people, like Lance Armstrong, have been cured with them.[11]

- **Pineoblastomas**
  These are malignant, rare and belong to a completely different family, called *primitive neuroectodermal tumors* (PNETs).[12] The name is similar, and they can originate near the pineal gland,[13] so this could cause confusion in terms. They are discussed separately in Chapter 11.

- **Pineocytoma tumors**
  These are rare, usually slow growing, and if completely removed they usually do not require additional therapy. If pineocytoma tumors are malignant or have spread into the spinal fluid, then radiation is the current treatment of choice.

- **Pineal cysts**
  Pineal cysts without tumor are common and occur in about 2 to 5 percent of the normal population. This is different from a pineocytoma. Sometimes a tumor also can have a cystic component. Your specialist should be able to evaluate this condition and tell which one you have.

RADIATION THERAPY

Radiation therapy has been the most extensively used treatment for all germ cell tumors. It is certainly effective, even curative for germinomas, although there is always a trade-off between effectiveness and serious long-term side effects (memory problems, dementia, vascular disease, and stroke). Its advantage, however, in treating low-grade germ cell tumors, or teratomas, is not agreed upon by cancer specialists. Recent studies suggest only local radiation may be needed for localized pure germinomas.[14] Used alone, radiation is less effective in long-term control of malignant teratomas and endodermal sinus type tumors. Chemotherapy has been used to delay or omit radiation therapy for both adults and children.

What Are the Different Types of Radiation Therapy for Germ Cell Tumors?

There are several different techniques used to irradiate germ cell tumors that all have advantages and disadvantages. Your radiotherapist should discuss with you the pros and cons specific to your tumor's location and stage.

Clinical trials are currently underway to study newer techniques of giving radiation that may overcome some former problems with brain injury. For example, instead of radiation to the whole brain, only the tumor site plus ventricles may receive radiation. (See Radiation section in Chapter 17)

CHEMOTHERAPY

Chemotherapy has been used successfully in the following settings:
- To shrink the tumor for later surgical removal
- As combinations to delay radiation treatment or limit radiation exposure
- For recurrent tumors, after radiation or first-line chemotherapy have failed
- Simultaneously with radiation to "sensitize" the tumor and destroy it more completely
- As the only therapy in young children or adults on a clinical trial
- For recurrent tumors, there are many Phase 2 clinical trials for both children and adults that can be accessed through the National Cancer Institute and www.virtualtrials.com websites (Table 13-2)

Chemotherapy in combination with radiation therapy has benefited all patients *except* those with pure germinomas.

Chemotherapy has been mentioned in standard protocols and recent textbooks. In both the young child and adult, many oncologists have been using combinations of platinum drugs (carboplatin or cisplatin), etoposide (VP-16) from may-apple extract (mandrake), vincristine (derived from the vinca plant), and cyclophosphamide as first line therapy before radiation. The "best therapy" is still controversial and several candidate combinations are being studied in clinical trials. See also two international studies, one being conducted by the International Pediatric Oncology Society (SIOP) in Europe and the other by Dr. John Finlay's group in Los Angeles.

EFFECTIVE TREATMENT FOR SIDE EFFECTS OF CHEMOTHERAPY

Lastly, a note on the importance of effective treatment for side effects of chemotherapy. There is a growing tendency for insurance companies and HMOs to refuse payments for these supportive medications.

I will never forget Jimmy, an 18-year-old honor student with a large, supportive family from China; he was my first patient as a Fellow in training. He had a

Bottom line: Germ Cell tumors can be cured!

germ cell tumor that completely responded to the new (in 1978) "Einhorn" protocol of cisplatin, bleomycin and vinblastine chemotherapy.[15,16] Jimmy suffered terribly from severe nausea and vomiting caused by cisplatin. I had taken a hypnosis course and offered my new skill to him, which seemed to help for one treatment, but he decided to stop chemotherapy because of the uncontrolled nausea. The tumor returned in four months, and he died. I know that if we had had effective anti-nausea drugs like Zofran™ or Kytril™ then, he would be alive today.

Many people receiving these drugs do not know how fortunate they are, compared with patients 25 years ago. Many insurance companies and HMOs still refuse to authorize these effective medications to prevent or treat side effects. (See Chapter 23 for advice on insurance coverage.)

Table 13-2 Internet Resources for Germ Cell Family of Brain Tumors

Subject	Website or Contact Information
Metastases To Brain	http://www.emedicine.com/radio/topic101.htm
Germ Cell Tumors (general)	http://intl-theoncologist.alphamedpress.org/cgi/content/full/5/4/312 http://neurosurgery.mgh.harvard.edu/newwhobt.htm#Other http://www.emedicine.com/med/topic2246.htm http://www.emedicine.com/med/topic863.htm
Pineal Region Tumors	http://www.stjude.org/disease-summaries/0,2557,449_2167_7407, 00.html?source=overture&kw=germ+cell+tumors http://neurosun.medsch.ucla.edu/diagnoses/braintumor/ braintumordis_11.html
Germ Cell Tumors, Metastases	http://www.emedicine.com/med/topic759.htm http://tcrc.acor.org/lance.html
Germ Cell Tumors -Clinical trials	http://www.centerwatch.com/patient/studies/cat564.html http://www.virtualtrials.com/new.cfm (newer trials) http://www.virtualtrials.com/mmenu.cfm http://www.cancer.gov/clinicaltrials/finding http://www.virtualtrials.com/trialdetails.cfm?id=61800391
Pituitary Network Association	http://www.pituitary.org or pna@pituitary.org mail: P.O. Box 1958, Thousand Oaks, CA 91358 phone: (805) 499-9973, Fax: (805) 480-0633 http://www.pituitary.com

Tabel 13-2 continued

Pituitary, General References	http://www.graphmed.com/Movies/anatomie.html (active cartoon) http://www.thedoctorsdoctor.com/diseases/pituitary_adenoma.htm http://www.clevelandclinicmeded.com/diseasemanagement/ endocrinology/pituitary/pituitary.htm#anatomy (Extensive review) http://www.iis.com.br/~jgcc/chiasm1.htm (optic chiasm)
Pituitary, Cushing's Disease and Effects	http://www.uic.edu/depts/mcne/homepage/neurofounders.html http://www.niddk.nih.gov/health/endo/pubs/cushings/ cushings.htm

CHAPTER 14

Brain Lymphomas - Tumors Originating in the Head

Hope is an invaluable asset to all of us in coping with illness, as well as with the frustration of not being able to identify a single best treatment option. And hope becomes even more vital when affirmation as to the most appropriate measures for managing your disease does not exist.

Neal Levitan, Executive Director, Brain Tumor Society

BRAIN LYMPHOMAS

Key search words

- lymphomas
- staging
- immunophenotype
- radiation
- internet resources

- metastases
- T and B cells
- steroids
- Rituxan™ antibody therapy

- MRI
- tumor markers
- chemotherapy
- therapy options

GENERAL QUESTIONS

WHAT IS A LYMPHOMA? IS THE TYPE IMPORTANT?

Lymphoma is a tumor that comes from immune cells. There are two types: the Hodgkin and non-Hodgkin lymphoma. The former is extremely rare in the head. Lymphomas usually grow in lymph glands, bones, or bone marrow anywhere in the body. Those starting in the brain are called *primary* central nervous system lymphomas (PCNSLs). The brain has no lymph nodes, so we do not know where they originate in the brain.

HOW COMMON ARE PRIMARY CENTRAL NERVOUS SYSTEM LYMPHOMAS?

Twenty-five years ago, a PCNSL was a rarity; today they are more common. The frequency of lymphomas has increased ten-fold from 0.5 percent to about 5 percent of all brain tumors. Why? The increase is due to three groups: a) patients with compromised immune systems who are now living longer (e.g., cancer and AIDS patients), b) patients with lupus, rheumatoid arthritis, and bone marrow transplantation who are receiving immune suppressive therapies; and c) patients who are having (more frequent) biopsies. The latter has led to diagnoses that are more accurate.

> A lymphoma metastasis is more common than a primary in the brain.

DOES THE LOCATION MAKE A DIFFERENCE?

Yes. Location can affect the diagnostic tests and therapy.
- Lymphomas originating in the brain are still unusual, so it's imperative that a search begin in all lymph node areas (neck, groin, chest, abdomen), since lymphomas usually start there.
- It is more suspicious for typical PCNSLs to appear in the frontal lobes, while metastases from elsewhere can be in any location.
- Tumors in the spine will require chemotherapy into the spinal canal, chemotherapy into a reservoir in the brain, or radiation along the spine.
- The location alone will usually not affect obtaining a biopsy or the effectiveness of later therapy (see the story of Gerald below).

DIAGNOSIS

WHAT ARE SYMPTOMS OF A LYMPHOMA IN THE BRAIN?

Typical symptoms reflect the area affected by the tumor. Most lymphomas in the brain grow in the frontal and temporal lobes. Symptoms include headache, vomiting, forgetfulness, difficulty in finding words, confusion, double vision, wobbliness (ataxia), weakness of a leg or arm, and sometimes facial weakness.

WHAT ARE THE DIFFERENCES BETWEEN A "T" AND A "B" LYMPHOMA?

These non-Hodgkin types are named after types of normal immune lymphocytes from which they develop. In normal lymph nodes, the outer area produces T cells that seek out and destroy germs, while B cells, produced in the inner area, are programmed (by the T cells) to make antibody proteins that protect against future attacks. This is what happens, for example, with successful immunization to tetanus or polio. Normal *and* tumor cells from these areas bear similar "marker" proteins (called the immunophenotype) for T or B cells. The T and B lymphomas respond to different chemotherapy and radiation combinations.

Correct lymphoma typing is mandatory for correct therapy.

WHAT TESTS ARE NEEDED FOR THE INITIAL EVALUATION OF A LYMPHOMA?

Most neurooncologists (brain tumor specialists) and other physicians will evaluate a patient with a suspected brain lymphoma in the following manner with:
1. Thorough medical history, general physical and neurological examination.
2. Brain and spine MRI with/without contrast to visualize the brain and tumor.
3. CT scan of the chest, abdominal MRI, or ultrasound including lymph node chains, liver, and spleen (to exclude primary lymphoma elsewhere).
4. Complete blood counts, sedimentation rate, liver and kidney function tests, serum and spinal fluid levels of lactic acid dehydrogenase (LDH).
5. Biopsy (almost always indicated).
6. Analysis of cells in spinal fluid, when a biopsy is dangerous (rare).
7. Evaluation of the tissue specimen or spinal fluid by a hematopathologist (a pathologist who specializes in diseases of the blood and lymph glands).
8. Immune marker analysis (immunophenotype) on the lymphoma tissue.

TREATMENTS

WHY DO I NEED A TEAM OF DOCTORS TO TREAT MY LYMPHOMA?

Remember: Lymphomas in the brain are uncommon. They require complex management with chemotherapy first, followed by radiation and possibly immune therapy (see below). Evaluation should take place in a comprehensive cancer center where physicians with different areas of expertise can work together. This team might include neurooncologists, neuroradiologists, neurosurgeons, neuropathologists, hematopathologists, neurologists, oncologists, radiation oncologists, endocrinologists, and neuropsychologists. (See Chapter 5.) Due to its rarity, families should be encouraged to participate in clinical trials in an attempt to improve and optimize therapy. Below is a case example of what might happen when a team is not involved:

> Gerald is a 49-year-old southern Californian executive who two years earlier had a mild stroke. He was treated with steroids and then rehabilitation. Gerald was told that he had a "brain tumor" that caused arm weakness. His local oncologist told him that the tumor could be either a glioma or "secondary" lymphoma (originating from elsewhere). Their team said that a biopsy was unnecessary, as he would need radiation therapy anyway. In the meantime, Gerald had received a week of steroids to lessen the swelling in the brain and return function to his arm.
>
> Gerald came to see me for a second opinion. We took an MRI scan and the tumor was gone! This disappearance after steroids is almost proof of a lymphoma. We waited eight weeks, took another scan, and sure enough the tumor had inched back near his brain stem (pons), next to the spinal cord. Dr. Keith Black performed careful biopsies around the brain stem area and on the fourth "pinch" sample of tumor, a B-cell-type lymphoma was diagnosed. Gerald received high dose intravenous methotrexate and Rituxan antibody therapy, followed by radiation. He is well four years later.

What can we learn from Gerald's story? Other neurosurgeons did not want to perform a biopsy because they considered it dangerous and *unnecessary*. Without the biopsy, however, Gerald would have received only radiation, which was not the correct therapy.

Do I Have Options Before Deciding on Surgery?

The option for surgery depends upon the severity of your symptoms. Emergency neurosurgery can be lifesaving to remove pressure and/ or insert a shunt to relieve pressure or obstruction.

Accurate diagnosis is paramount. If surgery is considered too dangerous, a diagnosis sometimes can be made by analyzing tumor cells in the spinal fluid that are obtained from a spinal tap.

> Steroids before biopsy can make a lymphoma disappear and confuse the diagnosis.

NEUROSURGERY FOR A LYMPHOMA – DOES IT HELP?

The role of neurosurgery for lymphomas is different from other tumors in the brain. For most brain tumors, the more tumor tissue that can be removed (for diagnosis and treatment) by the surgeon, the better the prognosis for longer life. Lymphomas are the exception to this rule.

We know that the amount of lymphoma removed at surgery has little effect on survival.[1] This was known even before our more effective combined chemotherapy and radiation approach. Surgery still remains important for three reasons:
- Biopsy to confirm the diagnosis and define the exact type of lymphoma
- Preservation or improvement of neurological function
- Insertion of a shunt to decrease pressure that cannot be managed by other means

One current approach to diagnosis is by stereotactic, closed biopsy. This should provide enough tumor for an accurate diagnosis 90 percent of the time.[2] This convenient, less traumatic method of biopsy avoids an open operation. Most patients go home in 24 hours or less. If needed after the diagnosis, a short course of steroids quickly reduces any swelling (often in less than 24 hours) with return of functions.

If My Lymphoma Is Removed or Reduced by Surgery, Are Other Therapies Needed?

Yes!

We know that even the best surgeon cannot completely remove all cancer cells; this is even truer for lymphomas. Thus, the after-surgical therapies are critical to your treatment and longer life. I recommend a Tumor Board evaluation or referral to a medical center that specializes in lymphoma treatment. Then an entire team can discuss the diagnosis, review tests, and make recommendations for the next sequence of treatments. This usually occurs after surgery, but it might also take place beforehand. Many centers offer experimental approaches that can include radiation, chemotherapy, and immunotherapy. (See Chapter 17: Treatments.[3]) There are few website resources for brain lymphomas.

> The major neurosurgical goal is biopsy rather than complete removal.

What Is a Shunt Operation, and Why Is It Necessary?

See section on shunts in Chapter 11 and Table 14-1.

What Medications Will I Receive Before or During Surgery?

See Chapter 9, Medications.

RADIATION THERAPY

How Has the Role of Radiation Therapy Changed in the Treatment of Lymphoma?

Twenty years ago, all patients with lymphomas of the brain or spine received immediate radiotherapy and showed dramatic tumor shrinkage within days. The problem was that the tumor returned in weeks to months.[3,4] Then, sensitivity of PCNSLs to chemotherapy was not understood. Now, chemotherapy, usually methotrexate, is the initial treatment at most centers. Irradiation is initiated *after* chemotherapy has been completed. One exception might be use of emergency irradiation to shrink a spinal tumor that causes paralysis.

> **Sequence of therapies:**
> 1) Chemotherapy first
> 2) Possible immune therapy (Rituxan)
> 3) Radiation is last.

WHAT ARE THE DIFFERENT TYPES OF RADIATION THERAPY FOR LYMPHOMAS?

There are several different techniques used to irradiate lymphomas. They all have advantages and disadvantages. Your radiotherapist should discuss with you the pros and cons specific to your particular tumor. Generally, the techniques that provide laser-like precision are less important because lymphomas are diffuse with poorly defined borders. The precise timing of radiation, whether after chemotherapy or immunotherapy, is still an evolving science. If used correctly, radiation continues to contribute to the cure of many patients with primary central nervous system lymphomas.

CHEMOTHERAPY AND OTHER DRUGS

WHY IS CHEMOTHERAPY GIVEN BEFORE RADIATION THERAPY FOR LYMPHOMA?

Primary central nervous system lymphomas illustrate of how poorly planned therapy can affect survival. There is a reason for the specific sequence of therapies. Radiation to the human brain causes changes in brain cells and blood vessels, which render them exquisitely sensitive to the toxic effects of methotrexate, the best chemotherapy we have for lymphoma. And when methotrexate is given *after* radiation, brain cells die and calcium deposits and dead tissue appear on scans. Unfortunately, dementia also may follow. We first noted this disastrous finding in children being treated for leukemia and lymphoma in the 1970s. When it was later reported in adults, it was called *demineralizing leukoencephalopathy* because of its effect on white matter tracts as well as neuron cells. This is why chemotherapy is now given *before* radiation.

WHAT IS THE ROLE OF CHEMOTHERAPY AND OTHER DRUGS FOR LYMPHOMAS?

Chemotherapy has evolved into the major component of successful treatment, paralleling the success of lymphoma therapy in other locations of the body. Fortunately, most lymphomas interrupt the blood-brain-barrier, so drug delivery to the tumor in the brain is not the problem. Since 1990, more than 10 trials have shown that either high dose methotrexate[6] or a combination of cyclophosphamide-adriamycin-vincristine (CAV) can double or triple *average* survival times by seven to more than 44 months!

No one combination has proven more effective than the other has, so choices still need to be made. For example, if you have received radiation, then a non-methotrexate combination could be tried initially. Finally, high-dose chemotherapy followed by stem cell infusion, harvested from the patient's own bone marrow, also has shown promising results. Several adult and pediatric clinical trials of new chemotherapies and immunotherapies are underway (Table 14-1).

Dr. Lisa DeAngelis in New York has described a fairly standard "chemotherapy first" approach.[7] This combination uses high-dose intravenous and intrathecal (direct administration into the spinal fluid) methotrexate, followed by the rescue drug called leucovorin, that protects the bone marrow and skin cells. This is followed by a combination of vincristine, procarbazine, and ara-C for several months. Only then does radiation commence. We know that over 50 percent of patients treated appropriately with chemotherapy first, sometimes followed by anti-lymphoma antibodies (Rituximab-Rituxan) – and then radiation – will be alive five years later; some will be cured (Chapter 19: Medications, section on regional chemotherapy).

IMMUNOTHERAPY – HOW IS IT USED TO TREAT LYMPHOMAS?

Immunotherapy uses the immune system to recognize, target, and kill tumor cells. Human lymph cells are the best studied and characterized in the body. Scientists know that one protein called CD-20 is on the surface of B-lymphoma cells and not on other normal tissues. A drug-antibody called Rituxan is an anti-CD-20 that is injected into a vein and targets the tumor cells and kills them.[8] Rituxan has been used successfully against lymphomas outside the central nervous system for more than seven years. It has been used sporadically for lymphomas of the brain and spine.[9] My colleagues and I have treated patients who showed disappearance of PCNSLs by MRI scan after only four intravenous injections of Rituxan. They are alive, and tumor-free more than four years later.

> Immune therapy with Rituxan may follow chemotherapy.

STEROIDS – HOW ARE THEY USED IN TREATMENT OF LYMPHOMAS?

Dexamethasone (Decadron) is the strongest steroid drug in clinical practice, and it is frequently administered to brain tumor patients to reduce swelling and "tightness". It has a unique role in diagnosis and therapy of lymphomas. Decadron can cause lymphomas to melt away in days or weeks, which is why lymphomas have disappeared on MRI scans "without cancer therapy." This post-steroidal effect can make diagnosis difficult or impossible. Under these circumstances, it is common to wait one to six months or more for the tumor to reappear, so that a biopsy can be obtained. Unfortunately, dexamethasone has significant side effects (See Chapter 9).

WHAT ARE MY CHANCES OF CURE WITH A LYMPHOMA?

Cure depends upon a variety of factors, some of the most important include:
- Accurate diagnosis of lymphoma.
- Accurate subtyping of lymphoma, B or T cell? T cell lymphomas have different surface receptor proteins and lack the CD-20 protein, excluding the use of Rituxan.
- AIDS-associated or not. Generally, non-AIDS associated lymphomas are more responsive.
- Location: Lymphoma only in the central nervous system or metastasis from elsewhere? The other sites may require surgery and separate radiation fields.
- Development while on or off chemotherapy. Those that recur while off chemotherapy have a wider range of therapies available to them.
- Receipt of correct therapy (e.g. the correct sequence of treatments) will determine not only outcome but also toxicity (radiation and methotrexate).
- Response to the previous and current therapies – the more responsive, the better the outcome.

Bottom line: You need to know the correct lymphoma immune type to receive correct therapy.

Table 14-1 Internet Resources for Lymphomas

Subject	Website or other resource
General Information	http://www.emedicine.com/RADIO/topic100.htm
Metastases to brain	http://www.emedicine.com/radio/topic101.htm
Clinical Trials	http://www.centerwatch.com/patient/studies/CAT95.html www.virtualtrials.com
Lymphoma and Rituxan™	http://www.rituxan.com/rituxan/index.jsp
Surgery- Shunts/ Hydrocephalus	http://www.yoursurgery.com/proceduredetails.cfm?br=4 &proc=44
Books	Houston, Lori (1999) *Non-Hodgkin's Lymphomas Making Sense of Diagnosis, Treatment & Options: Patient-Centered Guide* ; Sebastopol, O'Reilly & Associates, Inc: Zeltzer P.M. (2005). *Brain Tumors and Finding The Ark: – Meeting the Challenges of Treatment Choices, Side Effects, Healthcare Costs & Long Term Survival.* Encino: Shilysca Press

CHAPTER 15

Brain Metastases – Tumors from Other Areas of the Body

It has become, in my view, a bit too trendy to regard the acceptance of death as something tantamount to intrinsic dignity. Of course, I agree with the preacher of Ecclesiastes that there is a time to love and a time to die – and when my skein runs out, I hope to face the end calmly and in my own way.

For most situations, however, I prefer the more martial view that death is the ultimate enemy and I find nothing reproachable in those who rage mightily against the dying of the light.

Stephen J. Gould (cancer survivor)

⌐⊶ **Key search words**

- metastases
- breast carcinomas
- radiosurgery
- radiation sensitizers
- anti-angiogenesis

- colon cancer
- melanoma
- chemotherapy
- RSR13

- lung cancer
- radiation therapy
- experimental therapy
- Xcytrin™

GENERAL QUESTIONS

What Is a Metastasis?

A brain tumor *metastasis* (also called a "met" or secondary tumor) is a malignant tumor that has spread from cancer originating elsewhere in the body. As cancer treatment has become more effective, people with cancer are living long enough to allow metastasis to occur. About 25 percent of adult cancer patients will develop brain metastases at some time in their life. In contrast, less than 2 percent all children with cancer develop brain metastases.

> About 25% of adult cancer patients will develop a brain metastasis.

Where Do Metastases Originate?

In adults, brain metastases (150,000+ persons per year in the U.S.) are more common than tumors that originate in the brain. Metastases to the brain come from any cancer, but most frequently from the lung, breast, skin, colon, and prostate. Melanoma, a rare but aggressive form of skin cancer, has the highest frequency of brain metastasis (Table 15-1).

Table 15-1 Most Common Primary Tumors With Metastases to Brain (U.S.)[1]

	Frequency (%) of mets for each type of tumor	Total number people affected/year
Lung	32	45,500
Breast	21	9,300
Skin (melanoma)	48	4,200
Colon	6	3,200
Liver	5	1,800
Prostate	6	1,800
Kidney	11	1,100
Lymphoma	5	1,000
All other tumor types	*Not available*	80,000

The following Internet message illustrates the worry and uncertainty about whether there has been metastasis to the brain:

Hello, everyone. My name is Carol. I'm 48 and a breast cancer survivor (5 yrs, June 8, '02). I was recently told by my oncologist that I have a brain lesion in the pons (brainstem). I've undergone two brain MRIs previously and a third one in May, and will follow up with my new neurosurgeon on June 14th. There is no diagnosis as of yet and I am not sure what any of this means. Hoping it is not metastatic breast cancer to my head. Those of you who've been through cancer can relate to my "waiting period." I've read a few posts from this list today and see some very courageous people. Just wanted to introduce myself and perhaps meet some new friends, and maybe even encourage someone else in their own trials. Life is good... not always fair.

Carol. Salem, OR

DIAGNOSIS

ARE THERE TYPICAL SIGNS OR SYMPTOMS OF A BRAIN OR SPINAL METASTASIS?

Suspicion of a metastatic tumor may arise as a result of new symptoms, findings from the neurological exam, or routine CT or MRI scans. Symptoms usually indicate the tumor's location within the brain, but do not indicate the originating location of the primary tumor.

- Tumors in or near motor areas (frontal-parietal lobes) cause weakness on the body's opposite side.
- Tumors around the language areas (located on the left side of the parietal and temporal lobes in 90 percent of adults) can cause difficulties with understanding of speech or verbal communication.

For anyone previously diagnosed with cancer, the following symptoms should raise suspicion (Table 15-2):

> Nervous system or behavioral changes in anyone with cancer could be caused by a brain metastasis.

Table 15-2 Typical Signs and Symptoms for Brain & Spinal Metastasis

1. Persistent headache, with or without vomiting
2. Change in type or frequency of seizures
3. Partial loss of (or double) vision, mental changes, strange behavior, speech difficulty
4. Stroke or brain hemorrhage (more common with melanoma, renal carcinoma, choriocarcinoma)
5. Confusion
6. *Numbness, arm or leg weakness, back pain, difficulty in walking
7. *Loss of bowel or bladder control

* more common with spinal metastases

WHAT TESTS ARE NEEDED TO DETECT AND STAGE A METASTASIS?

Most important for therapy is knowledge of the tumor type, affected location(s) and tumor stage. This will let you and your doctors know which part of the brain needs treatment and whether attention needs to be given to the spine as well. The gold standard requires both enhanced and unenhanced MRI scans of the head or spine, depending on your symptoms or the particular tumor. Either single or multiple metastatic tumors can be present. At a minimum, the following tests should be performed in patients with a brain metastasis:

> MRI scan is the "gold standard" to diagnose the number and location of brain metastases.

- Brain and spinal MRI (spinal MRI may not be required in all patients)
- Spinal fluid analysis in some patients (if spinal MRI is negative)
- Search for the primary tumor, if one is not already known to exist

METASTASIS CLASSIFICATION OR GRADING – IS BIOPSY IMPORTANT?

The original tumor type and grade are analyzed by a pathologist and are critical to your treatment. These results could determine your therapy options. Without this information, you may not receive the most appropriate therapy. For example, a lymphoma can "look" like a metastasis on a scan, but successful treatment programs for each are very different. No one should make assumptions about your tumor type without a biopsy. Sometimes, what looks like cancer on the MRI or CT scan is not even a tumor. (See Chapter 1.) However, when a cancer diagnosis is known, and multiple lesions that look like metastases are seen on MRI, there is usually no need for a biopsy. This is especially true if the time interval from the original diagnosis to the onset of metastases is less than five years.

Pathologists who study metastases under the microscope assign "family" types (such as breast, colon, lung, lymphoma, or thyroid) following biopsy or removal. Rarely do a primary brain tumor and secondary tumor co-exist at the same time.

TREATMENTS

WHAT OPTIONS SHOULD MY TREATMENT CENTER PHYSICIANS OFFER?

There is no single standard treatment for all patients with brain metastases. Recommendations need to be tailored to each patient's own circumstances and hinge upon tumor type and number of brain metastases. For example, surgery is often followed by radiation therapy. Radiation can be whole brain, partial brain or radiosurgery (fractionated or single dose). The pros and cons of these approaches depend on the number and location of metastases, the extent of disease elsewhere in the body, and your overall condition. (See also Chapter 17: Traditional Treatments.[2]) It is important that you consult a major brain tumor center that has considerable experience, preferably one that offers clinical (research) trials and has the following areas of expertise:

> There is no single standard treatment for all patients with brain metastases.

Surgery

- For a single brain metastasis
- For an undiagnosed primary tumor
- For brain metastases developing more than five years after diagnosis of the initial tumor

Radiation Therapy

- For rapid relief of symptoms in patients with multiple metastatic nervous system tumors or when surgery is not indicated
- Tumor specific therapy, such as radioactive iodine for thyroid metastases

Chemotherapy

- For cancers that are sensitive to it, such as small-cell of lung, breast, or lymphoma.

Antibody Therapy

- Rituximab (Rituxan) in combination with chemotherapy has promising results for lymphomas.

EMERGENCY SITUATIONS AND THERAPIES

Surgery Is Helpful to Immediately Reverse the Following:

- Pressure-induced symptoms within 48 hours of onset
- Symptoms from pressure due to bleeding or tumor
- Arm or leg pain or paralysis
- Bowel or bladder paralysis
- Speech or visual problems
- Headache, nausea and/or vomiting
- Obstruction of cerebrospinal fluid

Radiosurgery Has Been Used for a Single Metastasis

Medication:

- Dexamethasone (16-48 mg/ day) quickly relieves pressure and reverses symptoms of paralysis, pain, speech arrest, nausea and vomiting due to brain or spinal cord pressure.
- Seizure medicines may be necessary to treat seizures. In rare instances, management requires hospitalization.

SURGICAL ISSUES

Options Before Deciding on Surgery

Whether or not to have surgery depends upon several factors. Emergency neurosurgery can be lifesaving and reverse symptoms for some patients. Sometimes, the main reason for surgery is to obtain tissue to make a correct diagnosis.

After any emergency is resolved, I recommend that your case be presented to the Tumor Board at the hospital where your neurosurgeon is based. Then, your team can make suggestions for the next sequence of treatments. For example, if there are multiple brain tumors, it can be challenging to decide which tumors should be surgically removed and which should receive radiation.

There is usually time to get a consultation at a major medical center that specializes in brain tumor treatment. (For more information on second opinions see Chapter 5: Your Team; Chapter 6: Getting to an Expert; and Chap 7: Academic Centers, University Hospitals & Institutes).

Goals of Surgery as Important Initial Therapy

- Preserve or improve your neurological function
- Improve mobility and function along with radiation (for spinal metastases)
- Remove the tumor, completely or partially
- Obtain a piece of the tumor for confirmation of the diagnosis (biopsy)

Developments that Have Made Surgery Safer

- Functional imaging and intra-operative brain mapping

These modalities have improved the safety of brain tumor surgery. Functional MRI (fMRI) uses MRI to map areas associated with vision, hearing, speech, taste, touch, and movement, whose locations in the brain vary from one person to the next. The map then allows the surgeon to plan precisely and avoid disrupting important areas, thus preserving your quality of life. (See Chapter 17: Treatment.)

Importance of Tumor Location

- Metastases to the brain have one advantage. They tend to be near the surface and thus easier to access, in contrast to primary brain tumors that originate deeper within the brain. Typically, there is some separation between the tumor and surrounding normal brain tissue in metastatic tumors.
- Spinal surgery is indicated to relieve pressure from the tumor
  - Effects of metastases to the spine can be alleviated, even when complete surgical removal is not possible.
  - Surgery plus radiation improves functional outcome. In one study of 32 patients who entered the trial unable to walk, 56 percent of those receiving surgery plus radiation regained mobility. This contrasted with only 19 percent of patients who received radiation alone.[3]

> Whole brain versus focused beam radiation are the main issues affecting quality of life.

Bottom line: Successful therapy to remove metastases is dependent upon exact location and skill of your neurosurgeon.

RADIATION THERAPY

Generally, the best option for unresectable brain metastases is radiation therapy. The decision-making can be complex and may require input from different specialists. The choice of which type of radiation therapy depends upon tumor location, number of metastases, and whether it is spinal and in a thin layer, or spinal and "bulky." Additional details can be found in Chapter 17: Treatments and in Chapter 21: Clinical Trials.

Types of Radiation Therapy for Metastases

There are basically four main options for radiation to treat metastases. These are discussed in detail in Chapter 17 of the next book.

1. Local and focal, external beam radiotherapy
2. Whole brain radiotherapy, with or without stereotactic radiation
3. Stereotactic radiation – fractionated (split up) or radiosurgery (one time).
4. Locally inserted radiotherapy (brachytherapy, GliaSite- , new and unproven)

Whole Brain or Focused (Partial) Radiation Therapy – What Are the Issues?

Choice of radiation technique can greatly affect tumor control and your quality of life... *after* treatment! There are very basic questions to ask about your *quality of life.* Certainly, there are situations where none of the choices is

> **Treatment choices depend upon tumor location and stage:**
> • Single metastasis near the surface • Six or more metastases
> • Diffuse tumor spread all along the spinal cord.

to your liking; but every individual deserves the right to determine if the (side effects of) therapy will be acceptable to his or her lifestyle (Table 15-3).

The individual technique can involve greater or lesser areas of brain tissue. This is a hot topic among specialists. A major debate exists as to whether people with fewer than four to six metastases should receive whole brain radiation or individual radiation beams to each tumor. Tumor type, size and number, location, and your age are the variables in this equation. There are several clinical trials in North America that are studying this question. Most major treatment centers understand these issues and can present the trade-offs to you. Then you can make an informed decision about which treatment to choose, rather than have someone else make this decision for you.

The anecdote below illustrates why therapy choices must be tailored to individual needs. A person who is retired and plays golf, but does not work, may choose the option for whole brain radiation. This physician's brain needed to function at a very high level, so his needs were different. His initial physicians didn't acknowledge his needs and they recommended whole brain radiation, which resulted in a poor first choice.

> A 58-year-old cardiologist from a large Health Maintenance Organization (HMO) in California consulted me. He had been recently diagnosed with a single metastasis from a lung cancer within the right temporal lobe. He became aware of the tumor after having the sensation of music playing in his head. His ability to function as a physician was very important to him. Radiation oncology colleagues at his HMO started him on "glioblastoma" doses (6000cGy) of radiation with 3 cm. margins. (This amounted to almost 75 percent of his brain receiving radiation). His radiation oncologist did not warn him of any potential neuropsychological side effects before starting treatment; his case was never presented to a Tumor Board. In addition, the option of chemotherapy (now considered initial therapy for lung cancer metastases) was never explained to him. Only after the radiation was almost half completed did he seek outside consultation. Three months after completing radiation, the tumor area was clear. But he became too incapacitated to work.

Table 15-3 Questions About Side Effects to Ask Before Starting Radiation Therapy

1. Will my brain work as it does now? If not, what changes will I notice?
2. Will I be able to continue my current work or hobbies?
3. Will my memory be affected?
4. Will I recognize my spouse or friends?
5. Will I be able to care (unassisted) for my daily needs like getting dressed, fixing a cup of coffee, and going to the toilet?

Make sure you ask any other questions that are most important to *You*!

Can Radiation Cause Harm?

Recent conflicting studies show both harm and safety of radiation for low-grade brain tumors in adults.[4] Now, some major centers offer experimental approaches that involve reduced or highly focused radiation, customized to the exact shape of the tumor, such as use of intensity modulated radiation therapy (IMRT). There is little data on this subject for survivors of metastases.

Bottom line: Clinical trials will determine if single, focused beams to each metastasis or whole brain radiation is more effective with least side effects.

I am not suggesting that you should avoid all radiation therapy because of the potential for long term side effects. Ask all doctors involved in your care very directly about the likelihood that any therapy could render you or your loved one unable to perform basic daily functions (Table 15-3). This is tough stuff, but it's critical to be fully informed when making difficult decisions about how you may want to live, or how you may *not* want to die. (Consequences of treatment is discussed in Chapter 20: Side effects and Later Effects of the tumor or Treatment; and Chapter 25: Your Legacy.[2])

What Medications Will I Receive Before or During Radiation?

See this section under traditional therapies in Chapters 9 and 17.

Radiation Therapy to *Prevent* Metastases?

The general conclusion is that for small-cell lung cancer, *preventative* cranial irradiation does improve survival for the patients who are in complete remission. For non-small-cell lung cancer, this question is still under investigation. The long-term effects on brain function and quality of life are not well established.[5]

SPECIFIC RECOMMENDATIONS

The Stanford Protocol for Multiple Metastases

For decades, treatment choices have been a product of regional belief and practice. Over the last 10 years, large clinical trials have sought answers to these important questions, but many remain unanswered. One example of local experience (for me, a California doctor) that is commonly used, but not always universally agreed upon, is based on the experience of Stanford University radiation therapists. It is meant to be a general approach, a format to ask questions of your radiation oncologist, but not necessarily a specific recommendation for you to follow (Table 15-4).

Table 15-4 Stanford University Protocol for Multiple Brain Metastases[6]

1. Progressive systemic disease, poor performance status, or more than four tumors: • Conventional radiotherapy • If there is MRI scan-documented reduction in the number of metastases, then possibly a stereotactic radiosurgical boost, if four or fewer tumors.
2. Patients with stable systemic disease and a good performance status but with tumor-related pressure or symptoms by one or more tumors: • Surgical resection of the symptomatic tumors • Radiosurgery or radiotherapy to treat the remaining smaller tumors
3. Patients with stable systemic disease, a good performance status, and no pressure effects related to their brain metastases (four or fewer tumors): • Optimum candidates for stereotactic radiosurgery • Most patients will eventually receive conventional radiotherapy. Patients with a single brain metastasis often undergo radiosurgery alone. • Conventional radiotherapy is reserved for tumor recurrence/progression and new brain tumors associated with a poor performance status or progressive systemic disease. • Unlike conventional brain radiotherapy, radiosurgery can be repeated months to years after initial treatment.

The basis for the decisions in Table 15-4 comes in part from a broad historical experience, not always from clinical trial results. Specifically, patients who were treated with whole brain radiation plus a radiosurgical boost lived an average of 36 months without recurrence, or six times longer than a *historical* reference to people who received only whole brain radiation (six months). Control of the cancer elsewhere in the body also plays an important role.[6]

What Are the Options for a Solitary Metastasis?

The specific recommendation depends upon many factors such as your current health, metastasis location, and previous therapies. The choices include the following:

- Surgery
- Radiosurgery
- Radiation (whole brain)
- GliaSite (new and unproven)
- Chemotherapy
- Clinical Trial

Bottom line: Patients who have a single metastasis, which is completely (surgically) removed, should have radiation therapy too, as individual tumor cells always remain after surgery.

What are Other Therapy Options With and Without Radiation?

a) Surgery could be helpful to reverse acute symptoms from a bleed or pressure from one or more metastases.

b) Internal, local or regional chemotherapy (Gliadel wafers, new and unproven).

c) GliaSite: This is an implantable, *local* radiation treatment which is FDA-approved for metastases. The procedure involves placing a balloon inside the tumor cavity, after the surgeon has prepared the area to receive it. The balloon is later inflated with a radioactive liquid that irradiates or "cooks" the tumor from the inside. This technique prevents damage from radiation beams passing through normal scalp, bone, and brain tissues. This has not been proven effective for any one type of metastasis; but it remains an option for treatment.

d) Systemic chemotherapy.

e) Antibodies or other immune therapies – new and unproven.

f) Radiation sensitizers RSR-13 and Xcytrin™ – new and unproven.

Chemotherapy for Metastases from Lung, Colon, Ovary, Breast, Kidney, or Melanoma?

Whether chemotherapy can be used to treat metastases from distant sites depends upon answers to the following questions (see also Table 15-5):

- Was the tumor in the original site sensitive to chemotherapy? If so, then chemotherapy is more likely to shrink the tumor.
- Was the tumor in control? Had the original tumor either disappeared or gotten smaller when the brain metastasis was diagnosed? If so, it might be controlled more easily.
- Did the metastasis appear when you were off your chemotherapy for more than a year? If so, then it is more likely to respond to chemotherapy.
- Did the metastasis appear while you were actively receiving chemotherapy? If so, then it is unlikely that the tumor is sensitive, and other drugs or approaches should be considered.
- How is your overall health; do you have any other medical problems?

What are Newer, Experimental Approaches?

Anti-angiogenesis

Avastin, formerly known as anti-VEGF, is designed to bind with and inhibit vascular endothelial growth factor (VEGF), a protein that plays a critical role in the formation of new blood vessels that feed the tumor and maintain established tumor blood vessels. This is called an "anti-angiogenesis" approach.

- In May 2003, Genentech announced that a Phase III clinical trial of Avastin had improved overall survival in metastatic colorectal cancer patients. Clinical trials are being developed for use with late-stage cancer, evaluating its potential use in metastatic colorectal, breast, non-small-cell lung and renal cell cancers. Ask about its status at your center.
- The Cancer and Leukemia Group B (CALGB) and National Cancer Institute will be initiating a Phase III study of Avastin for RCC (renal cell cancer) by the end of 2004. This trial will study first-line therapeutic approaches to metastatic tumors as well.

Radiation sensitizers

- Radiation sensitizers, such as RSR13 (or efaproxiral) and Xcytrin® have gained a "fast track" status to enter clinical trials (Table 15-6). They are drugs that enhance or multiply the radiation damage to cancer cells. Recent clinical trials show that RSR13 may improve the average survival time for women with breast cancer metastases to the brain.[8] Furthermore, Xcytrin delayed the progression of neurological symptoms, when added to standard whole brain radiation therapy in patients with lung cancer.

This study has identified major new clinical issues for the evaluation of treatments for brain metastases. It is the first study to demonstrate... neurological and neurocognitive deficits exist in patients with brain metastases and... that the natural progression of these defects can be positively impacted by treatment.

Dr. Minesh Mehta.[9]

You might want to consult with a radiation oncologist, neurooncologist or oncologist who treats at least 25 patients a year with brain tumors to be sure that you are receiving up-to-date options.

CHANCES OF LONGER LIFE WITH A METASTASIS

Having a brain metastasis is a serious complication, but being in expert hands can increase your chances for longer survival. Yes, many people will die from tumor progression. However, it's also fair to say that people with a solitary or fewer metastases, which can be removed completely, will usually live longer and have a better quality of life. I have patients who are alive and well five years later, after having had brain metastases. Read about Lance Armstrong[10] and others who are survivors of brain metastases.[11] The more you know, the more choices you will have. (Table 15-5).

The most important elements in predicting a successful result are the following:
- Location and number of tumors
- Type of tumor
- Tumors in other areas of the body
- Your age
- Tumor development while on or off chemotherapy
- Amount of the tumor that can be removed (skill of the neurosurgeon)
- Response of the tumor to the new therapy
- Other medical conditions or complications
- Functional state (Karnofsky score) before and after surgery

Table 15-5 Important Factors in Treating Metastatic Brain Tumors

Factor	Considerations
Location	Symptoms (brain and/ or spinal cord)
Tumor type and site of origin	Lung, breast, colon, prostate, melanoma, lymphoma, other
Timing of recurrence (off or on therapy)	Previous drugs or new agents Patient's clinical conditions Emergency or elective setting Location and thickness of disease (leptomeningeal or bulky) Number of metastases, steroid treatment dependence
Therapy options, standard and experimental	Surgery Radiation • whole brain • local • radiosurgery • stereotactic radiation implant or sensitizers Chemotherapy • chemotherapy wafer • systemic chemotherapy • intrathecal/ other Immunotherapy • local or systemic

Other Sources of Information- National Guidelines Clearinghouse

With advice of experts, the National Guideline Clearinghouse developed "best practice" guidelines for treatment of many medical conditions, including brain tumors. Treatment guidelines for single metastases can be found on the Internet.[12] (See Table 15-6.) I have some opinions on this source that I will share with you:

- The listed case examples on the website have rating scales for the appropriateness of various forms of therapy. "No therapy" was not listed but "observation" was a last choice option! But it might be a choice for some people and they deserve the chance to make that choice.
- Interestingly, not one guideline mentions "quality of survival" when whole brain radiation is compared with focused radiosurgery. This question has not been answered as yet by researchers. But you deserve to know, in your case, if the chances of withholding whole brain radiation and treating four or less individual tumors with radiosurgery or SRT, might allow for a better quality of life, even if it *might* be less effective.
- The fact that these are government-sponsored guidelines, with the authority this might carry, does not ensure that they represent sound advice… for you. Ask, Ask, Ask questions.

Remember, no matter how severe the situation, no one, physicians included, can predict what will happen with treatment. Predictions can be made for populations of patients but never for individual patients.

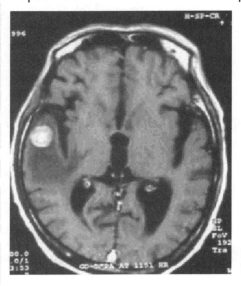

Figure 15-1
MRI: Single metastasis to the right tempora lobe

Table 15-6 Internet Resources for Brain Metastases

Subject	Website
General Information	http://cancerweb.ncl.ac.uk/cancernet/103854.html (options) http://www.emedicine.com/radio/topic101.htm http://www.braintumor.org/patient_info/publications/ brochures/documents/brainmetsbrochure.pdf
Clinical Trials	http://www.clinicaltrials.gov/ct/show/NCT00016211?order=34 lung cancer http://www.clinicaltrials.gov/ct/show/ NCT00030628?order=18 +/ - whole brain http://www.virtualtrials.com/MetastaticBrainTumor.cfm (all types and over 150 clinical trials are listed as of 10-15-04) http://www.centerwatch.com/patient/studies/stu47665.html (Whole brain + Radisurg. http://www.mskcc.org/mskcc/html/2270.cfm?IRBNO=01-088 (chemotherapy) http://www.yale.edu/opa/newsr/03-12-09-04.all.html (Phase 3- radiosensitizer)
Experimental Radiation Sensitizers	http://www.biospace.com/news_story.cfm?StoryID=1455012 0&full=1 http://www.docguide.com/news/content.nsf/news/85256977 00573E1885256DF0004C7967?OpenDocument&id=48DDE 4A73E09A969852568880078C249&c=Lung%20Cancer&co unt=10
National Guideline Clearinghouse	http://www.guideline.gov/ (search under "brain metastasis")

CHAPTER 16

Epilogue

There have been many times - I admit - that I desperately wanted to surrender, but through the strength of my family, I battled as hard as the "beast" was battling me. Education is my power, my source of control. If you know your enemy, you can fight.

Sheryl R. Shetsky, Founder & President,
South Florida Brain Tumor Association

EPILOGUE

EPILOGUE

Brain Tumors - Finding the Ark Can Help with Choices

A lot has happened since your diagnosis. You have learned much about your specific type of brain tumor and the importance of how knowledge can help... and how what you don't know can cause problems. I hope to have clarified the link between the stories from Genesis and how different interpretations of those same stories can free you to obtain more knowledge, effective treatments, and better healthcare. I also hope that you may see that you are not alone - many people quoted in this book have faced similar struggles on this same journey. Most seem to have benefited from becoming more knowledgeable; and many began to see this situation as less a punishment than a way to embrace the rest of their lives.

The companion book, *Brain Tumors – Finding the Ark: Meeting the Challenges of Treatment Choices, Side Effects, Healthcare Costs & Long Term Survival,* will take you more into active treatment options and important issues that affect your treatment choices and long term survival. In that book, I discuss the following subjects that follow in sequential chapters to this book:

Chapter 17: Traditional Approaches to Treatments (including Radiation Therapy, Chemotherapy, Immunotherapy, Newer Therapies).

- Neurosurgery – Are all Neurosurgeons created equal?
- Radiation Therapy – Are the rumors true?
- Radiosurgery- what is it?
- What questions do I need to ask before I receive it?
- Chemotherapy: Different types for different tumors?

Chapter 18: Complementary and Alternative Therapies for Brain Tumors

Over 50% of people with cancer take non-traditional medications to help them feel better or help fight their cancer. There are some data for their role in fighting brain tumors. Here are the explanations for how they work and to help you decide if they are for you:
- What are CAM, TCM, Ayurvedic medicine? Can they help fight my tumor?
- How can I get information on herbs- the pros and cons of using them?
- How can acupuncture help me?

- Spiritual counseling and healing- how can they...or do they help?
- How do support groups contribute to longer and better quality and length of life?

Chapter 19: Medications (to fight cancer and prevent chemotherapy-related complications)

You may be on one or many medications. Here is what they are for and possible side effects to look out for and advise your doctor:
- What can I do to prevent life threatening errors with my meds?
- Where to get info on herb and drug interactions?
- Is everyone ill with chemo?
- Minimizing and eliminating side effects like pain and nausea?
- Steroids- benefits and perils
- A guide to blood counts?
- Regional chemotherapy- what is it?
- Financial help with meds?

Chapter 20: Side Effects and Late Effects of Treatment

Long term side effects are a luxury of being alive. Some are unavoidable, others can be lessened or avoided. Some are specific to the type of treatment or location of the tumor:
- Effects on activities of daily living.
- Effects on sugar, salt, and sex.
- Radiation and the your pituitary gland.
- Frontal lobe and cerebellar mutism symptoms.
- Neuropsychological consequences of treatment.
- Resources for assistance: How, where, and what are the questions?
- The new normal: coping with everyday problems.

Chapter 21: Clinical Trials – Are They for You?

Improvements over standard therapy are made with carefully controlled clinical trials. Here are the rules on how they work, where you can get specific information about them and help on deciding what advantages/ disadvantages they might offer you.
- What are the Phases of a clinical trial?
- Where do I find one right for me?
- Will I be a guinea pig?
- What are my rights? Can I withdraw?

- What are the important questions to ask?
- Will my health insurance or HMO pay for the medications and treatments?

Chapter 22: Children with Brain Tumors – Special Considerations

Children are not just miniature adults. Their bodies and brains are growing, changing, and have different reactions to medicines compared with adults. Very special precautions must be taken, from the dose of x-rays in a CT scan to doses of radiation and medications:
- Common types of brain tumors in children.
- Why did my child get a brain tumor? What did I do wrong?
- Should I consult a Pediatric Neurosurgeon for my child's tumor?
- Pain control in hospital or after surgery.
- Successful school re-entry after diagnosis and treatment.
- Legal rights of every child with a brain tumor.
- Camps for Children with brain tumors.

Chapter 23: Managing Costs, Benefits, Insurance Companies, Medicare, and HMOs

How insurance can affect your care - the good and the bad. Many people do not realize that their doctor may not be the final decision-maker on the care they can receive. These are the ground rules you must know in order to get the care you need and deserve:
- Steps to obtain your rightful benefits.
- What are HMOs, PPOs POS's, indemnity and ….?
- Negotiating effectively with your provider: what you need to know.
- Guidelines for challenging denials.
- What is Medicare, Medicaid. Who is eligible?
- SSI, SSDI and SDI- what is the difference? Money…
- The Family Medical Leave Act- to what am I entitled?
- Health insurance language- a glossary.

Chapter 24: Heredity and Other Causes of Brain Tumors

The genes we inherit are responsible for much of what we are. Surprisingly, a cancer in one family member can be the first step in prevention or early diagnosis of cancer in other family members, both children and adults:

- Can I catch a brain tumor from someone else?
- Genetics and heredity- what is the difference?
- What is a gene?
- Are most brain tumors inherited?
- Can my brain tumor help others in my family prevent cancer?
- What is gene therapy?
- Do cell phones cause brain tumors?

Chapter 25: Your Legacy: The Personal Experience You May Want to Share About Having a Brain Tumor

Your legacy must seem like an unusual name for a chapter in a book about brain tumors. Here you can reflect about what this experience has taught you and what you want to tell the people you care about what you have learned:

- Completing your Life-Things to do.
- What are the stories I need to tell?
- How do I want to live? How do I want to die?
- What happens if I do not think about dying? A *Living Will*.
- Doctors and patients look at "End of Life" differently.
- Palliative Care and Hospice- What is the difference?
- Hospice and Insurance coverage.
- "The Good Side To Having A Brain Tumor"?

Continue on to more knowledge and empowerment!

Glossary

GLOSSARY

Anticipatory Nausea and Vomiting

Anticipatory means vomiting at the thought of the drug, or even before arriving at the clinic or hospital. This can affect compliance with taking the drug.

Astrocyte

A brain cell that provides support, structure, and nutrition to other brain cells.

Astrocytoma (Juvenile Pilocytic)

This is a type of low-grade astrocytoma which occurs in young children, most commonly near the cerebellum or 4th ventricle. Surgery is usually curative. When it occurs in other locations (near the hypothalamus or optic nerves or cerebrum) or in adults, it can be difficult to completely remove and may recur.

Astrocytomas (Astro-sigh –TOE- maz)

The most common types in the brain tumor family are called "gliomas." They develop from star-shaped glial cells called astrocytes. Pathologists assign grades to an astrocytoma following biopsy.

Low-grade, well differentiated: Also called, grade I and II astrocytomas. Their cells look relatively normal and are less malignant than the other two grades. They grow more slowly and sometimes can be completely removed. They can still be life threatening, if they are deep within vital locations.

Mid-grade, anaplastic: or Grade III astrocytomas grow more rapidly than well-differentiated astrocytomas and contain cells with malignant traits. Surgery followed by radiation and chemotherapy contribute to very long survivals.

High-grade, grade IV or glioblastoma multiforme (GBM): These tumors grow rapidly, invade nearby tissue, and contain cells that are very malignant. GBMs are among the most common and serious primary brain tumors that strike adults. Doctors usually treat glioblastomas with surgery followed by radiation therapy. Chemotherapy may be used before, during, or after radiation. There are many experimental studies available.

Benign Cancer

A tumor that tends to grow slowly, if it grows at all.

Brain Stem Gliomas (BSG) or Gliomas of the Brain Stem

Named by their location at the base of the brain rather than the cells they contain. BSGs are more common in children and young adults. There are two types: *intrinsic* and *extrinsic* or *exophytic.* Each behaves very differently. Surgery usually is not helpful for the intrinsic types because of their critical location but has a role for the exophytic types. Radiation therapy often reduces symptoms and improves survival.

Cancer

Any tumor that has the potential to grow without treatment.

Chordomas

More common in people in their 20s and 30s, develop from remnants which should have dissolved early in fetal development and is later replaced by the spinal cord. The tumors are often slow growing but can spread to other areas in the spine and brain. They typically are treated with surgery and radiation.

Choroid Plexus Carcinoma (CPC)

A rare and malignant tumor that is not curable with surgery alone but is treated with chemotherapy and sometimes radiation.

Choroid Plexus Papilloma (CORE-oid PLEX-us PAH-pee-LO-muh) (CPP)

CPP is a rare, benign tumor most common in children under the age of 12 years. CPPs grow slowly and eventually block the flow of cerebrospinal fluid causing hydrocephalus and increased intracranial pressure. CPP is most effectively treated with surgery which resolves the hydrocephalus in half of the patients. Remaining patients can require a shunt in addition to re-section.

Clinical Nurse Specialist

Has expertise in subspecialty areas such as Neurosurgery or Neurooncology. Can assist physicians.

CNS

Central Nervous System

Craniopharyngioma

It is not cancer and technically is not a "brain" tumor, though it occurs inside the head. They commonly affect infants and children. Developing from cells left over from early fetal development, they are located just behind the nose, near the pituitary gland. Pressure from the tumor can cause headache or disturbance in the pituitary gland's function. Treatment usually includes surgery and, in some patients, radiation therapy.

CT or CAT scan (Computerized Axial Tomography)

An x-ray device linked to a computer that produces an image of a cross-section of the brain. A special dye material may be injected into the patient's vein prior to the scan to help make any abnormal tissue more evident.

Cyst

A fluid filled sac. When not attached to a cancer, it is considered "benign." Benign cyst is different from a benign tumor. Cysts can be associated with a tumor.

DNET

Dysembryoplastic neuroepithelial tumor or desmoplastic cerebral astrocytoma. This is a variety of astrocytoma or mixed tumor, occurs in infancy or childhood and is extremely rare (less than 1 %). DNETs are often confused with a GBM by pathologists not familiar with childhood brain tumors. Surgery is often curative.

Ependymoma

Ependymomas usually affect children and develop from cells that line the hollow cavities of the brain (ventricles) and the canal inside the spine. About 85% of ependymomas are low grade but often are locally invasive. The pathologist's grade is not always predictive of their growth potential. Treatment usually includes surgery and then radiation therapy. Chemotherapy has been used in several clinical trials, especially for recurrent tumors.

Fellow

A graduate physician who has completed medical school, and residency training in an area of specialty such as internal medicine, pediatrics, or neurosurgery. The Fellow is the professor's right hand man.

Ganglioglioma

This is the rarest form of (mixed) glioma and contains both glial cells and mature nerve cells (neurons). They grow slowly in the brain or spinal cord. Gangliogliomas are usually treated with surgery. See MIXED GLIOMAS.

Germinoma

This family of tumor types that can occur anywhere in the body, usually in the midline (chest, ovaries, testicles, brain)as opposed to one side or the other. It can spread to the brain from anywhere else, or actually start to grow from there. Over the last 75 years, various names have been used for the different types: seminomas, germ cell tumors, teratomas, endodermal sinus tumor, choriocarcinoma (from the placenta), and non-germinomatous germ cell tumor.

In the brain, most do develop from the pineal gland and are called pineal region tumors (location). The tumor is made up of very primitive embryonic cells and sometimes can even contain teeth, muscle tissue or other glands (teratoma). Knowledge of the exact type is critical for your treatment success, as the different types require very specific therapies.

Glioma

A tumor from glial or astrocyte cells. Astrocytoma and glioma are interchangeable words in this book. There are a few gliomas that are called "benign," but they are more accurately named "low grade" (slow growing). High-grade gliomas are more malignant (faster growing).

About half of all primary brain tumors are gliomas. Within the brain, gliomas usually occur in the lobes of the upper part of the brain; but they may also grow in other areas, especially the optic nerve, the brain stem, and particularly among children in the cerebellum. Gliomas are classified into several groups because there are different kinds of glial cells. See also ASTROCYTOMA and OLIGODENDROGLIOMA, MIXED GLIOMA

Glioma of the Brain Stem

See Brain Stem Glioma.

Hemangioblastoma

A rare, non-cancerous tumor which arises from the blood vessels of the brain and the spinal cord. The most common form is linked in a small number of people as an inherited, genetic disorder called von Hippel-Lindau disease. Hemangioblastomas do not usually spread. Surgery can be curative. Kidney cancer, adrenal tumors and retinal abnormalities can also be present so a screening evaluation is recommended.

(Derived from Brain Tumor Society, Bruce Cohen, & www.virtualtrial.com)

Insurance Terms

See Chapter 23

Karnofsky Score

It is a measure of your ability to perform activities of daily living like getting dressed, feeding your self. It is used to see how you are responding to treatments and to determine your eligibility and strength to enroll on a clinical trial.

Lesion

A catch-all "doctor speak" term for any tissue mass ("lump") in question.

Malignant Cancer

A tumor that has grown or is growing, usually rapidly, and will not stop without some type of therapy.

Medical Student

In medical school, but is not part of the house staff and is not a hospital employee.

Medulloblastoma

Represents more than 25% of all childhood brain tumors. Other more rare PNETS include *Neuroblastomas, Pineoblastomas, Medulloepitheliomas, Ependymoblastomas.* Because their malignant cells can spread by the spinal fluid, PNETs can be difficult to remove totally through surgery. Doctors usually remove as much tumor as possible with surgery, and then prescribe radiation and chemotherapy.

Meningioma

Meningioma is not a true brain tumor. It develops from thin membrane, or meninges, that cover the brain and the spinal cord. Meningiomas account for 25% of all brain tumors. They affect people of all ages, but are most common among those in their 40s. Meningiomas grow slowly, generally do not invade surrounding normal tissue, and rarely spread to other parts of the nervous system; most are benign. Surgery is the preferred treatment for meningiomas. Recurrent meningiomas may require additional treatment including radiation therapy.

Metastasis

A tumor that spread from some other part of the body.

Metastatic Tumor

A tumor that has spread (to the brain) from elsewhere. Most frequently, the original sites are lung, colon, and breast cancer as well as melanoma. Therapy depends on the number of tumors, their size, and whether the primary tumor is under control or not. There are many clinical trials using new treatments and several look promising.

Mixed Glioma

Contains more than one type of glial cell, usually astrocytes and oligo-dendroglial cells. Neuropathologists do not always agree on the difference between mixed gliomas and anaplastic oligodendrogliomas. New tests detecting lost genes (1p/ 19q) help predict which of these tumors will respond to chemotherapy and radiation. See also oligodendroglioma and ganglioglioma.

Nurse Practitioner (CNP)

They are certified and licensed to examine, diagnose, and make independent treatment decisions in the absence of a physician.

Oligodendroglioma (O-lee-go-den-dro-glee-oma.)

This tumor, a form of glioma (5-8% of all brain tumors) can often present with a seizure or a bleed inside the brain. They arise from the special glial cells called oligodendroglia, which wrap around the nerves and insulate them. They occur most often in adults 30-55 years old and start within the brain's cerebral hemispheres. These tumors are treated with surgery. If completely removed and are low grade or benign, no further therapy is needed. The more malignant and recurring types can be very responsive to chemotherapy and radiation. Long term survivals are common.

Optic Nerve Gliomas

These astrocytomas or gliomas are found on or in the optic nerve and are particularly common in persons with Neurofibromatosis 1, also called NF-1. Treatment may include observation, surgery, radiation or chemotherapy. The most important factors affecting therapy decisions are vision preservation and damage to other parts of the brain.

Physician's Assistant (PA)

May have been a medic in the Armed Forces, an emergency medical technician (EMT) who has received two to three years of training and is licensed by the state. Physician's assistants work under the supervision and direction of a physician.

Pineal Tumor

The pineal gland is a small structure deep within the center of the brain. Pineal tumors are very rare, about 1% of brain tumors. Surgery for a biopsy to confirm the tumor type is very important. Different types of tumors requiring different therapies can all look identical on the CT and MRI scans. The three most common pineal region tumors are gliomas, germ cell tumors, and primitive neuroectodermal tumors (PNETs). Radiation or chemotherapy, or both can be used for malignant pineal tumors.

Pineocytoma

A rare tumor of the pineal gland which is usually removed by surgery and requires no additional therapy. A few are mixed with cells that are more immature and can re-grow and spread. The tumors which cannot be resected are commonly treated with radiation. Little data exists for any reliable chemotherapy. (See supratentorial PNETs)

Pituitary Adenoma

Tumor that affects the pituitary gland account for about 10% of tumors in the head. Doctors classify pituitary adenomas into two major groups: A) secreting Vs. non-secreting and B) micro adenomas (<1.5 cm) and macroadenomas (>1.5cm). Secreting tumors release unusually high levels of pituitary hormones, triggering one or many symptoms. These can include a) decreased sexual function or desire (impotence), b) loss of menstrual periods (amenorrhea), c) milk production in male or female breast (galactorrhea caused by prolactin), d) abnormal body growth (acromegaly), e) high blood pressure, f) sugar diabetes and fat deposits in the face and neck (Cushing's syndrome), or g) hyperthyroidism. Surgery and / or the drug bromocriptine or its newer successors are used to treat prolactin-secreting pituitary adenomas. Larger, non-secreting adenomas are treated with surgery and radiation therapy.

Pituitary or "master gland,"

A small oval-shaped structure located at the base of the brain, is just behind the nose. This "master gland' releases several chemical messengers called hormones, which control the body's other glands and influence the body's growth, metabolism, and sexual function and maturation.

Primitive Neuroectodermal Tumor or PNET

Primitive neuroectodermal tumors (PNETs) usually affect children and young adults. Their name reflects the belief held by many scientists that these tumors spring from primitive cells left over from early development of the nervous system. PNETs are very malignant, grow rapidly and about 35% spread easily within the brain and spinal cord. In rare cases, they spread outside the CNS. They used to be called *Medulloblastoma* when they occurred in the back of the brain, near the cerebellum.

Professor or consultant

Also called attending physicians (attendings). He/ she is at the "top of the ladder" for responsibility.

Schwannoma

A tumor that comes from the cells that form a protective sheath around the body's nerve fibers. They're usually benign and surgically removed when possible. One of the more common forms of this tumor affects the eighth cranial nerve, which contains nerve cells important for balance and hearing. Facial paralysis may occur if the tumor involves the adjacent seventh nerve. Also known as *vestibular schwannomas* or *acoustic neuromas*, these tumors may grow on one or both sides of the brain and are potentially curable with stereotactic radiosurgery. People with a different form of inherited Neurofibromatosis, NF-2, can have these and benign meningiomas as well.

Teaching Hospital

Has a nationally approved educational program for Nursing or Medicine.

Teratoma, Malignant Teratoma

A member of the family of germ cell (germinoma) tumors. It is composed of two or more cell types and can contain teeth, skin and hair. The more slow growing ones are called teratomas. The malignant teratomas often secrete "marker" proteins called AFP, and B-hG which can be detected in the blood and spinal fluid. They are treated with a combination of chemotherapy and radiation.

Tumor or Neoplasm

A solid "anything" that should not be there, before or after it is actually diagnosed.

UBO

Doctor-speak for "unidentified bright objects" on an MRI scan.

Vascular Tumor

A rare, non-cancerous tumor arising from the blood vessels of the brain and the spinal cord. The most common vascular tumor is the *hemangioblastoma*, often linked with a genetic disorder called *von Hippel-Lindau disease*. Hemangioblastomas do not usually spread and surgery provides the cure. A screening is recommended to rule out renal cancer, adrenal tumors and retinal abnormalities.

References

PREFACE

1 Bill Moyers, Genesis: A Living Conversation (New York: Doubleday, 1996).
2 Arthur Frank, *The Wounded Storyteller: Body, Illness and Ethics* (Chicago: University of Chicago Press, 1995).

CHAPTER 1

1 M. Fouladi, et al., "Outcome of children with centrally reviewed low-grade gliomas treated with chemotherapy with or without radiotherapy on Children's Cancer Group high-grade glioma study CCG-945," *Cancer*, 2003 Sep 15;98(6): 1243-52.
2 http://www.tumorfree.com/survivors.htm.
3 Ben Williams, *Surviving "Terminal" Cancer: Clinical Trials, Drug Cocktails, and Other Treatments Your Oncologist Won't Tell You About* (Minneapolis: Fairview Press, 2002).
4 Virginia Stark-Vance, and M. L. Dubay, *100 Questions & Answers About Brain Tumors* (Boston: Jones & Bartlett Publishers, 2003).

Figure 1-1 Hans Baldung Grien: The Flood, 16th Century, Giraudon/ Art Resources NY

CHAPTER 2

1 Paul Zeltzer, *Brain Tumors - Finding the Ark - Meeting the Challenges of Treatment Choices, Side Effects, Healthcare Costs & Long Term Survival* (Encino, CA: Shilysca Press, 2004).
2 P. Kaatsch, et al. "Population-based epidemiologic data on brain tumors in German children," *Cancer*, 2001 Dec 15;92(12):3155-64. This article can be viewed at http://info.imsd.uni-mainz.de/Michaelis/m55.pdf.
3 Stephen Jay Gould, "The Median Isn't the Message," *Discover*, June 1985. This essay can be accessed online at http://www.stat.berkeley.edu/~rice/stat20_98/ GouldCancer.html and at http://www.cancerguide.org/median_not_msg.html.
4 S. M. Russell, and P. J. Kelly, "Incidence and clinical evolution of postoperative deficits after volumetric stereotactic resection of glial neoplasms involving the supplementary motor area," *Neurosurgery*, 2003 Mar; 52(3):506-16.
5 J. A. Cowan Jr., et al., "The impact of provider volume on mortality after intracranial tumor resection," *Neurosurgery*, 2003 Jan;52(1):48-53; discussion 53-4.
6 D. M. Long, et al., "Outcome and cost of craniotomy performed to treat tumors in regional academic referral centers," *Neurosurgery*, 2003 May;52(5):1056-63.

Figure 2-4 Mind Body Connection. Turkey 19th Century, Private collection of Paul and Lonnie Zeltzer
Figure 2-5 Sistine Chapel Ceiling. Adam and Eve Leaving the Garden, Scala/ Art Resource, NY.
Figure 2-6 Mosaccio. Adam and Eve. Leaving the Garden, Scala/ Art Resource, NY.
Figure 2-7. van Leyden. Adam and Eve Leaving the Garden

Chapter 3

1 Dylan Thomas, *The Poems of Dylan Thomas*, published by New Directions. Copyright © 1952, 1953.
2 N. S. Kadan-Lottick, et al., "Childhood cancer survivors' knowledge about their past diagnosis and treatment: Childhood Cancer Survivor Study," *JAMA*, 2002 Apr 10; 287(14):1832-9.
3 Virginia Stark-Vance, and M. L. Dubay, *100 Questions & Answers About Brain Tumors* (Boston: Jones & Bartlett Publishers, 2003).
4 Paul Zeltzer, *Brain Tumors - Finding the Ark - Meeting the Challenges of Treatment Choices, Side Effects, Healthcare Costs & Long Term Survival* (Encino, CA: Shilysca Press, 2004).

Chapter 4

1 http://www.nightflight.com/foldoc.
2 Adapted from J.S. Schneider, PhD: http://www.tbts.org/virtual_html/Internetsearch.htm.

Chapter 5

1 M. W. Rabow, J. M. Hauser, and J. Adams, "Supporting family caregivers at the end of life: 'They Don't Know What They Don't Know'," *JAMA*, 2004 Jan 28; 291(4):483-91.
2 E. Farace, and M. E. Shaffrey, "An intervention with caregivers improves QOL for malignant brain tumor patients," *Neurooncology* 3 (4): 338, 2001 (Abstract).
3 J. Illardo, and C. Rothman, *I'll Take Care of You: A Practical Guide to Family Caregivers* (New York: New Harbinger Publications Inc., 1999).
4 Books for Family Caregivers of the Elderly or Disabled retrieved May 20, 2004, http://media.seniorconnection.org/?doc=booklist.inc.
5 S. M. Russell, and P. J. Kelly, "Incidence and clinical evolution of postoperative deficits after volumetric stereotactic resection of glial neoplasms involving the supplementary motor area," *Neurosurgery*, 2003 Mar; 52(3): 506-16.
6 F. G. Barker, et al., "Survival and functional status after resection of recurrent glioblastoma multiforme," *Neurosurgery*, 1998 Apr;42(4):709-20; discussion 720-3.
7 J. A. Cowan Jr., et al., "The impact of provider volume on mortality after intracranial tumor resection," *Neurosurgery*, 2003 Jan; 52(1):48-53; discussion 53-4
8 D. M. Long, et al., "Outcome and cost of craniotomy performed to treat tumors in regional academic referral centers," *Neurosurgery*, 2003 May;52(5):1056-63.
9 A. L. Albright, et al., "Effects of medulloblastoma resections on outcome in children: a report from the Children's Cancer Group," *Neurosurgery*, 1996 Feb;38 (2):265-71.
10 P. M. Zeltzer, et al., "Metastasis stage, adjuvant treatment, and residual tumor are prognostic factors for medulloblastoma in children: conclusions from the Children's Cancer Group 921 randomized phase III study," *J Clin Oncol*, 1999 Mar;17(3):832-45.
11 C. L. Armstrong, et al., "Radiotherapeutic effects on brain function: double dissociation of memory systems," *Neuropsychiatry Neuropsychol Behav Neurol*, 2000 Apr;13 (2):101-11.
12 P. Salander, A. T. Bergenheim, and R. Henriksson, "How was life after treatment of a malignant brain tumour?" *Soc Sci Med*, 2000 Aug; 51(4):589-98.
13 M. Klein, et al., "Effect of radiotherapy and other treatment-related factors on mid-term to long-term cognitive sequelae in low-grade gliomas: a comparative study," *Lancet*, 2002 Nov 2;360 (9343):1361-8.

14 Paul Zeltzer, *Brain Tumors - Finding the Ark - Meeting the Challenges of Treatment Choices, Side Effects, Healthcare Costs and Long Term Survival* (Encino, CA: Shilysca Press, 2004).

15 Ibid. Refer to Chapter 23: Managing Costs, Benefits, and Healthcare with Insurance, HMOs and More.

CHAPTER 6

1 P. M. Zeltzer, et al., "Metastasis stage, adjuvant treatment, and residual tumor are prognostic factors for medulloblastoma in children: conclusions from the Children's Cancer Group 921 randomized phase III study," *J Clin Oncol*, 1999 Mar;17(3):832-45.

2 MD Anderson's CancerWise newsline, Sept 2002.

3 J. A., Cowan, et al., "The impact of provider volume on mortality after intracranial tumor resection," *Neurosurgery*, 2003 Jan; 52(1):48-53; discussion 53-4.

4 I. F. Pollack, et al., "The influence of central review on outcome associations in childhood malignant gliomas: results from the CCG-945 experience," *Neurooncol*, 2003 Jul;5(3):197-207.

5 Paul Zeltzer, *Brain Tumors - Finding the Ark - Meeting the Challenges of Treatment Choices, Side Effects, Healthcare Costs and Long Term Survival* (Encino, CA: Shilysca Press, 2004). Refer to Chapter 21: Clinical Trials.

6 M. Glantz, et al., "Temozolomide as an alternative to irradiation for elderly patients with newly diagnosed malignant gliomas," *Cancer*, 97; 2262-66, 2003.

7 Paul Zeltzer, *Brain Tumors - Finding the Ark - Meeting the Challenges of Treatment Choices, Side Effects, Healthcare Costs and Long Term Survival* (Encino, CA: Shilysca Press, 2004). Refer to Chapter 23: Managing Costs, Benefits and Healthcare with Insurance, HMOs and More.

CHAPTER 7

1 Arthur Frank, *The Wounded Storyteller: Body, Illness and Ethics* (Chicago: University of Chicago Press, 1995).

CHAPTER 8

1 V. Vallejos, et al., "Use of 201Tl SPECT imaging to assess the response to therapy in patients with high grade gliomas," *J Neurooncol*, 2002 Aug;59(1):81-90.

2 Paul Zeltzer, *Brain Tumors - Finding the Ark - Meeting the Challenges of Treatment Choices, Side Effects, Healthcare Costs and Long Term Survival* ((Encino, CA: Shilysca Press, 2004). Refer to chapters on treatments.

3 I. F. Pollack, et al., "The influence of central review on outcome associations in childhood malignant gliomas: results from the CCG-945 experience," *Neurooncol*, 2003 Jul;5(3):197-207.

4 S. W. Coons, et al., "Improving diagnostic accuracy and inter-observer concordance in the classification and grading of primary gliomas," *Cancer*, 1997 Apr 1;79 (7):1381-93.

CHAPTER 9

1 Accessed July 1, 2004 at http://www.davidmbailey.com.

2 Paul Zeltzer, *Brain Tumors - Finding the Ark - Meeting the Challenges of Treatment Choices, Side Effects, Healthcare Costs & Long Term Survival* (Encino, CA: Shilysca Press, 2004).

3 L. T. Kohn, J. M. Corrigan, and M. S. Donaldson, "To Err Is Human: Building a Safer Health System," Committee on Quality of Health Care in America, Institute of Medicine, Washington DC, 1999, http://www4.nationalacademies. org/news.nsf/isbn/0309068371?OpenDocument.

4 Retrieved May 21, 2004 at http://www.ptsafety.org.

5 Adapted from *20 Tips to Help Prevent Medical Errors in Children*, Patient Fact Sheet, (Agency for Healthcare Research and Quality, September, 2002), AHRQ Publication No. 02-P034, Rockville, MD, http://www.ahrq.gov/consumer/20tipkid.com.

6 Paul Zeltzer, *Brain Tumors - Finding the Ark - Meeting the Challenges of Treatment Choices, Side Effects, Healthcare Costs & Long Term Survival* (Encino, CA: Shilysca Press, 2004).

7 *Brain Cancer*, ed. Michael Prados, (London: B. C. Decker, 2002).

8 *Brain Tumors*, ed. A. H. Kaye and Laws Jr. (New York: Churchill-Livingston, 1995).

9 E. Bruera, et al., "Methylphenidate associated with narcotics for the treatment of cancer pain," *Cancer, Treat Rep*, 1987 Jan; 71 (1):67-70.

10 Adapted in part from http://www.stat.washington.edu/TALARIA/table10.html.

11 C. A. Meyers, et al., "Methylphenidate therapy improves cognition, mood, and function of brain tumor patients," *J Clin Oncol*, 1998 Jul; 16(7):2522-7.

12 F. Fernandez, et al., "Methylphenidate for depressive disorders in cancer patients: An alternative to standard antidepressants," *Psychosomatics*, 1987 Sep;28(9):455-61.

13 T. Akechi, et al., "Efficacy of methylphenidate for fatigue in advanced cancer patients: a preliminary study," *Sugawara Palliat Med*, 2002 May;16 (3):261-3.

14 T. Batchelor, and L. M. DeAngelis, "Medical management of cerebral metastases," *Neurosurg Clin N Am*, 1996 ;7(3):435-46.

15 H. S. Friedman, et al., "Irinotecan therapy in adults with recurrent or progressive malignant glioma," *J Clin Oncol*, 1999 May; 17(5):1516-25.

CHAPTER 10

1 Paul Zeltzer, *Brain Tumors - Finding the Ark - Meeting the Challenges of Treatment Choices, Side Effects, Healthcare Costs and Long Term Survival* (Encino, CA: Shilysca Press, 2004).

2 Ibid.

3 C. B. Scott, et al., "Validation and predictive power of Radiation Therapy Oncology Group (RTOG) recursive partitioning analysis classes for malignant glioma patients: a report using RTOG 90-06," *Int J Radiat Oncol Biol Phys*, 1998 Jan 1; 40(1): 51-5.

4 M. Glantz, et al., "Temozolomide as an alternative to irradiation for elderly patients with newly diagnosed malignant gliomas," *Cancer*, 2003 May 1;97(9): 2262-6.

5 C. Leighton, et al., "Supratentorial low-grade glioma in adults: an analysis of prognostic factors and timing of radiation," *J Clin Oncol*, 1997;15(4):1294-301.

6 C. C. Leighton, "A meta-analysis of radiation therapy in adult low-grade glioma," 39th ASCO Annual Meeting, Chicago, IL, May 31-June 3, 2003 (Abstract No. 442).

7 P. D. Brown, et al., "The neurocognitive effects of radiation in adult low-grade glioma patients," *Neuro-oncol*, 2003 Jul;5(3):161-7.

8 T. J. Postma, et al., "Radiotherapy-induced cerebral abnormalities in patients with low-grade glioma," *Neurology,* 2002 Jul 9; 59(1): 121-3. Comment in: *Neurology,* 2002 Jul 9;59(1):8-10.

9 G. Bauman, et al., "Pretreatment factors predict overall survival for patients with low-grade glioma: a recursive partitioning analysis," *Int J Radiat Oncol Biol Phys,* 1999 Nov 1; 45(4): 923-9.

10 M. Fouladi, et al., "Survival and functional outcome of children with hypothalamic/chiasmatic tumors," *Cancer,* 2003 Feb 15;97(4):1084-92.

11 M. Glantz, et al., "Temozolomide as an alternative to irradiation for elderly patients with newly diagnosed malignant gliomas," *Cancer,* 2003 May 1;97(9):2262-6.

12 P.S. Mischel, and T. F. Cloughesy, "Targeted molecular therapy of GBM," *Brain Pathol,* 2003 Jan; 13(1): 52-61.

13 E. R. Laws, et al., "Survival following surgery and prognostic factors for recently diagnosed malignant glioma: data from the Glioma Outcomes Project," Glioma Outcomes Investigators, *J Neurosurg,* 2003 Sep;99(3): 467-73.

14 R. Stupp, et al., "Promising survival for patients with newly diagnosed glioblastoma multiforme treated with concomitant radiation plus temozolomide followed by adjuvant temozolomide," *J Clin Oncol,* 2002 Mar 1; 20(5): 1375-82. Comment in: *J Clin Oncol,* 2002 Jul 15;20(14):3179-80; author reply 3181-2, *J Clin Oncol,* 2002 Jul 15;20(14):3180-1; author reply 3181.

15 S. B. Tatter, et al., "New Approaches to Brain Tumor Therapy Central Nervous System Consortium, An inflatable balloon catheter and liquid 125I radiation source (GliaSite Radiation Therapy System) for treatment of recurrent malignant glioma: multicenter safety and feasibility trial," *J Neurosurg,* 2003 Aug; 99(2): 297-303.

16 C. N. Chang, et al., "High-dose-rate stereotactic brachytherapy for patients with newly diagnosed glioblastoma multiforme," *J Neurooncol,* 2003 Jan; 61(1):45-55. Review.

17 M. Westphal, et al., "A phase 3 trial of local chemotherapy with biodegradable carmustine (BCNU)wafers (Gliadel wafers) in patients with primary malignant glioma," *Neuro-oncol,* 2003 Apr; 5(2): 79-88.

18 M. Esteller, et al., "Inactivation of the DNA-repair gene MGMT and the clinical response of gliomas to alkylating agents," *N Engl J Med,* vol: 343, no. 19: pages 1350-4, Nov 9, 2000.

19 E. C. Nwokedi, et al., "Gamma knife stereotactic radiosurgery for patients with glioblastoma multiforme," *Neurosurgery,* 2002 Jan; 50(1): 41-6; discussion 46-7.

20 M. D. Walker, et al., "Randomized comparisons of radiotherapy and nitrosoureas for the treatment of malignant glioma after surgery," *N Engl J Med,* 1980 Dec 4;303(23):1323-9.

21 A. A. Brandes, et al., "A prospective study on glioblastoma in the elderly," *Cancer,* 2003 Feb 1; 97(3): 657-62.

22 E. S. Newlands, T. Foster T, and S. Zaknoen, "Phase I study of temozolamide (TMZ) combined with procarbazine (PCB) in patients with gliomas," *Br J Cancer,* 2003 Jul 21; 89(2): 248-51.

23 S. A. Grossman, et al., "Phase III study comparing three cycles of infusional carmustine and cisplatin followed by radiation therapy with radiation therapy and concurrent carmustine in patients with newly diagnosed supratentorial glioblastoma multiforme: Eastern Cooperative Oncology Group Trial 2394," *J Clin Oncol,* 2003 Apr 15;21(8):1485-91.

24 R. A., Kristof, et al., "Combined surgery, radiation, and PCV chemotherapy for astrocytomas compared to OLIGOdendrogliomas and OLIGOastrocytomas WHO grade III," *J Neurooncol,* 2002 Sep;59(3):231-7.

25 J. G. Cairncross, et al., "Specific genetic predictors of chemotherapeutic response and survival in patients with anaplastic oligodendrogliomas," *J Natl Cancer Inst,* 1998 Oct 7;90(19):1473-9.

26 V. A. Levin, et al., "Phase III randomized study of postradiotherapy chemotherapy with combination alpha-difluoromethylornithine-PCV versus PCV for anaplastic gliomas," *Clin Cancer Res,* 2003 Mar;9(3):981-90.

27 T. Watanabe, et al., "Phenotype versus genotype correlation in oligodendrogliomas and low-grade diffuse astrocytomas," *Acta Neuropathol* (Berl), 2002 Mar;103(3):267-75.

28 J. C. Buckner, et al., "Phase II trial of procarbazine, lomustine, and vincristine as initial therapy for patients with low-grade oligodendroglioma or oligoastrocytoma: efficacy and associations with chromosomal abnormalities," *J Clin Oncol*, 2003 Jan 15;21(2):251-5.

29 G. S. Bauman, et al., "Allelic loss of chromosome 1p and radiotherapy plus chemotherapy in patients with oligodendrogliomas," *Int J Radiat Oncol Biol Phys*, 2000 Oct 1;48(3):825-30.

30 J. G. Cairncross, D. R., Macdonald, and D. A. Ramsay, "Aggressive oligodendroglioma: a chemosensitive tumor," *Neurosurgery*, 1992 Jul;31(1):78-82.

31 M. J. van den Bent, et al., "European Organization for Research and Treatment of Cancer Brain Tumor Group. Phase II study of first-line chemotherapy with temozolomide in recurrent oligodendroglial tumors: the European Organization for Research and Treatment of Cancer, Brain Tumor Group Study 26971," *J Clin Oncol*, 2003 Jul 1; 21(13): 2525-8.

32 P. M. Zeltzer, et al., "PCV or Temozolomide for Oligodendroglioma: Toxicity and Response to dose intensive 42 day TMZ prior to PCV in newly diagnosed or TMZ prior to Carboplatin-VP-16 in recurrent oligodendroglioma. A Phase 2 study," *Neurooncology*, 2003 October; TA-43, p 358.

33 M. J. van den Bent, et al., "Second-line chemotherapy with temozolomide in recurrent oligodendroglioma after PCV (procarbazine, lomustine and vincristine) chemotherapy: EORTC Brain Tumor Group phase II study 26972," *Ann Oncol*, 2003 Apr; 14(4): 599-602.

34 K. Peterson, et al., "Salvage chemotherapy for oligodendroglioma," *J Neurosurg*, 1996 Oct; 85(4): 597-601.

35 Adapted from V. A. Levin, et al., *Cancer: Principles & Practice of Oncology*, 2001:2100-2160.

CHAPTER 11

1 http ://w w w.jncicancerspectrum.oupjournals.org /cgi /pdq /jncipdq ;CDR000006 2775.

2 L. Harisiadis, and C. H. Chang, "Medulloblastoma in children: a correlation between staging and results of treatment," *Int J Radiat Oncol Biol Phys*, 1977 Sep-Oct;2(9-10):833-41.

3 P. M. Zeltzer, et al., "Metastasis Stage, Adjuvant Treatment, and Residual Tumor Are Prognostic Factors for High Stage Medulloblastoma in Children: Conclusions from the Children's Cancer Group 921 Randomized Phase 3 Study," *J Clin Oncol*, 1999 March, 17(3):832-845.

4 A. L. Albright, et al., "Correlation of Neurosurgical subspecialization with outcomes of children with malignant brain tumors," *Neurosurgery*, 47:879-887,2000.

5 Ed. P. Zeltzer, and C. Pochedly, *Medulloblastoma in Children: New Concepts in Tumor Biology, Diagnosis, and Treatment* (New York: Praeger, 1986).

6 P. R. Thomas, et al., "Low-stage medulloblastoma: final analysis of trial comparing standard-dose with reduced-dose neuraxis irradiation," *J Clin Oncol*, 2000 Aug;18(16):3004-11.

7 R. J. Packer, et al., "Treatment of children with medulloblastomas with reduced dose craniospinal radiation therapy and adjuvant chemotherapy: a Children's Cancer Group Study," *J Clin Oncol*, 1999 Jul;17(7):2127-36.

8 M. D., Ris, et al., "Intellectual outcome after reduced-dose radiation therapy plus adjuvant chemotherapy for medulloblastoma: a Children's Cancer Group study," *J Clin Oncol*, 2001 Aug 1;19(15):3470-6.

9 P. L. Robertson, et al., "Survival and prognostic factors following radiation therapy and chemotherapy for ependymomas in children: a report of the Children's Cancer Group,"*J Neurosurg*, 1998: 88(4):695-703.

CHAPTER 12

1 Yann Martel, *Life of Pi* (New York: Harcourt, 2001), 161.
2 http://www.cancerbacup.org.uk/Treatments/Chemotherapy/Individualchemotherapydrugs/ Hydroxyurea.
3 http://www.c3.hu/~mavideg/jns/4.html.
4 http://www.ghorayeb.com/TransSphenoidAnatomy.html.
5 http://www.neurosurgery.org/focus/may03/14-5-9.pdf.
6 Paul Zeltzer, *Brain Tumors - Finding the Ark* - Meeting the Challenges of Treatment Choices, Side Effects, Healthcare Costs and Long Term Survival (Encino, CA: Shilysca Press, 2004).
7 W. Friedman, and K. Foote, "Linear accelerator-based radiosurgery for vestibular Schwannoma," *Neurosurg Focus*, 14 (5):Article 2, 2003.

CHAPTER 13

1 http://neurosurgery.mgh.harvard.edu/newwhobt.htm
2 http://neurosurgery.mgh.harvard.edu/newwhobt.htm.
3 R. J. Packer, B. H. Cohen, and K. Cooney, "Intracranial Germ Cell Tumors," *The Oncologist*, vol. 5, no. 4, 312-320, 2000.
4 mailto:jallen@bethisraelny.org.
5 Int. Coordinator and Registration Centre, Clinic of Pediatric Haematology and Oncology, Children's Hospital, Heinrich Heine University Düsseldorf, P.O. Box 10 10 07, D-40001 Düsseldorf, Germany. E-mail: calaminus@med.uniduesseldorf.de.
6 jfinlay@chla.usc.edu.
7 M. Kochi, et al., "Successful treatment of intracranial non-germinomatous malignant germ cell tumors by administering neoadjuvant chemotherapy and radiotherapy before excision of residual tumors," *J Neurosurg*, 2003 Jul;99(1): 106-14.
8 Paul Zeltzer, *Brain Tumors - Finding the Ark* - Meeting the Challenges of Treatment Choices, Side Effects, Healthcare Costs and Long Term Survival (Los Angeles, CA: Shilysca Press, 2004).
9 A. C. Paulino, B. C. Wen, and M. Najeeb-Mohideen, "Controversies in the Management of Intracranial Germinomas," *Oncology*, 13(4):513-521, 1999. Retrieved online June 4, 2004 at http://www.cancernetwork.com/journals/oncology/o9904c.htm.
10 D. A. Haas-Kogan, et al., "Radiation therapy for intracranial germ cell tumors," *Int J Radiat Oncol Biol Phys*, 2003 Jun 1;56(2):511-8. Erratum in: *Int J Radiat Oncol Biol Phys*, 2003 Sep 1;57(1): 306.
11 http://tcrc.acor.org/lance.html.
12 B. H. Cohen, et al., "Prognostic factors and treatment results for supratentorial primitive neuroectodermal tumors in children using radiation and chemotherapy: a Childrens Cancer Group randomized trial," J Clin Oncol, 1995 Jul; 13(7): 1687-96.
13 R. I. Jakacki, et al., "Survival and prognostic factors following radiation and/or chemotherapy for primitive neuroectodermal tumors of the pineal region in infants and children: a report of the Childrens Cancer Group," J Clin Oncol, 1995 Jun;13(6):1377-83.
14 D. A. Haas-Kogan, et al., "Radiation therapy for intracranial germ cell tumors," Int J Radiat Oncol Biol Phys, 2003 Jun 1;56(2):511-8. Erratum in: Int J Radiat Oncol Biol Phys, 2003 Sep 1;57(1): 306.

15 L. H. Einhorn, "Curing metastatic testicular cancer," Proc Natl Acad Sci, 2002 Apr ;99(7):4592-5. E-pub 2002 Mar 19.
16 Refer to the testicular cancer website: http://tcrc.acor.org/index.html.

Chapter 14

1 K. Murray, "Primary malignant lymphoma of the central nervous system. Results of treatment of 11 cases and review of the literature," J Neurosurg, 1986 Nov;65(5):600-7.
2 M. E. Sherman, et al., "Stereotactic brain biopsy in the diagnosis of malignant lymphoma," Am J Clin Pathol, 1991 Jun;95(6):878-83.
3 Paul Zeltzer, Brain Tumors - Finding the Ark - Meeting the Challenges of Treatment Choices, Side Effects, Healthcare Costs and Long Term Survival (Encino,CA: Shilysca Press, 2004).
4 D. F. Nelson, et al., "Non-Hodgkin's lymphoma of the brain: can high dose, large volume radiation therapy improve survival? Report on a prospective trial by the Radiation Therapy Oncology Group (RTOG): RTOG 8315," Int J Radiat Oncol Biol Phys, 1992;23(1):247-8.
5 S. A. Leibel, and G. E. Sheline, "Radiation therapy for neoplasms of the brain," J Neurosurg, 1987 Jan;66(1):1-22.
6 A. Calderoni, and S. Aebi, "Combination chemotherapy with high-dose methotrexate and cytarabine with or without brain irradiation for primary central nervous system lymphomas," J Neurooncol, 2002 Sep;59(3):227-30.
7 L. E. Abrey, J. Yahalom, and L. DeAngelis, "Treatment for primary CNS lymphoma: the next step," J Clin Oncol, 2000 Sep;18 (17):3144-50.
8 http://www.rituxan.com/rituxan/index.jsp.
9 H. Pels, et al., "Intraventricular and intravenous treatment of a patient with refractory primary CNS lymphoma using rituximab," Neurooncol, 2002 Sep;59(3):213-6.

Chapter 15

1 A. H. Kaye, and E. R. Laws, Brain Tumors (New York: Churchill-Livingstone, 1995), 924.
2 Paul Zeltzer, Brain Tumors - Finding the Ark - Meeting the Challenges of Treatment Choices, Side Effects, Healthcare Costs and Long Term Survival (Encino, CA: Shilysca Press, 2004).
3 W. F. Regine, et al., "Metastatic spinal cord compression: a randomized trial of direct decompressive surgical resection plus radiotherapy vs. radiotherapy alone," Int J Radiat Oncol Biol Phys, 2003 Oct 1;57(2 Suppl):S125.
4 P. D. Brown, et al., "The neurocognitive effects of radiation in adult low-grade glioma patients," Neuro-ncology, 2003 Jul;5(3):161-7.
5 A. Auperin, et al., "Prophylactic cranial irradiation for patients with small-cell lung cancer in complete remission. Prophylactic Cranial Irradiation Overview Collaborative Group," N Engl J Med, 1999 Aug 12;341(7):476-84.
6 S. D. Chang, and J. R. Adler, "Current treatment of patients with multiple brain metastases," Neurosurg, Focus 9 (2):Article 5, 2000.
7 D. Kondziolka, et al., "Decision making for patients with multiple brain metastases: radiosurgery, radiotherapy, or resection?" Neurosurg Focus 9 (2):Article 4, 2000.
8 J. Suh, et al., "A Phase 3 randomized open label comparative study of standard whole brain radiation therapy with supplemental oxygen (O2) with or without RSR-13 in patients with brain metastases," Neuro-oncology, (2003) 5, Abstract RT-13: 354.

9 Professor and Chairman, Department of Human Oncology, University of Wisconsin Medical School.

10 http://www.laf.org/lance/lance_diagnosis.html.

11 http://www.tumorfree.com/survivors.htm.

12 http://www.guideline.gov/, s. v. "brain metastasis."

Index

INDEX

I

Immortality *45*
Immunophenotype *326*
Immunotherapy *102, 270, 327, 330, 331*
Inability to look upward *312*
Incomplete resection *281*
Inflammation *206, 213*
Information *72, 162*
Infratentorial *284*
Initial evaluation *236*
Initiation of labor *299*
Innocence *45*
Inside rules *152*
Instruction *92*
    quality of life *92*
Insurance *51, 107, 152, 321*
Intensity modulated radiation therapy (IMRT) *344*
Intensive chemotherapy *313*
Interferons *219, 266*
Internet *60, 62, 71, 73, 74, 81, 129, 199, 283*
    dark sides *81*
    Rip-offs *83*
Interns *153, 155*
Intravenous and intrathecal (direct administration into the spinal fluid) methotrexate *331*

J

Jump sites *78*
Juvenile pilocytic astrocytomas (JPA) *40, 235, 243, 263, 267*

K

Kaiser Plan *142*
Karnofsky score *248, 349*
Keppra *227*
Kytril *321*

L

Laboratory reports *53*
Lactate *192*
Lance Armstrong *349*
Language *35, 338*
Lesion *38*
Leucovorin *331*
Leyden, van *47*
Local radiation *318, 319*
Location *43*
Lomustine *282*
Low-grade *33*
Lowered radiation doses *281*
Low thyroid stimulating hormone (TSH) *303*
Lung *340*
Lung cancer *40*
Luteinizing hormone *302*
Luteinizing hormone [LH]) *300*
Lymphoma *194, 238, 340*
    after-surgical therapies *329*
Lymph glands *325*

M

M-3 PNET *278*
M-stage *276*
Macroadenomas *300*
Magnetic resonance imaging *191*
    MRI *191*

Morbidity   *239*
Morphine   *210*
Mosaccio   *46*
Motor/ sensory strips   *35, 338*
   Left Side   *35*
   Right Side   *35*
MRI   *39, 54, 99, 130, 189, 190, 260, 267, 269, 277, 278, 280, 285, 302, 305, 315, 326, 338, 339*
   enhanced   *339*
   unenhanced   *339*
MR Spect   *97, 192, 237, 315*
Multidisciplinary team   *89, 237*
Muscle-wasting   *207*
Mutism syndrome   *243*
Myelin   *190*
Myelogram   *193*
Myths   *208*
   pain   *208*

N

N-acetylaspartate   *192*
Narcotics   *209*
   side effects   *209*
National Brain Tumor Foundation (NBTF)   *58, 60, 138*
National cancer institute   *320, 348*
National guideline clearinghouse   *350*
Nausea   *217, 284*
Neck pain   *284*
Necrosis   *97, 134, 193, 194, 195, 238, 268*
Neoplasm   *38*
Netscape   *74*
Network   *143*
Neuro-ophthalmologic evaluation   *302*
Neurofibromatosis type 1 (NF-1)
239, 242, 266
Neurofibromatosis type 2 (NF-2)
293, 306
Neurological function   *328*
Neurologist   *104, 262, 270, 279, 327*
Neuronal tumors   *311*
Neurooncologist   *102, 261, 270, 279, 327, 348*
Neurooncology   *131, 141, 194*
Neuropathologist   *99, 262, 270, 276, 279, 327*
Neuropathology   *100*
Neuropsychological
   assessment   *113*
   side effects   *344*
   testing   *237, 315*
Neuropsychologist   *112, 279, 327*
Neuropsychology   *110*
Neuroradiologist   *97, 262, 270, 279, 327*
Neuroradiology   *194*
Neurosurgeon   *44, 94, 95, 130, 189, 196, 262, 270, 279, 295, 327*
   expertise   *44*
   general   *95*
   how do I choose   *95*
Neurosurgery   *264, 270, 328*
New Approach to Brain Tumor Treatment (NABTT)   *266*
NF-1   *120*
Noah and the Ark   *293*
Non-AIDS associated lymphomas *332*
Non-germinomatous germ cell tumors *311, 318*
Non-Hodgkin lymphoma   *325, 326*
Non-hormone secreting   *300*
Nonsteroidal anti-inflammatory agents *221*

Norman Cousins   *123, 127*
North american brain tumor consort
271
Notebook   *51*
No therapy   *350*
Nurse   *121, 156*
   Practitioner   *156*

O

Observation   *256, 296, 297, 306, 350*
Obstructive hydrocephalus   *264, 280*
Occipital   *35*
Occupational therapy (OT)   *110*
Octreotide, Sandostatin   *303*
Older adult   *248*
Oligiodendroglioma   *41, 53, 234, 236,
249, 251, 254, 256, 258, 260, 272*
   adults   *251*
   children   *251*
   low-grade   *256*
Oligodendrocytes   *234*
Oligodendrogliomas
   recurrent lower-grade   *260*
Ombudsman   *142, 143*
Oncogenes   *269*
Oncologist   *102, 131, 262, 270, 327,
348*
Oncology   *131*
One day at a time   *63*
Open biopsy   *197*
Open skull surgery   *238*
Ophthalmologist (eye doctor)   *120*
Optic nerves   *300, 303, 312*
Optic pathway   *233, 242*
Oregon Health Sciences University
Hospital   *162*
Organization   *51*
Osteoporosis   *207, 218*

Outside consultation   *143*
Ovaries   *118, 311*
Overwhelmed   *59*
Oxycodone   *210*

P

Pain   *164, 206, 207, 208, 209, 210,
211*
   complication of surgery   *207*
   ladder   *209*
   monitoring   *211*
Paralysis   *294, 341*
Parent   *90*
Parietal & Occipital   *35, 36*
Parietal lobe   *34*
Pathologist   *52, 131, 140, 189, 198,
339*
Pathology report   *52, 99*
Patient safety institute   *203*
PCV   *60, 241, 248, 259*
Pediatric neurosurgeon   *279, 280*
Pediatric neurosurgery   *95*
Pediatric oncologist   *41*
Pediatric oncology society (SIOP)   *313*
Peptic ulcers   *217*
Percocet percodan   *210*
Peripheral vision   *300*
PET   *97, 193, 267*
Pharmacist   *109*
Physiatrist   *110*
Physical therapy   *110*
Physician assistant (PA)   *157*
Pineal   *118*
   cysts   *319*
   gland   *312, 319*
   gland tumors   *311*
   region tumors   *41, 288, 321*
Pineoblastoma   *314, 319*
Pineocytoma   *314, 319*

NOTES

What Leading Brain Tumor Specialists Are Saying About the Book

...well-written, authoritative, comprehensive "how-to" guide...immensely useful to patients with brain tumors, their families, and everyone...entrusted with the care of patients with brain tumors. Steven Brem, MD H. Lee Moffitt Cancer Center & Research Institute,Tampa, FL

...an extraordinarily useful tool for patients and families to navigate the confusing and frightening brain tumor experience. The index and glossary make the information easily accessible. Joseph V. Simone, MD Chair, National Cancer Policy Board, Institute of Medicine

...thoughtfully written by someone who has clearly the experience and the compassion to care about patients afflicted by these diseases. Ray Sawaya, MD, Chairman of Neurosurgery, MD Anderson, Houston, TX

...should be mandatory reading for all health care professionals who care for patients with brain tumors. Reid Thompson MD, Director of Neurosurgical Oncology, Vanderbilt University, Nashville, TN

an important resource for patients. Keith Black MD, Director, Maxine Dunitz Neurosurgical Institute, Los Angeles, CA

This is a must read for anyone ...trying to cope with a brain tumor. It should be read as soon as the diagnosis is made or even suspected. Dr. Zeltzer draws on his vast experience...at the world's most prestigious brain tumor centers to dig out questions...concerns that many patients are afraid to - or just don't know enough to - discuss with their own doctors. Al Musella, DPM, President, Musella Foundation For Brain Tumor Research & Information, Inc., www.virtualtrials.com

"Meaty" and practical" - this book is the antidote for patients who spend too much time traveling around the country, becoming paralyzed with fear and indecision. Dr Jonathan Finlay MD, Children's Hospital, Los Angeles, CA

...an excellent resource for brain tumor patients in North America... valuable to health care professionals with a special interest in brain tumors...adds significantly to the current available literature. Dr. Rolando Del Maestro, Clinical Director, Brain Tumour Research Centre, Montreal, Canada

Brain Tumors: Finding the Ark: *Meeting the Challenges of Treatment Choices, Side Effects, Healthcare Costs & Long Term Survival. (2005) (390 pages)* Paul M. Zeltzer M.D.

In this latest sequel to *Brain Tumors: Leaving the Garden of Eden*, "Dr. Paul" continues to guide you through the brain tumor minefield so that you have the best chances for quality survival. In nine chapters are the key answers to questions about medications, CAM, late effects of treatment, clinical trials, HMOs, Medicare & insurance, role of heredity, & brain tumors in children.

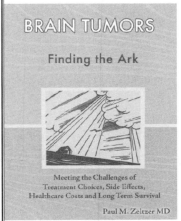

BRAIN TUMORS

Finding the Ark

Meeting the Challenges of
Treatment Choices, Side Effects,
Healthcare Costs and Long Term Survival

Paul M. Zeltzer MD

Finding the Ark will help you find the answers to your questions like:

- Are all Neurosurgeons created equal?
- Radiation Therapy–Are the rumors true? Radiosurgery–What is it? (Chap 17); What questions do I ask before I receive it?
- What is CAM, TCM, Ayurvedic medicine? Can they help me to fight my tumor? Spiritual counseling and healing- how they can help (Chap 18)?
- Can I prevent life threatening medication errors (Chap 19)?

Long term side effects are a luxury of being alive. Some are unavoidable, others can be lessened or avoided. (Chap 20).
- What are the effects on activities of daily living?
- The effects on sugar, salt, and sex?

Clinical trials. Here are the rules on how they work, where you can get specific information about them (Chap 21)?
How does insurance affect my care? The good and the bad. (Chap 22)
- Many people don't realize their doctor may not be the final decision-maker on the care they can receive.
- Children & Brain Tumors- over 20 special considerations: Legal rights, camps, school re-entry, pain control.

See www.braincancersurvivors.com or www.survivingbraincancer.com for more information.

I am deeply grateful to the Brain Tumor Society
for facilitating funding for

Brain Tumors - Leaving the Garden of Eden.

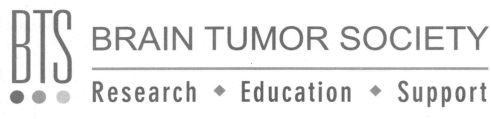

BRAIN TUMOR SOCIETY

Research ◆ Education ◆ Support

800.770.TBTS (8287)
www.tbts.org

I also acknowledge the financial support of
Schering-Plough Oncology.

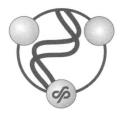